Early Vision and Beyond

Editor-in-Chief
Thomas V. Papathomas
Associate Editors
Charles Chubb, Andrei Gorea,
and Eileen Kowler

Early Vision and Beyond

A Bradford Book
The MIT Press
Cambridge, Massachusetts
London, England

This book was set in Palatino by Asco Trade Typesetting Ltd., Hong Kong and
was printed and bound in the United States of America.

Library of Congress Cataloging-in-Publication Data

Early vision and beyond / edited by Thomas V. Papathomas ... [et al.].
    p.   cm.
"A Bradford book."
Includes bibliographical references and index.
ISBN 0-262-16146-X
 1. Vision. 2. Visual perception. I. Papathomas, Thomas V.
QP475.E16   1994
152.14—dc20   94-3117
                                                                  CIP

Contents

Foreword

A glance at the contents of this book should convince anyone of the enormous progress our field of vision research is making. A most interesting development over the past few years is the increasing dialogue, indeed the blurring of much of the distinction, between neurophysiological and psychophysical approaches. Gradually we are coming to understand each other's languages and are mastering each other's techniques. The field has become immeasurably richer.

The computer has contributed enormously to both fields, especially perhaps to psychophysics, where it has played a role comparable to the microelectrode in neurophysiology: it has replaced the strings and pulleys and relay racks, much as the electrode and associated electronics have supplanted strain gauges and string galvanometers.

No example of the fruitful use of computers coupled with brilliant imagination can surpass the invention of the random-dot stereogram by Béla Julesz. This is surely the biggest step in depth perception studies since Wheatstone, and constitutes the most important tool in that field for physiologists and psychologists alike. To take just an example, it is hard to think of many experiments that have allowed us to localize an event in a neural pathway without physically invading the nervous system.

We are still a long way from a complete understanding of stereopsis, just as we are far from understanding color, form, or movement. But it is hard to think of a better example of a flourishing field than stereopsis between 1960, when the random-dot stereogram was invented, and the present. For this Béla Julesz is largely responsible.

David H. Hubel

Preface

We are astonished at thought, but sensation is equally wonderful.

Voltaire, "Sensation," Philosophical Dictionary (1764)

The average person takes vision for granted. After all, it does not seem to take any effort or learning to perceive the world around us. Even babies are "grandmasters of vision," to use one of Bela Julesz's favorite expressions. The degree to which people underestimate the sophisticated processes of vision becomes obvious when you ask them a question that I often ask my audience of educated nonspecialists when I am invited to give a lecture on vision. "What computer program do you think is more difficult to design: One that analyzes images and recognizes faces and objects, or one that can play chess at a world-class level?" There is a strong preference to answer that the chess program is a lot harder to design, and some people are astounded to hear that today's computer programs play chess at a formidable mid- to strong-grandmaster level, whereas our progress with machines that perform generic vision tasks has been relatively slow. Early workers in artificial intelligence were overoptimistic for progress in vision. One anecdotal story is that a student was assigned to "solve vision" as a summer project some decades ago! It is perhaps because people take vision for granted that even simple concepts and discoveries had to wait until relatively recently. Thus it took as late as the seventeenth century for the blind spot to be discovered, whereas the stereoscope's invention had to wait until the nineteenth century.

Vision researchers, on the other hand, take nothing about vision for granted. The complex issues encountered in the study of vision have forced researchers to attempt to isolate simpler modules and processes for detailed examination. Some of the most successful attempts have been in early, or low-level, visual processes. Indeed, much progress has been made in recent years in the areas of depth, motion, texture perception, and visual attention. The nature of the problems is such that interdisciplinary approaches offer the most effective plan for solutions. In recent decades, experimental psychologists, neurophysiologists, and scientists in computational vision have made remarkable progress in studying perceptual issues, understanding neuronal mechanisms and pathways, and developing mathematical models that begin to predict the response of biological vision processes. The choice of material in this book and its organization were based on the above considerations. The book is divided into four main sections, each covering an important low-level visual process: binocular vision and stereopsis, the perception of movement, visual texture segregation, and attention and learning in early vision. Within each section, we have included chapters by leading researchers who represent the following three main disciplines: visual psychophysics, cognitive neuroscience, and computational vision. It is our hope that this book will emphasize to the student of vision the need to form interdisciplinary links for addressing common problems, obtaining evidence, and enriching each other's understanding.

Even though the chapters have been divided into the four sections mentioned above, there are other common threads that run through the chapters' themes and across section boundaries. For example, there are several chapters in which "psychoanatomical" techniques are used. Purely psychophysical experiments with carefully selected stimuli are conducted to probe the information flow in neural pathways, or to locate the neural sites of perceptual processes (see the chapters by Blake, Kulikowski and Walsh, Nakayama, and Zanker). Such techniques emphasize the need for interdisciplinary knowledge, in this case psychology and physiology. Another subset of chapters shares the property of examining the role of color in various visual tasks (see the contributions by Cavanagh; Farell; Kulikowski and Walsh; Nakayama and He; Schiller; Victor et al.; Wolfe, Chun, and Friedman-Hill). Researchers in color vision can thus find color-related work in diverse areas of early visual processing. Finally, the chapters by Sagi, by Schiller, by Desimone et al., and by Ahissar and Hochstein share the theme of perceptual learning, a relatively new area of research in early vision. The apparent contradiction between these two chapters regarding interocular transfer in perceptual learning, probably explainable by different experimental conditions, is indicative of the richness of issues that need to be addressed in this area.

This book is primarily aimed at three types of readers: First, vision researchers may benefit from the material in the above four areas, especially from the contributions of disciplines other than their own. Second, graduate or advanced undergraduate students in any field of vision research will find the level particularly suited to their needs. Finally, the nonspecialist scientist who is interested in vision can read the chapters to gain a good understanding of the issues involved.

The idea for this book grew from an international conference that took place on April 30 and May 1 of 1993, to honor Bela Julesz, on the occasion of his sixty-fifth birthday, for his many seminal contributions in vision.[1] To emphasize the interdisciplinary interactions in vision, we selected as speakers 20 leading researchers from three main disciplines: visual psychophysics, cognitive neurosciences, and computational vision. About 200 people from all over the world converged to Rutgers University in Piscataway, New Jersey, and participated in a lively exchange of ideas. It is difficult for me to separate my activities as an organizer of the conference and as the editor of the present volume. The two are so inextricably intertwined that, in my mind, it would be a serious omission not to acknowledge in this volume those who played a role in the conference.

My most important acknowledgment is to Bela himself. I consider myself extremely fortunate to be closely associated with Bela Julesz. Naturally, I have known all along that he enjoys an enviable reputation among researchers not only in vision, but also in many other scientific fields. However, in the course of organizing the conference, I had several young colleagues tell me that they were inspired by Bela in their careers, and I believe that this is the tribute he appreciates most. Personally, I have been transformed by Bela Julesz from a Bell Labs supervisor and designer of multiprocessor systems to a researcher in vision. What made the transformation smooth and pleasurable was Bela's patience and understanding. After all, he himself began his career as an electrical engineer, so at least I had an "existence proof!" Was it worthwhile to change? To use his criterion, "you know someone likes his job when he whistles while he works." Well, I have never stopped "whistling" since I got involved in vision, and my gratitude to Bela is deeply felt.

The words of Demosthenes are as true today as they were when he uttered them more than two millennia ago: "Δεῖ, δεῖ χρημάτων καί, ἄνευ τούτων, οὐδέν ἐστιν γενέσθαι," which translates into "We need, we need money and, without them, nothing is to be done." It is fitting, therefore, to thank the sponsors of the conference for their generous support: Willard Vaughan and Harold

1. Bela was motivated to write some notes, on the occasion of his sixty-fifth birthday, with the idea of presenting them to the many postdoctoral students and close collaborators whom he worked with over the years. This project eventually grew into a volume of scientific monograph: *Dialogues on Perception,* also published by MIT Press, is a book in which Bela, in his inimitable style, has some lively discussions with his alter-ego, who plays the devil's advocate, on very important and interesting issues on perception that cannot be covered in scientific papers or in textbooks.

Hawkins of the U.S.A. Office of Naval Research, Peter Katona of the Whitaker Foundation, Carver Mead of the California Institute of Technology, Per Uddén and Curt von Euler of the Rodin Foundation, and Joe Giordmaine of the NEC Research Institute.

Rutgers, the State University of New Jersey, supported us in many ways; it was only after we secured their backing that we could ask others outside the University for sponsorship. The following entities supported us generously: The Offices of the Provost and the Dean, the Research Council, the Departments of Psychology and of Biomedical Engineering, and the Center for Cognitive Sciences. Our thanks to Joseph Seneca, Andrew Rudczynski, Peter Loeb, Paul Leath, Joseph Potenza, Richard Foley, Ellis Dill, Charles Flaherty, Evangelia Micheli-Tzanakou, and Zenon Pylyshyn for their help and encouragement.

All the speakers and authors agreed to contribute to this effort with enthusiasm. It would be almost impossible to bring together such a constellation of workers in vision research had it not been for Bela's sake. Many thanks to all, with special thanks to our keynote speaker, David Hubel. In addition to the conference speakers whose chapters appear in this volume, we also thank some speakers who were unable to contribute chapters for various reasons. Let me mention them here for the record: E. H. Adelson, J. R. Bergen, P. Burt, E. Hildreth, J. Krauskopf, and T. A. Poggio.

Each member of the organizing committee (Charlie Chubb, Eileen Kowler, Zenon Pylyshyn, Paula Tallal, Evangelia Micheli-Tzanakou, Jerry Lettvin, Bishnu Atal, and Ira Black) contributed in their own way to the success of the conference. The first two, along with Andrei Gorea, were also session chairs and are section editors in the present volume. A decision was made, early on in the planning stages, not to include the editors' contributions, since we wanted to act as "hosts" for the authors both at the conference and in the present volume. This is the reason for the absence of chapters by the section editors, whom I thank of help, advice, and encouragement. I also acknowledge Joe Lappin and Ralph Siegel for co-chairing two sessions at the conference. We were blessed with a competent and tireless support staff. Particular thanks to Carol Esso, our secretary at the Laboratory of Vision Research, whose organizational skills made it possible to plan and coordinate the many activities for the conference and the preparation of the book.

I appreciate the help I received from my colleagues at the Department of Biomedical Engineering and from the members of the Laboratory of Vision Research, which Bela founded at Rutgers in 1989: Bart Anderson, Itzhak Hadani, Ilona Kovacs, Jih Jie Chang, Akos Feher, and K. S. Ramanujan. The first three, along with Ralph Siegel, also served as reviewers for some of the manuscripts, as did several of the authors (each chapter was reviewed typically by two people). Akos helped me with the book jacket's design and, more important, he did the lion's share in preparing the index. Michael Cooper and Barbara Walsh of the University of Medicine and Dentistry of New Jersey did a fine job implementing my ideas for the book jacket. My apologies to numerous others who helped with the many details of the conference and this book for not mentioning them by name.

I am pleased to acknowledge Fiona Stevens and Katherine Arnoldi of MIT Press for their advice, guidance and professionalism, which made it a real pleasure to work together. The credit for the fine format and appearance of this book belongs entirely to them.

Finally, I am now indebted even more than before to my wife Georgia for being gracefully patient as a (working) "married parent without partner," as she put it, whenever deadlines had to be met. It is because she has been so generous in so many ways that this book is published right on schedule.

Thomas V. Papathomas

Part I

Binocular Vision and Stereopsis

Thomas V. Papathomas

Without doubt, two of the most important inventions that shaped the psychophysics of depth perception were the stereoscope by Wheatstone (1838) and the random-dot stereogram (RDS) by Julesz (1960). The first established binocular disparity as one of the stimulus cues that are utilized by the visual system to arrive at a three-dimensional percept from the two eyes' inputs. The second succeeded in isolating binocular disparity from all other depth cues and demonstrated that monocular form recognition is not a prerequisite to stereoscopic fusion. The introduction of RDS techniques not only enabled psychophysicists to study the role of binocular disparity in depth perception for cyclopean and hypercyclopean (e.g., Tyler, 1975) stimuli (for a review, see Julesz 1986; see also Tyler's chapter [chapter 1] in this section), it also provided a method whereby neurophysiologists could isolate disparity-tuned units in the visual cortex (e.g., Poggio et al., 1985; Hubel, 1988; Poggio, Gonzalez, and Krause, 1988; see also Poggio's chapter [chapter 5] in this volume). Furthermore, computational models of stereopsis are based, to a large extent, on research with RDS (Julesz, 1971; Dev, 1975; Marr and Poggio, 1976, 1979) and the use of RDS as a benchmark for stereo algorithms is a standard practice (Weinshall, 1989; Pollard, Mayhew, and Frisby, 1985; Jones and Malik, 1992). Beyond binocular vision, the RDS may have provided the inspiration for the random-dot cinematogram (RDC) (Julesz and Payne, 1968; Anstis, 1970; Braddick, 1974), which played a very important role in motion perception; for more on the use of RDC, see the section on motion (part III).

From the psychophysical and the computational perspectives, one of the central issues in depth perception is concerned with the *correspondence problem*, that is, the computation of the appropriate disparities for corresponding points and regions across the two-dimensional retinal images. Beyond this, the richness of the binocular and especially stereopsis-related processing of monocular images in constructing a final percept is considered in the chapter by Tyler. He proposes a very complex heterarchical stereopsis model, which is motivated by a great deal of important work on depth perception that he and his co-workers have done over the years (for a review, see

Tyler 1991). The model is very general and it accommodates a remarkably wide range of phenomena in stereoscopic perception. It has relevance to psychophysics and to neurophysiology. The author discusses several such phenomena and presents reasonable arguments for the validity of the model's architecture, which may be relevant for future work on computational modeling.

In the natural world, the great majority of surfaces and regions in the monocular images are visible to both eyes and the correspondence process must compute the disparities of these common regions (of course, occlusions give rise to areas that are visible only to one of the two eyes, and there is evidence that the processing of these areas takes place in parallel with correspondence matching [Anderson and Nakayama, 1994]). The phenomenon of *binocular rivalry*, which arises when corresponding areas of the two retinae are stimulated by entirely different stimuli, occurs rarely in everyday life, but it can be used to study binocular vision in the laboratory. Blake and his colleagues have studied this phenomenon extensively and have gained a great deal of insight into visual processes (for a review, see Blake, 1989). His chapter in this section (chapter 2) provides an excellent brief review of the psychophysics and modeling of binocular rivalry. In addition, it presents some experiments with judiciously selected binocularly rivalrous stimuli, which enable one to answer important psychoanatomical questions.

The role of color in binocular vision and stereopsis is still not clear. Although early evidence seemed to indicate that stereopsis is "color-blind," recent experiments have shown that the chromatic pathway does contribute to depth perception (e.g., Grinberg and Williams, 1985; Jordan, Geisler and Bovik, 1990; Kovacs, Papathomas and Julesz, 1991; Kovacs and Julesz, 1992). Despite some recent progress, much work remains to be done to arrive at a good understanding of the processes involved. Neurophysiological experiments are essential in settling the issue, but computational models can incorporate color in stereo-matching algorithms independently of how the issue is resolved. Kulikowski and his collaborators have been working on color vision lately, examining both psychophysical and neurophysiological issues in this area (Mullen and Kulikowski, 1990; Walsh, Kulikowski, and Butler, 1992; Kulikowski and Walsh, 1993). The chapter by Kulikowski and Walsh (chapter 3) presents results with a simple set of chromatic stimuli, and it offers another example of psychoanatomical techniques on the role of color in binocular rivalry and stereopsis.

In the area of modeling, Weinshall and Malik, both of whom have worked extensively on computational vision and have developed ideas on models of stereopsis (Weinshall, 1989; Jones and Malik, 1992), join forces to present a brief review of progress in this area. They start with a discussion of the correspondence problem and the constraints of similarity, uniqueness, epipolar geometry, ordering, and smoothness. After presenting the circumstances under which these constraints fail, they briefly review a few matching algorithms. They consider what can be inferred from the geometric interpretation of the disparity field about the three-dimensional structure of the world, and which computation should be carried out based on considerations of robustness and efficiency. They first discuss the vertical disparities question: does human vision use only the horizontal component of the disparity field, or does it use both components? They then discuss what should be computed from the disparity field: is it necessary to recover the camera geometry, or can we do without it? Need we compute depth, relative depth, or just depth ordering? The feature that makes this chapter especially relevant in a book that attempts to cover issues from a multidisciplinary perspective is that the authors relate the above computational issues to available psychophysical data.

Finally, Gian Poggio's chapter (chapter 5) offers an important, interesting, and comprehensive review of research in neurophysiology that focused on the properties of disparity-tuned neurons that appear as early as area V1 in the visual cortex of monkeys. He is among the best qualified to write such a chapter, because he and his coworkers have had a far-reaching involvement in the neurophysiology of stereopsis in monkeys. He was among the first physiologists to employ stimuli with random-dot stereograms and correlograms for recording from disparity-tuned neurons and to study their properties. In his chapter, he reviews the accomplishments of the past three decades or so, concentrating on studies and results of his own team of collaborators. His reference to psychophysical results that closely agree with physiological data is a prime example of what motivated us to emphasize interdisciplinary interactions in this volume.

References

Anderson, B. L., and Nakayama, K. (1994). Towards a general theory of stereopsis: Binocular matching, occluding contours, and fusion. *Psychol. Rev. 101*.

Anstis, S. M. (1970). Phi movement as a subtraction process. *Vision Res. 10*, 1411–1430.

Blake, R. (1989). A neural theory of binocular rivalry. *Psychol. Rev. 96*, 145–167.

Braddick, O. (1974). A short-range process of apparent motion. *Vision

Res. 14, 519–527.

Dev, P. (1975). Perception of depth surfaces in random-dot stereograms: A neural model. *Int. J. Man-Machine Stud. 7*, 511–528.

Grinberg, D. L., and Williams, D. R. (1985). Stereopsis with chromatic signals from the blue-sensitive mechanism. *Vision Res. 25*, 531–537.

Jones, D. G., and Malik, J. (1992). A computational framework for determining stereo correspondence from a set of linear spatial filters. *Proceedings ECCV*, Genova, Italy.

Jordan III, J. R., Geisler, W. S., and Bovik, A. C. (1990). Color as a source of information in the stereo correspondence process. *Vision Res. 30*, 1955–1970.

Julesz, B. (1960). Binocular depth perception of computer generated patterns. *Bell Syst. Tech. J. 39*, 1125–1162.

Julesz, B. (1971). *Foundations of Cyclopean Perception*. Chicago: University of Chicago Press.

Julesz, B. (1986). Stereoscopic vision. *Vision Res. 26*, 1601–1612.

Julesz, B., and Payne, R. A. (1968). Differences between monocular and binocular stroboscopic movement perception. *Vision Res. 8*, 433–444.

Hubel, D. H. (1988). *Eye, Brain, and Vision*. New York: Scientific American Library.

Kovacs, I., and Julesz, B. (1992). Depth, motion, and static-flow perception at metaisoluminant color contrast. *Proc. Natl. Acad. Sci. U.S.A. 89*, 10390–10394.

Kovacs, I., Papathomas, T. V., and Julesz, B. (1991). Interaction of color and luminance in stereo perception. *Opt. Soc. Am. Tech. Dig. 17*, 202.

Kulikowski, J. J., and Walsh, V. (1993). Color vision: isolating mechanisms in overlapping system. *Prog. Vision Res. 95*, 417–426.

Marr, D., and Poggio, T. (1976). Cooperative computation of stereo disparity. *Science 194*, 283–287.

Marr, D., and Poggio, T. (1979). A computational theory of human stereo vision. *Proc. R. Soc. Lond. (B) 204*, 301–328.

Mullen, K. T., and Kulikowski, J. J. (1990). Wavelength discrimination at detection threshold. *J. Opt. Soc. Am. A 7*, 733–742.

Poggio, G. F., Motter, B. C., Squatrito, S., and Trotter, Y. (1985). Responses of neurons in visual cortex (V1 and V2) of the alert macaque to dynamic random-dot stereograms. *Vision Res. 25*, 397–406.

Poggio, G. F., Gonzalez, F., and Krause, F. (1988). Stereoscopic mechanisms in monkey visual cortex: binocular correlation and disparity selectivity. *J. Neurophysiol. 40*, 1392–1405.

Pollard, S. B., Mayhew, J. E. W., and Frisby, J. P. (1985). A stereo correspondence algorithm using a disparity gradient limit. *Perception 14*, 449–470.

Tyler, C. W. (1975). Stereoscopic tilt and size aftereffects. *Perception 4*, 187–192.

Tyler, C. W. (1991). Cyclopean vision. In D. Regan (Ed.), *Vision and Visual Disorders, Vol. 9, Binocular Vision* (pp. 38–74). New York: Macmillan.

Walsh, V., Kulikowski, J. J., and Butler, S. R. (1992). The effects of lesions of area V4 on the visual abilities of macaques: colour categorization. *Behav. Brain. Res. 52*, 81–89.

Weinshall, D. (1989). Perception of multiple transparent depth planes in stereo vision. *Nature (Lond.) 341*, 737–739.

Wheatstone, C. (1838). Some remarkable phenomena of binocular vision. *Phil. Trans. Roy. Soc. 128*, 371–394.

Cyclopean Riches: Cooperativity, Neurontropy, Hysteresis, Stereoattention, Hyperglobality, and Hypercyclopean Processes in Random-Dot Stereopsis

Christopher W. Tyler

Although the concept of combination of the monocular images into a single cyclopean view image dates back over a century, it was the development of the random-dot stereogram by Bela Julesz in 1960 that revealed the richness of the cyclopean process. Over the next three decades, Julesz and co-workers explored a wealth of stereoscopic phenomena that revealed many principles of neural organization both within and beyond the binocular processes. A sampling of these perceptual principles includes the following:

• *globality* in the ability to solve the binocular correspondence problem, i.e., to identify a unified percept of a coherent depth image from the cloud of possible correspondences between all the dots projecting to one eye and all the dots projecting to the other eye;

• *cooperativity* between the processing of different regions of the stereo image, which also may be required for solving the correspondence problem effectively;

• *hyperglobality* in the ability to perceive multiple surfaces simultaneously in the same region of space;

• *catabolic hysteresis* in the formation and dissolution of the fused depth image from and to the state of zero binocular correlation. Both depth perception and interocular correlation detection experiments show that it is easier to dissolve than to build up the fused global depth image;

• *attentional* effects in the third dimension that can seed the perception of one of a multiple stack of ambiguous stereoplanes;

• *hypercyclopean* effects that indicate the existence of a higher level of processing specific for the form elements of the cyclopean depth image.

The aim of the present chapter is to consider these examples of challenging stereoscopic effects in the context of a model of neural processing developed in previous work (Tyler, 1983, 1993). In summary, these and other phenomena may be viewed in the context of a five-stage model of stereopsis as a serial-parallel heterarchy for combining information from the two eyes. First is the optical transform generating the differences between the two eyes' images, followed by a set of parallel processing mechanisms specialized for comparing the disparate information in the two eyes. The information from these mechanisms is combined in a third stage of cooperative interactions, resulting in a "cleaned" cyclopean depth image. The fourth stage represents the receptive fields of hypercyclopean mechanisms viewing this cyclopean stereo image. The final stage combines this sensory mapping with information from other sensory sources and from memory to assign distance information. The full model is designed to accommodate all known stereoscopic phenomena in a unified heterarchical scheme.

Modes of Cortical Processing and Binocularity

The current view of the visual cortex is that it consists of many separate visual representation areas, each organized along both a serial hierarchical principle and a parallel distributed principle (Van Essen and Zeki, 1978; Van Essen and Maunsell, 1983; Livingstone and Hubel, 1988). The hierarchical principle is that the neural representation is organized into layers, with the inputs from each layer converging so as to condense the information as it projects onto the neurons of the next layer. The fact that this hierarchical condensation of information is happening in each of a large number of visual representation areas conforms to a parallel distributed principle on a large scale. There is also a medium-scale parallel organization of neural processing in that the hypercolumns within each representation area process local areas of the visual field in parallel. Finally, there is a small-scale parallel organization of neurons into separate columns making up each hypercolumn, with each column processing a different attribute of the region of the visual image served by the hypercolumn. This overlapping organization of parallel hierarchies, which may be termed a multiscale serial-parallel heterarchy, appears to be a ubiquitous principle of neural organization. Actually, the brain is even more complicated, in that there are neural feedback connections between hierarchical levels and interconnections between the parallel representations at each level, making it an interconnected heterarchy. This might seem to be so complex that the organization should be viewed as a homogeneously interconnected neural net, but there is sufficient differentiation imposed by the specificities of the various connections that it is important to recognize underlying structure in the connectivity.

In summary, the general organization of the cortex may be described as a multiscale interconnected heterarchy. This organization is descriptive of the structure of cortical hypercolumns in each representation area in each of the sensory systems (with the possible exception of olfaction, which may be just a homogeneous neural net). The local connectivity forms the similar types of heterarchy within the visual system from the retina to the cerebellum. It would not be surprising, therefore, to find a heterarchical arrangement within a particular sensory modality such as stereopsis. Although stereopsis is generally modeled as a single unified processing system, there is significant evidence that it has a number of independent subsystems, each specialized for extracting depth in a different manner.

It should be emphasized that the subsystems discussed here all fall within the domain of stereopsis from binocular disparity (i.e., to depth perception arising solely from the differences between the images projecting to the two eyes). There are many other monocular depth cues that can be used to generate dramatic depth impressions, such as differential motion cues, perspective, shape-from-shading, blur, interposition and so on. There are also nonvisual depth cues from such possible sources as convergence, accommodation, object familiarity, auditory cues, and so on. These cues all feed into the overall sense of depth in the real-world situation. The present analysis, however, focuses specifically on the role of binocular disparities of various kinds in the array of depth phenomena constituting stereopsis. Blake's chapter in this volume (chapter 2) deals with the psychophysics and modeling of binocular rivalry processes, which are postulated to occur at the second stage of the scheme of figure 1.1.

Binocular Optics: The First Stage of Stereoscopic Processing

The first operation that the human visual system performs on the three-dimensional (3D) information of the visual world is the geometric projection that condenses the 3D world down to the two planar images projected on the two retinas. This operation imposes a basic structure for which the cortex must compensate before the information can be processed into its 3D object relations. The binocular projection geometry was first worked out by Helmholtz (1866) and is elaborated in Tyler (1991a). Breitmeyer, Julesz, and Kropfl (1976) provided the first stereoscopic evidence for the backward shift of the horopter (Helmholtz had relied on evidence of the difference in perceived monocular tilts). Figure 1.2A shows how the regions of binocular fusion spread around a basic construction (the zero-disparity horopter) consisting of two lines—a vertical horopter line that is inclined backward by an amount that varies with fixation distance and a circle (or conic section) that lies at an angle close to hori-

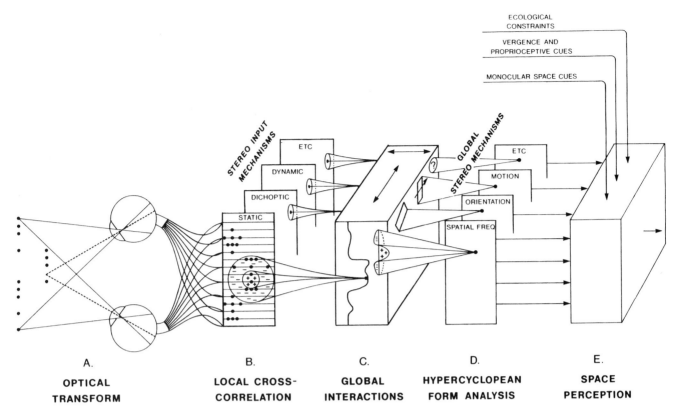

ECOLOGICAL
CONSTRAINTS

VERGENCE AND
PROPRIOCEPTIVE CUES

MONOCULAR SPACE CUES

STEREO INPUT
MECHANISMS

ETC
DYNAMIC
DICHOPTIC
STATIC

GLOBAL
STEREO MECHANISMS

ETC
MOTION
ORIENTATION
SPATIAL FREQ

A.	B.	C.	D.	E.
OPTICAL TRANSFORM	LOCAL CROSS-CORRELATION	GLOBAL INTERACTIONS	HYPERCYCLOPEAN FORM ANALYSIS	SPACE PERCEPTION

Figure 1.1

A model framework for stereoscopic depth perception in the form of a multistage serial-parallel heterarchy. (*A*) The binocular optical transform of spatial information. (*B*) Keplerian arrays of neural disparity processing. (*C*) Global cleaning of the refined depth image. (*D*) Hypercyclopean processing of the cyclopean forms. (*E*) Integration with nonbinocular depth cues to form the spatial map.

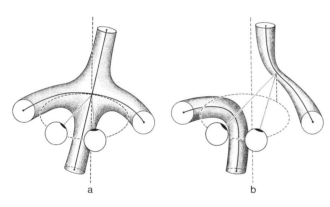

a

b

Figure 1.2

The fusion horopter, or region of points in space that are perceived as binocularly fused. (*a*) For fixation straight ahead and (*b*) for oblique fixation up and to the right. Note the complexity that the binocular optical transform imposes on the depth reconstruction task.

zontal. The fusion region will vary in thickness around them according to the distance from the fovea. Figure 1.2B shows how the horopter lines and the fusion "sausage" is modified when fixation is moved away from the straight-ahead position.

The horopter represents the zero positions for the binocular disparity metric, relative to which all other dispar-ities must be scaled to generate the depth map. This structure and its variation with fixation position must be built in and redressed by the depth reconstruction mechanism if a valid and reliable depth map is to be constructed. How the brain achieves this compensatory calibration is unknown, but it is interesting to recognize the complexity of the problem that needs to be solved.

Addressing the Correspondence Problem

The key problem for the perception of depth from the geometric projections onto the two retinas comes down to the problem of which point in one eye to consider as the "true" match for a particular point in the other; one of the most challenging problems for the understanding of vision. This "correspondence problem" did not arise from the invention of the random-dot stereogram, but was highlighted by their invention. Julesz (1962) pointed out that, in establishing corresponding details in disparate images, the ambiguity of which elements should be paired between the two eyes to give the appropriate depth image increases with the square of the number of points in each horizontal line, and felt that the solution of this problem required a cooperative process in the cortex. In fact, correspondences between dots with some vertical displacement must also be considered, so that the ambiguity problem actually increases with the fourth power of the matrix resolution, or linear dot density, up to the limits of neurally corresponding disparities. Tyler (1977) showed that the limiting foveal array size of 100×100 would have the astounding number of 25 million spurious correspondences, which would take a large proportion of brain cells just to represent them. Thus the processes by which the brain might reduce the ambiguity problem are of considerable interest. A precyclopean solution is one that utilizes processing (e.g., receptive field structure) before disparity identification to simplify the monocular inputs to the neural disparity array, whereas a post-cyclopean solution utilizes relationships between outputs from elements within that array (e.g., disparity inhibition).

Heterarchical Disparity Encoding Model

When reviewing the evidence for the variety of mechanisms contributing to stereopsis, I have concluded (Tyler, 1983) that it is not possible to accommodate all the diverse results within any single hierarchical model, which formed the basis for all stereopsis models that had been proposed both up to that time (e.g., Julesz, 1962; Sperling, 1970; Dev, 1975; Marr and Poggio, 1979) and subsequently (e.g., Pollard, Mayhew, and Frisby, 1985; Prazdny, 1985; Lehky and Sejnowski, 1990; Stevenson, Cormack, Schor, and Tyler, 1992). Depth perception has been demonstrated for diverse stimulus types that are incompatible with any single process for solving the binocular correspondence problem. The variety of stereoscopic mechanisms is described (Tyler, 1983) within the conceptual framework of a set of simple analyses by local cortical elements responsive to the disparity field, and similar local processing at higher levels, as opposed to the inherently cooperative models of such authors as Julesz (1971). It is assumed that the region of physical space that is processed by this system is optimized by means of both conjunctive (x, y) and vergent (z) eye movements. The organization of the neural components of the model has recently been described in detail with supporting evidence (Tyler, 1993). Only the main features of the neural model therefore will be summarized here.

This multilevel local approach has the advantage of breaking down the global nature of stereopsis (Julesz, 1978) into a sequence of processes (figure 1.1) that are empirically distinguishable. Within this serial structure, a further parallel organization is required for analyzing specialized global features of the stereoscopic image.

Philosophical Reflections on the Structure of Complex Models

The attempt to provide a model structure that can account for all known data on stereoscopic depth perception raises the philosophical question of whether such a model can be scientific, in the sense that it can be invalidated by empirical tests. Can any conceivable stereoscopic result be incorporated into the proposed modular heterarchy? If not, the approach is more of an analytic framework in which to develop particular models than a model in itself.

First, it should be stated that there is no attempt to develop a quantitative or computation model of any stereoscopic phenomena. The model structure to be presented is intended, rather, to highlight the shortcomings of previous models and sketch the kind of structure that might be required to account for the diverse range of depth perception effects. In doing so, the model has been constrained to have some features and not others. It has a modular structure at several of the stages, in which processing is discretely of one kind or another kind, as opposed to being a homogeneous neural net that can take any form within the N-dimensional space of processing options. The model also has a serial structure in which certain processes are assigned to early stages and others to late stages. These constraints predict particular experimental outcomes that could be, but have not yet been, tested. Examples of such predictions will be provided after the full model has been described.

Local Disparity-Selective Mechanisms

The point of departure of the neural model is a parallel array of cortical disparity "detectors," each responding to the presence of a stimulus with a particular location in x, y, z coordinates (represented by the rectangles in figure 1.1B, with the y axis omitted for clarity). The key feature of this approach is a reliance on arrays of specialized mechanisms of binocular matching to account for a variety of attributes of the stereoscopic process. Such mechanisms are represented by the sketched rectangles extending behind the first one in figure 1.1B. Examples of such attributes that will be discussed are the direction selectivity for motion in depth and selectivity for orientation of the elements making up the random-dot stereograms (RDS). Such selectivities are not predicted by inhibition or facilitation between simple disparity-selective neurons. Each specialized disparity array is assumed to operate in parallel with other such arrays at the same processing level, with the overall output being determined either by a combination of the processes or by the most sensitive process under particular stimulus conditions.

There are numerous indications that specialized arrays of local mechanisms might exist to process specific attributes of the field, in contrast to the unitary models that are often proposed for disparity processing. Classic examples of specialized mechanisms are provided by "feature-specific" neurons (or neural circuits) selectively sensitive to direction and velocity of retinal motion, color-opponent neurons, and neurons with orientation-specific excitation and inhibition (Hubel and Wiesel, 1962). Each specialized mechanism for stereopsis is assumed to operate in parallel with the others, in a manner analogous to such feature-specific neurons. (Note that it is the processing *arrays* of neurons that are proposed to operate in parallel in this model. Even unitary models postulate individual neurons that operate in parallel on the arrays of inputs from the retinas.)

Specialized disparity mechanisms may themselves exist in two classes according to whether specialization occurs at the local level (retinal-receptive-field characteristics) or global level (cortical interactions). Examples of local mechanisms that have been discussed are those specialized for the detection of stimuli with specific sizes and orientations, orientational disparities, motion in depth, and spatial frequency differences between the eyes.

As depicted in figure 1.1B, the initial stage of binocular combination is a disparity detection process that might be achieved by the various types of neurons with facilitatory responses to different disparities, as recorded in the visual cortex of cat and monkey (Barlow, Blakemore, and Pettigrew, 1967; Poggio et al., 1985; and Poggio, chapter 5 in this volume). This may be considered as a local cross-correlation process, performed by neurons tuned to different disparities, occurring at each location in the binocular visual field. As the eyes vary their vergence, cortical projections of the visual scene slide over one another to obtain the shift (or disparity) that produces the best match or correlation in each local region of the visual field. The images matched in this way are said to be in register. In practice there are, of course, two dimensions of field location, and there is no reason to suppose that the array is as regular as depicted here.

Mechanisms of Binocular Combination

The specialized mechanisms that have evolved in the human brain to accommodate the complexity of the binocular reconstruction process were categorized by Tyler (1993) into three classes (figure 1.3). The first consisted of *dichoptic mechanisms* for reconciling the essentially disjunctive information falling in corresponding points in the two eyes. Such dichoptic mechanisms included binocular fusion of similar images in adjacent dichoptic regions, interocular suppression and rivalry of strongly discrepant, high-contrast images at corresponding locations, binocular luster of areas with different local illumination levels, and the newly discovered process of linear binocular summation of discrepant images of low contrast or high spatial frequency (Tyler, 1993; Liu, Tyler, and Schor, 1992a).

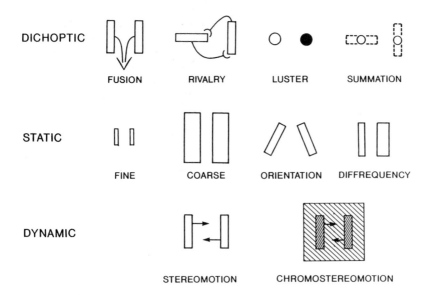

Figure 1.3
Types of binocular mechanisms. Each row diagrams a set of independent mechanisms of binocular combination in the form of its canonical binocular receptive field.

The next class was *static stereomechanisms* for the processing of horizontal disparities, which has been proposed to consist of fine and coarse spatial mechanisms (see review by Norcia, Sutter, and Tyler, 1985; Tyler, 1993). For an overview of the neurophysiological basis for such mechanisms, see chapter 5 by Poggio in this volume. In addition, there is evidence for specialized processing of orientational disparities between elongated receptive fields in the two eyes, which encode vertical inclinations in depth (Blakemore, Fiorentini, and Maffei, 1972; von der Heydt, Adorjani, and Hanny, 1977), and also for spatial frequency differences between the eyes, which encode lateral tilts in depth (Blakemore, 1970; Tyler and Sutter, 1979; see Tyler, 1993).

A distinction in this class that was not discussed in Tyler (1993) was whether static spatial disparity mechanisms operate on the basis of positional disparity or phase disparity (figure 1.4). This distinction arises on consideration of the retinal receptive fields of cortical neurons encoding the disparity signal. Such receptive fields are often well described by a Gabor sensitivity profile, which consists of a sinusoidal carrier windowed by a Gaussian envelope. This description raises the issue of whether the receptive field disparity between the two eyes is best represented by a disparity in the carrier alone (figure 1.4A, right) or both the carrier and envelope together (figure 1.4A, left). (There are other logical possibilities, but these examples represent the most likely types of organization.) A shift of both the carrier and the envelope together represents a positional disparity—the receptive field is shifted bodily to a noncorresponding position. This type is essentially the mechanism proposed by Barlow et al. (1967) to underlie stereopsis in cat cortex. A shift of the carrier alone represents a phase disparity—a mechanism that has been championed as the basis for cat stereopsis by Ohzawa, DeAngelis, and Freeman (1990). Liu, Tyler, Schor, and Ramachandran (1992b) pitted these two approaches against one another to predict contrast thresholds for human stereopsis when tested with *stimuli* with Gabor profiles that had either a phase disparity or a position disparity (which should have been optimal for the *receptive fields* with these respective organizations). The results clearly supported the positional disparity prediction and gave no hint of any contribution of a phase disparity mechanism in humans.

A further aspect that arises from consideration of these stimuli is the possibility of envelope disparity alone, with disparity information eliminated from the sinusoidal carrier signal. Liu et al. (1992b) ensured such elimination by (1) setting the carrier modulation to vertical (horizontal stripes) so that no horizontal disparity information was

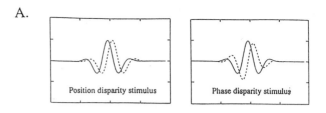

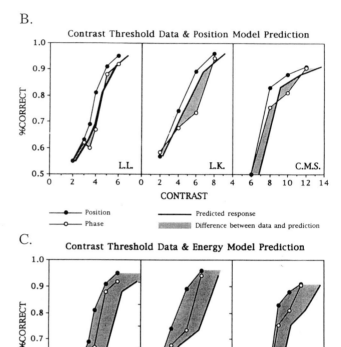

Figure 1.4

(*A*) Position and phase disparity stimuli used for contrast threshold measurements. (*B*) Psychometric functions for three observers for the contrast threshold for depth discrimination based on a 90° phase disparity (open circles) or the equivalent position disparity (filled circles). Hatched area shows the discrepancy between the position disparity data and the predictions of the disparity energy (phase) model. (*C*) Phase disparity data are well fitted by corresponding prediction from the position disparity model.

present, (2) doing the same but setting the interocular phase to 180° so that the stimuli were in phase rivalry, and (3) setting the two eyes' orientations to opposite obliques so that the stimuli were in orientation rivalry. In each case, depth was easily seen, although the disparity threshold was substantially higher than for carrier disparity and was in the range found for Gaussian luminance blobs of the same contrast and scale as the envelope information. Envelope disparity, even on stimuli that have both position and phase disparity blocked by rivalry, therefore appears to be a valid cue to depth. Although it is a second-order cue, in the sense that the information is unavailable to a linear (or first-order) mechanism, envelope disparity therefore is a valid candidate as an input cue to the stereoscopic processing heterarchy under discussion.

A final class of binocular mechanisms was that of *dynamic stereomechanisms* specialized for processing motion in depth. One reason for regarding these as separate mechanisms is that binocular receptive fields cannot logically be direction selective both for purely lateral motion and for purely depth motion. One requires the receptive fields to be selective for the same direction of motion in the two eyes, while the other requires opposite selectivities. There must therefore be a distinct class of dynamic stereomechanisms. Evidence has shown this class to include separate mechanisms with different properties for achromatic and chromatic depth motions (Tyler and Cavanagh, 1991), again as reviewed in Tyler (1993).

Global Interactions

The third cortical stage of the model is the site of the global interactions between the local disparity detectors that serve to refine the representation of the disparity image from its initial crude array of stimulated points to a coherent representation of the 3D surfaces present in the field of view (see figure 1.1C). A variety of such processes have been proposed by Julesz and others over the years, summarized in Julesz (1971, 1978) and Tyler (1983, 1991b).

Mechanisms in this class of global interactions use either conventional positional disparity information from the two retinas or specialized disparity information, but respond on the basis of some global aspect of the disparity field. The examples to be highlighted in this treatment are globality, cooperativity, hysteresis and hyperglobality.

Globality will be defined as the ability to solve the binocular correspondence problem, that is, to identify a unified percept of a coherent depth image from the cloud of possible correspondences between all the dots projecting to one eye and all the dots projecting to the other eye. The term is used in many different senses, but this definition follows that of Julesz (1978) in referring to the processes that embody a uniqueness constraint by restricting depth perception to a single perceived depth along any line of sight.

Cooperativity is the second type of global interaction discussed by Julesz in conjunction with random-dot stereogram perception. It is defined as any type of mutual interaction between the processing for different *spatial* regions of the stereo image. Such lateral cooperativity

may also be involved in solving the correspondence problem effectively; it may well include such interactions as lateral inhibition between disparity detectors (figure 1.5), disparity-specific pooling or facilitation, the disparity gradient limitation on the upper limit for depth reconstruction, coarse-to-fine matching processes for building up the depth image from the monocular information, and so on. These processes all may be conceived as taking place within the locus of global interactions following the interocular matching or disparity detection stage but preceding the generation of a unified global depth image from the plethora of available disparity information.

Hysteresis is a difference in sensitivity for a change between two states according to the direction of the change (figure 1.6). It may be termed catabolic hysteresis if the change is an order/disorder transition that occurs more readily for increases in disorder, or entropy, than for decreases in entropy. An example for the neural binocular system occurs in the formation and dissolution of the fused depth image from the state of zero binocular correlation. Both interocular correlation detection (Julesz and Tyler, 1976; Tyler and Julesz, 1976) and depth perception (Anderson, 1992) experiments show that it is easier to dissolve than to build up the perception of a fused global depth image.

Hyperglobality is defined as the ability to perceive multiple surfaces simultaneously in the same region of space (Julesz, 1978) (figure 1.7). This capability transcends the uniqueness constraint against such simultaneous perception of more than one surface which characterizes the simple globality principle. The uniqueness constraint is not, apparently, violated at any one spatial location; instead, the stereoscopic reconstruction process seems to be able to complete a perceived surface across neighboring elements attributable to each surface organization separately.

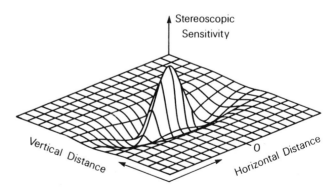

Figure 1.5
Cyclopean cooperativity in the form of the lateral interaction field between disparity detectors derived from data on the spatial frequency tuning to cyclopean corrugation stimuli. (From Tyler, 1991b.)

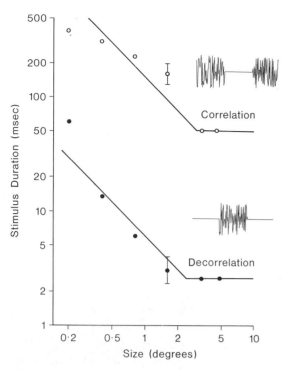

Figure 1.6
Demonstration of hysteresis in the detection of changes of binocular correlation. Decorrelation from a correlated state is much easier to detect than is correlation from a decorrelated state, for all field sizes. (From Tyler and Julesz, 1978.)

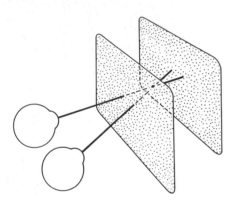

Figure 1.7
Depiction of the hyperglobal perception of two transparent surfaces in a random-dot stereogram.

Stereoscopic attention is another aspect of the stereoscopic reconstruction process that is raised by the perception of transparent surfaces. Whether both surfaces can be perceived simultaneously or whether there is an attentional alternation between the two (or more) possibilities is an open question. Julesz and Chang (1976) showed that the perception of ambiguous planes could be seeded by being preceded by a weak cuing stimulus that was invisible when presented alone. However, because the cue

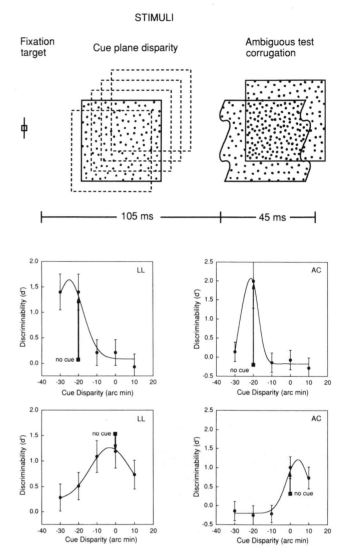

Figure 1.8
Demonstration of the operation of stereoscopic attention controlled by an exogenous cue plane, for two observers. The task is detection of the phase of depth corrugations presented ambiguously in one of a pair of transparent planes. Without the cue (squares) the corrugations are indiscriminable. The two different graphs for each observer show narrow disparity tuning of an attentional enhancement by the cue plane when it is proximal in depth to the test corrugation.

added information to the cued location, this result could be explained by subthreshold summation (a linear process) without recourse to an attentional enhancing mechanism. Kontsevich and Tyler (1992) performed a similar cueing experiment except that the task was to discriminate the phase of a stereo corrugation (figure 1.8). Subthreshold summation with the flat cue plane would then have reduced its discriminability, but performance was raised from chance levels to good discriminability when the cue plane was close to one of the test corrugations, but not otherwise. They therefore concluded that stereoattention could be attracted with 100 msec by the exogenous cue of a preceding test plane.

Hypercyclopean Perception

The concept of hypercyclopean analysis refers to the fourth level of processing of stereoscopic images described in figure 1.1. By analogy with the cortical neurons with receptive fields selective for particular properties of the retinal image, there could be neurons at a higher level in cortex having "receptive fields" at the level of the "cleaned" cyclopean depth image. These receptive fields would have a cyclopean basis, in the sense of having properties specific to the disparity selective neurons in the cyclopean retina, but would perform a hypercyclopean analysis of the spatial and temporal *form* of the depth image. Hypercyclopean receptive fields would have characteristics defined in terms of the figural properties of the cyclopean image, but independent of its specific disparity characteristics, that is, which particular disparity is stimulated at any given retinal location.

The existence of such a hypercyclopean level of processing can be demonstrated by means of a stereograting adaptation paradigm (Tyler, 1975) in which the stereograting is moved continuously across the retina, so as to avoid any stereoscopic depth afterimage. The obtained threshold elevation, which is specific to both spatial frequency and orientation of the adapting grating, therefore must be occurring at a higher level of form processing beyond that of the cyclopean processing for depth per se. Hypercyclopean specificities for adaptation to the spatial frequency content of the cyclopean image was demonstrated by Tyler (1975) and Schumer and Ganz (1979), orientation specificity in a cyclopean tilt aftereffect by Tyler (1975), and motion specificity in the form of a motion aftereffect to motion of the purely cyclopean depth image by Papert (1964).

Even beyond the hypercyclopean level there must be a further level of abstract spatial representation in which stereoscopic information is integrated with other spatial representations, such as those from the motion vector field (Gibson, 1950; Nakayama and Loomis, 1974), the texture gradient field (Gibson, 1950), and accommodation, vergence, vestibular, and other nonstereoscopic cues. Moreover, this integrated spatial representation is a likely site for the operation of "top-down" processes, where the spatial representation is configured to make sense in terms of object properties in the physical world. Stored knowledge of the object constraints operates to select between competing interpretations of the depth information up to this point, and to interdict aspects of the interpretations that are incompatible with object properties. This level of integration is indicated by figure 1.1E, but is not considered in detail in the present analysis.

Empirical Predictions of the Heterarchical Model Structure

Having completed the outline of the heterarchical model of stereoscopic processing, I will delineate the kinds of empirical tests that could be applied to assay its validity. With a model of this complexity, such tests should not be expected to be able to prove or disprove the model as a whole, but to help characterize the limits of its applicability. Nevertheless, there are aspects that, if not empirically supported, would seriously challenge the value of pursuing the modular heterarchical approach.

A simple way in which the parallel structure could be invalidated, for example at the early stage of monocular form recognition (figure 1.1B), would be a demonstration that the evidence for preprocessing into different stimulus features could be explained by a unitary mechanism. If, for example, the psychophysical evidence that orientation disparity plays a role in human vision were shown to be explained by some variety of nonlinear isotropic filtering within each retina, it could be that orientation disparity serves no detectable role in human depth perception (although I have been unable to generate such an explanation). Similar analytic demonstrations for each of the proposed modalities would imply that the early monocular processing was unitary rather than parallel in nature, rendering that stage of the model redundant.

Conversely, the global cleaning of the depth map at stage C is modeled as being a unitary process operating on the combined outputs of all the parallel modules at stage B. The model thus has a convergent/divergent structure that specifically does not postulate multiple depth maps for each monocular cue type. It further postulates that the nonstereoscopic depth cues enter to scale the depth representation late in the process (stage E), rather than modifying the scalings for each monocular cue type independently at stage B. In principle, these predictions are testable by experiments in which mixtures of different depth cues are presented with different time relations, but this is not the place to elaborate such paradigms in detail. The point is that the model has significant constraints that are empirically testable in future studies.

In conclusion, the comprehensive model framework that is proposed here is based on modules that are intended to be physiologically plausible. Nevertheless, much work remains to be done to specify the details of the processes to account for the psychophysical and electrophysiological data concerning binocular function. For an overview of specific computational schemes that address such details, mostly at the second stage of the model (figure 1.1B), see the chapter by Weinshall and Malik in this volume. It is hoped that my model framework will help to lay the groundwork for further efforts in developing a complete computational model of human stereopsis.

Acknowledgments

Supported by NIH grant EY 7890.

References

Anderson, B. L. (1992). Hysteresis, cooperativity, and depth averaging in dynamic random-dot stereograms. *Percep. Psychophy. 51*, 511–528.

Barlow, H. B., Blakemore, C., and Pettigrew, J. D. (1967). The neural mechanism of binocular depth discrimination. *J. Physiol. 193*, 327–342.

Blakemore, C. (1970). A new kind of stereoscopic vision. *Vision Res. 10*, 1181–1200.

Blakemore, C., Fiorentini, A., and Maffei, L. (1972). A second neural mechanism of binocular depth discrimination. *J. Physiol. 226*, 725–749.

Breitmeyer, B., Julesz, B., and Kropfl, W. (1976). Dynamic random-dot stereograms reveal up-down anistropy and left-right isotropy between cortical hemifields. *Science 187*, 269–270.

Dev, P. (1975). Perception of depth surfaces in random-dot stereograms. *Int. J. Man-Machine Stud. 7*, 511–528.

Gibson, J. J. (1950). *The Perception of the Visual World*. Boston: Houghton-Mifflin.

Helmholtz, H. von (1866). *Handbuch der physiologische Optik*. (Vol. III) Hamburg: Voss.

Hubel, D. H., and Wiesel, T. N. (1962). Receptive fields, binocular interaction and functional architecture in the cat's visual cortex. *J. Physiol. 160*, 106–154.

Julesz, B. (1960). Binocular depth perception of computer-generated patterns. *Bell Syst. Tech. J. 39*, 1125–1162.

Julesz, B. (1962). Towards the automation of binocular depth perception (AUTOMAP-I). In C. M. Popplewell (Ed.), *Proceedings IFIPS*. Amsterdam: North-Holland.

Julesz, B. (1971). *Foundations of Cyclopean Perception*. Chicago: University of Chicago Press.

Julesz, B. (1978). Global stereopsis: Cooperative phenomena in stereoscopic depth perception. In R. Held, H. W. Leibowitz, and H.-L. Teuber (Eds.), *Handbook of Sensory Physiology, Vol VII: Perception*. Berlin: Springer-Verlag.

Julesz, B., and Chang, J. J. (1976). Interaction between pools of binocular disparity detectors tuned to different disparities. *Biol. Cybern. 22*, 107–119.

Julesz, B., and Tyler, C. W. (1976). Neurontropy, an entropy-like measure of neural correlation in binocular fusion and rivalry. *Biol. Cybern. 22*, 107–119.

Kontsevich, L. L., and Tyler, C. W. (1992). The role of disparity cueing in depth perception. *Invest. Ophthalmol. Visual Sci. 33*, 1373.

Lehky, S. R., and Sejnowski, T. J. (1990). Neural model of stereoacuity and depth interpolation based on a distributed representation of stereo disparity. *J. Neurosci. 10*, 2281–2299.

Liu, L., Tyler, C. W., and Schor, C. M. (1992a). Failure of rivalry at low contrast: Evidence of a suprathreshold binocular summation process. *Vision Res. 32*, 1471–1479.

Liu, L., Tyler, C. W., Schor, C. M., and Ramachandran, V. S. (1992b). Position disparity is more efficient in encoding depth than is phase disparity. *Invest. Ophthalmol. Visual Sci. 33*, 1373.

Livingstone, M., and Hubel, D. H. (1988). Segregation of form, color, movement and depth: Anatomy, physiology and perception. *Science 240*, 740–749.

Marr, D., and Poggio, T. A. (1979). A computational theory of human stereo vision. *Proc. R. Soc. London 204*, 301–328.

Nakayama, K., and Loomis, J. M. (1974). Optical velocity patterns, velocity sensitive neurons and space perception: A hypothesis. *Perception 3*, 63–80.

Norcia, A. M., Sutter, E. E., and Tyler, C. W. (1985). Electrophysiological evidence for the existence of coarse and fine disparity mechanisms in human vision. *Vision Res. 25*, 1603–1611.

Ohzawa, I., DeAngelis, G. C., and Freeman, R. D. (1990). Stereoscopic depth discrimination in the visual cortex: Neurons ideally suited as disparity detectors. *Science 249*, 1037–1041.

Papert, S. (1964). Stereoscopic synthesis as a technique for localizing visual mechanisms. *MIT Quart. Prog. Rep. 73*, 239–243.

Pollard, S. B., Mayhew, J. E. W., and Frisby, J. P. (1985). PMF: A stereo correspondence algorithm using disparity gradient. *Proceedings of the 3rd International Symposium on Robotics Research*. (pp. 19–26). Cambridge, MA: MIT Press.

Poggio, G. F., Motter, B. C., Squatrito, S., and Trotter, Y. (1985). Responses of neurons in visual cortex (V1 and V2) of the alert macaque to dynamic random dot stereograms. *Vision Res. 25*, 397–406.

Prazdny, K. (1985). Detection of binocular disparities. *Biol. Cybern. 52*, 93–99.

Schumer, R. A., and Ganz, L. (1979). Independent stereoscopic channels for different extents of spatial pooling. *Vision Res. 19*, 1303–1314.

Sperling, G. (1970). Binocular vision: A physical and neural theory. *J. Am. Psychol. 83*, 461–534.

Stevenson, S., Cormack, L., Schor, C. M., and Tyler, C. W. (1992). Disparity tuning mechanisms of human stereopsis. *Vision Res. 32*, 1685–1694.

Tyler, C. W. (1975). Stereoscopic tilt and size aftereffects. *Perception 4*, 187–192.

Tyler, C. W. (1977). Spatial limitations in stereopsis. *Transact. Soc. Photo Opt. Instrum. Eng. 120*, 36–42.

Tyler, C. W. (1983). Sensory processing of binocular disparity. In C. M. Schor and K. J. Ciuffreda (Eds.), *Vergence Eye Movements: Basic and Clinical Aspects*. (pp. 199–295). London: Butterworths.

Tyler, C. W. (1991a). The horopter and binocular fusion. In D. Regan (Ed.), *Vision and Visual Disorders, Vol. 9, Binocular Vision.* (pp. 19–37). New York: Macmillan.

Tyler, C. W. (1991b). Cyclopean vision. In D. Regan (Ed.), *Vision and Visual Disorders, Vol. 9, Binocular Vision.* (pp. 38–74). New York: Macmillan.

Tyler, C. W. (1993). The development of the threshold nonlinearity, peripheral acuity, binocularity and complex stereoscopic processing. In K. Simons (Ed.), *Infant Vision: Basic and Clinical Research.* (pp. 38–74). New York: Oxford University Press.

Tyler, C. W., and Cavanagh, P. (1991). Purely chromatic perception of motion in depth: Two eyes as sensitive as one. *Percep. Psychophy. 49,* 53–61.

Tyler, C. W., and Julesz, B. (1976). The neural transfer characteristic (neurontropy) for binocular stochastic stimulation. *Biol. Cybern. 23,* 33–37.

Tyler, C. W., and Julesz, B. (1978). Binocular cross-correlation in time and space. *Vision Res. 18,* 101–105.

Tyler, C. W., and Sutter, E. E. (1979). Depth from spatial frequency difference: An old kind of stereopsis? *Vision Res. 19,* 859–865.

Van Essen, D. C., and Maunsell, J. H. R. (1983). Hierarchical organization and functional streams in the visual cortex. *Trends Neurosci. 6,* 370–375.

Van Essen, D. C., and Zeki, S. M. (1978). The topographic organization of rhesus monkey prestriate cortex. *J. Physiol. 277,* 193–226.

von der Heydt, R., Adorjani, C., and Hanny, P. (1977). Neural mechanisms of stereopsis: Sensitivity to orientational disparity. *Experientia 33,* 786.

2

Psychoanatomical Strategies for Studying Human Visual Perception

Randolph Blake

It is commonly acknowledged that the visual system consists of a hierarchically arranged series of processing stages. Most visual scientists believe that neurons at early stages of this hierarchy signal the presence of primitive features of the visual scene (e.g., contour orientation, edge polarity) at local regions of the retinal image, while higher stages register more abstract, global aspects of the visual scene. Over the last few decades, the cartography of the primate visual pathways has grown ever more complex (compare, for example, the map produced by Hubel, 1988, with that by Felleman and Van Essen, 1991), and there is every reason to believe that these advances will continue as neuroscientists move from well-charted visual areas (e.g., V1) into less familiar cortical territories (e.g., medial intraparietal, MIP).

As we learn more about the neural organization of the primate visual system and the receptive field properties of neurons at various processing stages, it becomes increasingly tempting to assign specific visual functions to particular stages. Indeed, this represents a key theme of the conference that sponsored this volume. To pursue this linkage between neuroscience and perception, however, also requires the deployment of psychophysical strategies for generating *functional* maps of visual processing. As will be illustrated in this chapter, this is possible using perceptual/psychophysical data to draw conclusions about stages of processing in human vision—collectively, the strategies for generating and interpreting these data constitute *psychoanatomy*. Stated succinctly, psychoanatomy involves the construction of flow diagrams of stages of perceptual processing based on psychophysical data.

Typically, psychoanatomical conclusions are of the form "process *A* precedes process *B*," where *A* and *B* refer to neural operations underlying perceptual phenomena. These ideas were introduced in Julesz's 1971 book on *Foundations of Cyclopean Perception*:

a process (or neural net) A is before another process B if B utilizes A. This directionality in the information flow is not affected if a process C is after process B and the output of C is utilized by A (feedback). Even if A and B are connected in a closed loop, B thus utilizing A and vice versa, we will regard

A *as being before* B *if* A *(and not* B) *utilizes a process* I *that utilizes neither* A *nor* B. *(p. 82)*

An analogy may clarify the basic idea. Suppose we wish to prepare one of the world's truly great culinary treats, Hungarian goulash. In the upper part of figure 2.1 are listed the ingredients, which constitute the "input" to the process. But in addition to this list of ingredients, one also needs the recipe, i.e., the hierarchically arranged series of stages through which the ingredients must pass on their way to becoming Hungarian goulash. As those ingredients pass through the early stages, they are combined to create new entities that constitute the input to even later stages. We can, in fact, construct a flow diagram representing the hierarchical stages involved in creating this dish, and that is shown in the lower part of figure 2.1.

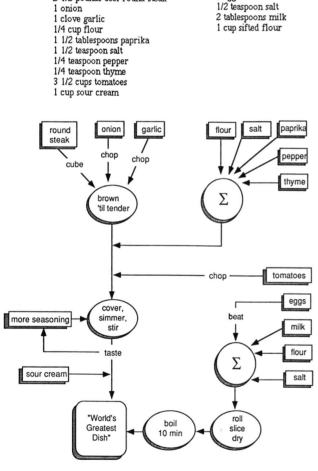

Figure 2.1
List of ingredients (*top*) and recipe in flow diagram form (*bottom*) for preparing Hungarian Goulash.

Visual perception, although staggeringly more complex than preparing goulash, can be conceptualized similarly. Physics and mathematics allow us to characterize the inputs, or ingredients, of perception. These inputs comprise objects and events in the visual world, definable in physical terms such as spatial frequency, wavelength, optic flow, and so on.[1] Using psychophysical techniques we can measure perceptual and behavioral responses to those inputs, i.e., the output, which corresponds to the completed dish in the cooking analogy. But how do we go about isolating and studying the intervening stages between input and final product, i.e., the recipe for seeing? What strategies can be devised for tracing the flow of visual information as it evolves from simple primitive features to the complex, rich product that guides our behaviors and populates our conscious experiences?

The following sections outline several complementary strategies for determining the ordering of functional stages of vision and, hence, for constructing the psychoanatomy of human vision. It should be stressed that the perception literature is replete with examples of psychoanatomical reasoning—the ones discussed here are merely illustrative. Moreover, interested readers are referred to the stimulating essays by Teller (1984, 1990)—these provide a very thoughtful analysis of reasoning patterns employed by visual scientists in their attempts to relate visual perception to underlying neural processes. Also of relevance is the chapter by Teller and Pugh (1983), who formalize the notion of "critical loci" in visual processing. It is strategies for isolating these critical loci that constitute the topic of this chapter.

Inferential Strategies

One class of strategies relies explicitly on anatomical and/or physiological data for inferring stages of processing. Recognizing that anatomy and/or physiology may impose limits at a given locus of visual processing—by filtering or condensing information available to subsequent stages of processing—one may ask whether visual performance on a given task is restricted by those limitations. If so, one may infer something about the relative ordering of processes. To give a trivially obvious example, the eye's optics limit the spatial detail in the retinal image, thereby imposing a ceiling on visual resolution. (Other, postoptical elements may, of course, lower that ceiling even further.) Another, more powerful exam-

---

1. The physical characterization of the effective stimulus for perception represents a fundamental, nontrivial problem in the study of visual perception, as underscored by the chapters in this volume by Lappin et al., by Watt, and by Victor et al.

ple of this line of reasoning comes from color matching: as a consequence of the univariance principle instantiated within the three cone types, physically different wavelengths can be appropriately mixed to yield indistinguishable color patches. Moving a little deeper into the visual pathways, it is known that falloff in vernier acuity with eccentric viewing scales with the human cortical magnification factor, not with variation in retinal ganglion cell density (Levi, Klein, and Aitsebaomo, 1985), implying that the neural interactions limiting fine positional discriminations arise within the cortex, not the retina. A comprehensive example of the application of this line of psychoanatomical reasoning can be found in Geisler (1989) and a critical analysis of the logical status of this line of reasoning can be found in Teller (1984).

While knowledge about actual anatomical/physiological limitations can promote psychoanatomical reasoning, such information is not necessary for the deployment of inferential strategies. It is possible to answer "before/after" questions by determining the effective stimulus for a given perceptual phenomenon. Specifically, has that effective stimulus been constrained or "colored" by prior visual processing? Without going into the details, the following represent just a few examples of psychoanatomical conclusions derived using this line of reasoning:

• Filling in of the blind spot occurs before visual search and pop-out (Ramachandran, 1992).

• Surface segmentation and representation of occlusion precede disambiguation of motion in a barber pole animation sequence (Shimojo, Nakayama, and Silverman, 1989).

• Neural events responsible for depth segregation precede those for disambiguation of plaid motion (Stoner, Albright, and Ramachandran, 1990).

• Neural adaptation responsible for the motion aftereffect occurs after registration of information about the shape of the aperture within which motion occurs (Power and Moulden, 1992).

Deployment of Unique Stimuli

Another, related category of psychoanatomical strategies involves using clever visual stimuli to reveal the relative ordering of perceptual processes. Included in this category are stimuli portraying object characteristics not explicitly represented in the retinal image. To illustrate, consider the following examples.

It is well known that half-images like those shown in figure 2.2a generate stereoscopic depth: the lines appear rotated about a horizontal axis out of the picture plane.

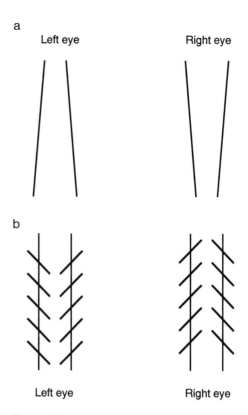

Figure 2.2
Two pairs of stereo half-images. The top pair (*A*), because of the differences in orientation, creates an impression of depth: the two lines appear rotated out of the picture plane. The bottom pair (*B*) consists of perfectly parallel vertical lines that *look* different in orientation. The perceptual, but not physical, conditions for stereo depth are present in this lower pair of half-images.

The disparity responsible for generating this sensation of depth is explicit in the images themselves. But consider the half-images in figure 2.2b—here the pairs of lines are, in fact, parallel but *appear* slightly tilted owing to the Zollner illusion. Upon fusion of these half-images, is stereo depth experienced? According to Lau (1922; cited in Julesz, 1971) the answer is yes. This result, if true, would imply that the neural process registering disparity (process B) receives contour information that has been colored by the neural events underlying the Zollner illusion (process A). Although Lau's observations are controversial (e.g., Ogle, 1952), the claim represents a clear instance of psychoanatomical reasoning.

Turning to another example of the use of one phenomenon to elicit another, Smith and Over (1975; see also Paradiso, Shimojo, and Nakayama, 1989) found that the tilt aftereffect could be generated by prolonged inspection of a subjective contour; the orientation selectivity of this aftereffect was comparable to that associated with adaptation to real contours. This implies that orientation-selective neurons subject to adaptation (process B) can be

Table 2.1
Some visual phenomena experienced with random-dot stereograms

Phenomena	Reference
Necker cube reversals	Julesz (1971)
Ebbinghaus illusion	Julesz (1971)
Vertical–horizontal illusion	Julesz (1971)
Zollner illusion	Julesz (1971)
Poggendorf illusion	Julesz (1971)
Müller–Lyer illusion	Julesz (1971)
Ponzo illusion	Patterson and Fox (1983)
Metacontrast masking	Patterson and Fox (1990)
Ternus effect	Patterson et al. (1991)
Apparent motion	Patterson et al. (1992)
Motion aftereffect	Fox et al. (1982, but see Papert, 1964)
Illusory contours	Julesz and Frisby (1975)
Optokinetic nystagmus	Fox et al. (1978)

activated by illusory contours (process A).[2] In a similar vein, illusory contours are effective maskers of real contours in a backward masking paradigm (Smith and Over, 1977).

The epitome of this strategy is the random-dot stereogram, and the pinnacle of its application may be found in Julesz's 1971 book. The idea is both simple and elegant. Shapes or objects can be created using random-dot stereograms, and any characteristics associated with those shapes or objects must be attributable to perceptual processes that arise after the stereoscopic combination of information from the two eyes. Thus, for example, we may create a cyclopean Necker cube, and we observe that this cube exhibits the same sort of bistability experienced upon viewing the textbook version. But, of course, the cyclopean Necker cube is literally the creation of binocular disparity, so we are forced to conclude that the bistability experienced in this cube results from neural actions that transpire after the registration of disparity information between the two monocular views—the requisite information literally does not exist prior to this level of processing. Table 2.1 provides a sample of classic visual phenomena (including references) that have been shown to exist in cyclopean forms generated by random-dot stereograms.

Binocular Interaction

In a sense, cyclopean stereoscopy is one member of a family of psychoanatomical strategies that exploit binocular vision. Another familiar binocular strategy involves interocular transfer of visual adaptation, which works like this. One eye is exposed to some visual display for a period of time, the so-called adaptation period. Immediately following this adaptation period, the aftereffects of adaptation are tested in the other eye. If an aftereffect is observed in this nonadapted eye, the aftereffect is said to "transfer" interocularly (i.e., between the eyes). Interocular transfer is taken as evidence that adaptation occurs at a central site, at or beyond the point where information from the two eyes has been integrated neurally (Blake, Overton, and Lema-Stern, 1981). For this conclusion to be definitive, however, interocular transfer must be paired with retinal pressure blinding (e.g., Blake and Fox, 1972). With this technique, pressure applied to an adapted eye induces ischemia in its retinal ganglion cells, thus blocking transmission of signals from that eye to the brain; if an adaptation aftereffect is still observed by the other eye while the adapted eye is pressure blinded, the locus of adaptation must be cortical, not retinal.

The rest of this chapter focuses on a phenomenon of binocular vision that, in a sense, constitutes the antithesis of stereopsis. This phenomenon is binocular rivalry, the repetitive fluctuations in monocular perception occasioned by dissimilar stimulation of the two eyes. Rivalry is fascinating, because it represents a striking dissociation between conscious visual perception and physical stimulation: a complex, intense monocular image may be suppressed from consciousness for many seconds at a time. What transpires within the visual nervous system to cause this temporary interruption of vision? And where in the chain of visual processing are the neural events responsible for this interruption occurring? Obviously, the optical image of the suppressed picture continues to impinge on the retina; the photoreceptors continue to function and, presumably, the ganglion cells of that eye convey their messages onto higher visual stages. But at some point in the normal chain of events, the neural messages associated with that eye's view are blocked or disrupted. In fact, it is possible to specify the neural site of the

2. Whether there is a *single* site of orientation-specific adaptation, activated either by real contours or illusory contours, remains to be learned. Some might argue that illusory contours—and their associated adaptation aftereffects—arise at a processing stage (e.g., V2—see von der Heydt et al., 1984) different

from the site of adaptation to real contours (e.g., V1). This does not undermine the logic of the psychoanatomical strategy, but it does qualify the conclusions derived from application of the strategy.

disruption relative to the neural events responsible for other visual phenomena. It is possible, in other words, to draw firm psychoanatomical conclusions, using binocular rivalry as a reference landmark. The following examples illustrate application of this strategy, and an additional example may be found in the chapter by Kulikowski and Walsh in this volume.

Size Constancy

Let us start with size constancy, the invariance in the perceived size of an object despite variations in image size with viewing distance. This invariance, or constancy, implies the existence of a mechanism that scales retinal image size by distance. With this in mind, consider next how the spatial extent of binocular rivalry depends on rival target size (Blake, O'Shea, and Mueller, 1992). Large rival targets tend to engage in piecemeal rivalry: one eye's view rarely dominates completely when targets are large and, instead, the observer experiences a dynamic mosaic consisting of bits and pieces of each eye's view. With small targets, however, rivalry tends to be complete: one eye's view or the other's dominates in its entirety. So, whether rivalry is piecemeal or complete depends on the size of the inducing targets. But is this dependence based on retinal image size or on perceived size? In other words, does rivalry operate before or after size constancy has scaled retinal images?

To answer this question, Blake, Fox, and Westendorf (1974) exploited Emmert's law, wherein the perceived size of an afterimage varies with viewing distance. The afterimage (whose angular subtense is fixed on the retina) looks small when viewed against a near surface but large when viewed against a far surface. We induced afterimages of rival targets and had observers view the ongoing rivalry between the afterimages on a near surface and on a far surface. As long as the angular size of the afterimages was small, rivalry was always complete, even though the targets looked quite large because of size/distance scaling. Large angular images always engaged in piecemeal rivalry, even when apparently small. Clearly, then, rivalry operates on images unscaled for distance; rivalry occurs prior to the process responsible for size constancy. But the output from rivalry does undergo size scaling, for rival afterimages do obey Emmert's law. Size constancy occurs after and receives input from rivalry.

Apparent Motion

Next consider apparent motion (AM). Imagine a two-frame AM sequence in which a rectangular cluster of dots

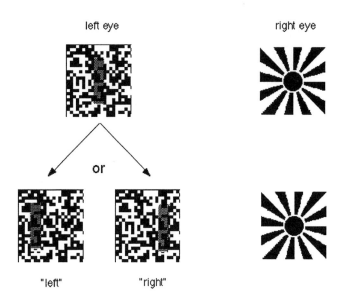

Figure 2.3
Schematic of stimulus conditions used to test for perception of apparent motion during binocular rivalry. The gray rectangles within the random-dot patterns merely denote clusters of dots and they were not present in the actual two-frame animation sequences. Clear apparent motion is experienced regardless of whether the initial frame (*top*) was dominant or completely suppressed by the other eye's rival target.

in the first frame is shifted either leftward or rightward in the second frame. Observers will experience a rectangle moving from the center to one side or the other. Using rival targets like those shown in figure 2.3, Wiesenfelder and Blake (1991) found that observers could still make this discrimination—left vs. right motion—even when the first frame of the AM sequence is suppressed during rivalry. The observers were instructed to depress a computer key whenever the "sunburst" target was completely dominant, with no trace of the random-dot pattern. This key press triggered the replacement of the first random-dot pattern with a second one, in which a subset of dots had been shifted in one direction or the other. Performance was essentially perfect, and no different from that measured when the transition occurred while the dot pattern was dominant. Evidently, the positional information in the first frame was registered during suppression and was available for integration with the information contained in the second frame.

Wiesenfelder and Blake also noted that the AM sequence initiated during suppression prematurely terminated suppression of the random-dot pattern; in this respect, AM behaves just like real motion, which can trigger an abrupt transition from suppression to dominance (Walker and Powell, 1979). This pattern of results implies that the output from the process responsible for AM feeds into the neural site of rivalry suppression; the two processes do not occur along parallel, noninteracting pathways.[3]

Motion Adaptation

Psychoanatomical reasoning has also been applied to another aspect of motion perception, visual adaptation. Everyone is familiar with the motion aftereffect (MAE): after staring at motion for a period of time, a subsequently viewed stationary object appears to drift in the opposite direction. This illusory motion presumably results from a temporary reduction in the responsiveness of neurons registering image motion in a given direction, such that following adaptation there is a temporary imbalance in opponently organized, direction-selective neurons. Lehmkuhle and Fox (1975) found that a robust motion aftereffect could be induced even when the monocular adapting motion was suppressed for a substantial portion of the time during binocular rivalry. This implies that

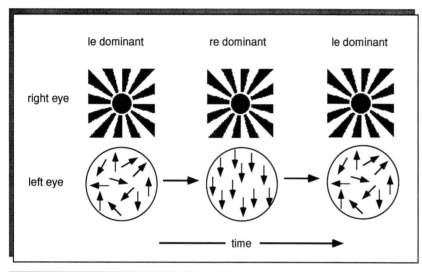

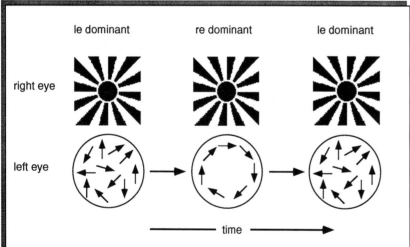

Figure 2.4
Schematic of rival displays used to adapt observers to coherent motion only during periods of suppression. The arrows denote motion vectors, and the top panel shows random motion during left eye dominance and downward motion during left eye suppression. In the lower panel, dots move randomly during left eye dominance but rotate clockwise during left eye suppression. Following adaptation, the upper adaptation sequence yields a vivid motion aftereffect: random motion appears to have an upward drift. The lower adaptation sequence, which under normal conditions produces a strong counterclockwise motion aftereffect, yields no rotational aftereffect. In the actual experiments, the diameter of the rival targets was 1 deg, and the dot density was approximately 40 dots deg^{-2}.

---

3. When it is found that process A is unaffected by process B, one cannot conclude that A precedes B in a chain of neural events; A and B could occur within parallel pathways. To conclude that A precedes B, one must also demonstrate that A affects B while B does not affect A.

the neural events underlying motion adaptation transpire prior to or in parallel with the site of rivalry suppression. Wiesenfelder and Blake (1990), however, found that adaptation to spiral motion *was* weakened by suppression, suggesting that this more complex type of motion (which entails expansion and rotation) is registered at a neural site *after* suppression. These complementary findings have been replicated and extended by van der Zwan, Wenderoth, and Alais (1993).

In the adaptation studies mentioned above, the adaptation motion was intermittently visible, owing to the inevitable alternations in rivalry dominance. Thus, observers periodically experienced motion during adaptation. Very recently Karen Yu and I developed a procedure for adapting an eye to either translational motion or to rotational motion, with this adapting motion always confined to suppression phases of rivalry (i.e., the adapting motion was always invisible). With our procedure (see figure 2.4), one eye viewed a small patch of dots moving randomly with no coherent direction of motion; the other viewed a "sunburst" pattern, which was contrast reversed a few times a second. The observer pressed computer keys to track periods of dominance of the two displays. Whenever the observer signaled complete dominance of the sunburst, the random motion was replaced with coherent motion—this constitutes the adaptation motion. This replacement nearly always went completely unnoticed, and the moment the observer released the key signaling dominance of the motion, the coherent motion reverted to random motion. So, in effect, the observer actually "saw" the adapting motion only momentarily before releasing the key—exposure to coherent motion was essentially confined to periods of suppression. Because the sunburst

is a strong stimulus, it tended to dominate much of the time, and because the rival targets were very small (recall the discussion of size constancy) even brief periods of partial dominance were very infrequent.

We interspersed brief test periods throughout this procedure. The tests consisted of 1-sec presentations of random or near-random motion, with nothing presented to the other eye. The observer was forced to judge the direction of motion of the test display (see Blake and Hiris, 1993, for details of this procedure). We found that suppression did not block adaptation to translational motion—a robust MAE is generated to a motion sequence that is never seen. But rotational motion is neutralized by suppression—no evidence was found for a rotational MAE following periods of adaptation to the suppressed rotary motion. This pattern of results, from two observers so far, implies that translational motion and rotational motion are registered at distinct neural sites, with rivalry suppression sandwiched between.

Concluding Ideas

Figure 2.5 shows a flow diagram summarizing results from my utilization of rivalry as an inferential, psychoanatomical tool. Without going through each of the connections, suffice it to say that the relative ordering has been established by determining the effect of rivalry on these various phenomena, and vice versa. Note that the flow is not strictly one-way and instead includes feedback connections (see Wiesenfelder and Blake, 1990, for discussion of feedback). Vision, after all, is not strictly serial in nature; rather, it involves an indefinite succession of

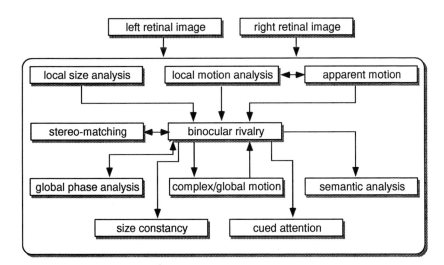

Figure 2.5
Schematic showing ordering of stages of processing, based on experiments using binocular rivalry as a neural reference site.

intertwined neural events, each influencing the other. Note also that this diagram is not comprehensive—many obvious aspects of vision are missing (e.g., color). The diagram simply illustrates the kind of ideas germinating from this particular psychoanatomical approach. Moreover, each functional stage denoted in this diagram may itself be decomposed into constituent processes. For example, stereopsis is commonly thought to involve feature matching of the two monocular images followed by disparity computation, and as Tyler's chapter in this volume details, these operations may be performed in multiple parallel pathways—see his figure 1.1 as well as the chapter by Poggio on the putative neural concomitants of stereopsis.

Ultimately we would like to know the relation between the kind of psychoanatomical diagram shown in figure 2.5 and the maps derived by neuroanatomists (e.g., Felleman and van Essen, 1991). At a minimum, these psychoanatomical data should provide the neurophysiologist with useful clues about the possible neural concomitants of these perceptual phenomena. In this spirit, psychoanatomy is complementary to the elegant localization techniques utilized in neuroscience. It seems altogether fitting that an overview of these strategies be included in a volume honoring one of the pioneer pscychoanatomists, Bela Julesz.

Acknowledgments

The author's work described in this chapter was supported by grants from the Eye Institute, National Institutes of Health, and the National Science Foundation. Karen Yu provided helpful comments on an earlier draft.

References

Blake, R., and Fox, R. (1972). Interocular transfer of adaptation to spatial frequency during retinal ischaemia. *Nature (London) 240*, 76–77.

Blake, R., and Hiris, E. (1993). Another means for measuring the motion aftereffect. *Vision Res. 33*, 1589–1592.

Blake, R., Fox, R., and Westendorf, D. (1974). Visual size constancy occurs after binocular rivalry. *Vision Res. 14*, 585–586.

Blake, R., Overton, R., and Lema-Stern, S. (1981). Interocular transfer of visual aftereffects. *J. Exp. Psychol. Hum. Percept. Perform. 7*, 367–381.

Blake, R., O'Shea, R. P., and Mueller, T. J. (1992). Spatial zones of binocular rivalry in central and peripheral vision. *Visual Neurosci. 8*, 469–478.

Felleman, D. J., and van Essen, D. C. (1991). Distributed hierarchical processing in the primate cerebral cortex. *Cerebral Cortex 1*, 1–47.

Fox, R., Lehmkuhle, S., and Leguire, L. E. (1978). Stereoscopic contours induce optokinetic nystagmus. *Vision Res. 18*, 1189–1192.

Fox, R., Patterson, R., and Lehmkuhle, S. W. (1982). Effect of depth position on the motion aftereffect. *Invest. Ophthalmol. Visual Sci. (Suppl.) 22*, 144.

Geisler, W. S. (1989). Sequential ideal-observer analysis of visual discriminations. *Psychol. Rev. 96*, 267–314

Hubel, D. H. (1988). *Eye, Brain and Vision*. New York: W. H. Freeman.

Julesz, B. (1971). *Foundations of Cyclopean Perception*. Chicago: University of Chicago Press.

Julesz, B., and Frisby, J. P. (1975). Some new subjective contours in random-line stereograms. *Perception 4*, 145–150.

Lehmkuhle, S. W., and Fox, R. (1975). Effect of binocular rivalry suppression on the motion aftereffect. *Vision Res. 15*, 855–859.

Levi, D. M., Klein, S. A., and Aitsebaomo, A. P. (1985). Vernier acuity, crowding and cortical magnification. *Vision Res. 25*, 963–977.

Ogle, K. N. (1962). The optical space sense. In H. Davson (Ed.), *The Eye* (Volume 4, pp. 211–232). New York: Academic Press.

Papert, S. (1964). Stereoscopic synthesis as a technique for localizing visual mechanisms. *M.I.T. Quart. Prog. Rep. 73*, 239–243.

Paradiso, M. A., Shimojo, S., and Nakayama, K. (1989). Subjective contours, tilt aftereffects, and visual cortical organization. *Vision Res. 29*, 1205–1213.

Patterson, R., and Fox, R. (1983). Depth separation and the Ponzo illusion. *Percept. Psychophys. 34*, 25–28.

Patterson, R., and Fox, R. (1990). Metacontrast masking between cyclopean and luminance stimuli. *Vision Res. 30*, 439–448.

Patterson, R., Hart, P., and Nowak, D. (1991). The cyclopean Ternus display and the perception of element versus group motion. *Vision Res. 31*, 2085–2092.

Patterson, R., Ricker, C., McGary, J., and Rose, D. (1992). Properties of cyclopean motion perception. *Vision Res. 32*, 149–156.

Power, R. P., and Moulden, B. (1992). Spatial gating effects on judged motion of gratings in apertures. *Perception 21*, 449–463.

Ramachandran, V. S. (1992). Filling in gaps in perception: Part 1. *Curr. Directions Psychol. Sci. 1*, 199–205.

Shimojo, S., Nakayama, K., and Silverman, G. H. (1989). Occlusion and the solution to the aperture problem for motion. *Vision Res. 29*, 619–626.

Smith, A. T., and Over, R. (1975). Tilt aftereffects with subjective contours. *Nature (London), 257*, 581–582.

Smith, A. T., and Over, R. (1977). Orientation masking and the tilt illusion with subjective contours. *Perception 6*, 441–447.

Stoner, G. R., Albright, T. D., and Ramachandran, V. S. (1990). Transparency and coherence in human motion perception. *Nature (London), 344*, 153–155.

Teller, D. Y. (1984). Linking propositions. *Vision Res. 24*, 1233–1246.

Teller, D. Y. (1990). The domain of visual science. In L. Spillman and J. S. Werner (Eds.), *Visual Perception: The Neurophysiological Foundations*, San Diego, CA: Academic Press.

Teller, D. Y., and Pugh, E. N., Jr. (1983). Linking propositions in color vision. In J. D. Mollon and T. Sharpe (Eds.) *Colour Vision: Physiology and Psychophysics*. (pp. 11–21). New York: Academic Press.

van der Zwan, R. Wenderoth, P., and Alais, D. (1993). Reduction of a pattern-induced motion aftereffect by binocular rivalry suggests the involvement of extrastriate mechanisms. *Visual Neurosci. 10*, 703–709.

von der Heydt, R., Peterhans, E., and Baumgartner, G. (1984). Illusory contours and cortical neuron responses. *Science 224*, 1260–1262.

Walker, P., and Powell, D. J. (1979). The sensitivity of binocular rivalry to changes in the nondominant stimulus. *Vision Res. 18*, 827–835.

Wiesenfelder, H., and Blake, R. (1990). The neural site of binocular rivalry relative to the analysis of motion in the human visual system. *J. Neurosci. 10*, 3880–3888.

Wiesenfelder, H., and Blake, R. (1991). Apparent motion can survive binocular rivalry suppression. *Vision Res. 31*, 1589–1600.

3

Demonstration of Binocular Fusion of Color and Texture

Janus J. Kulikowski and
Vincent Walsh

Normal observers perceive depth of a luminance contour by making use of the horizontal disparity of the images in both eyes (for review see Ogle, 1950; Julesz, 1971; Bishop, 1982; Regan, 1991; Poggio, this volume).

If the disparity is within a specific range, a single contour is seen. For a fine line this is Panum's area, which depends on the retinal eccentricity, but for other stimuli this range may be extended (Hyson et al., 1983; Fender and Julesz, 1967; Julesz, 1971). In particular, sinusoidal stripes (gratings) in spatial antiphase, i.e., with a half-cycle horizontal disparity, are seen as single patterns positioned in front of or behind the fixation point (Kulikowski, 1978).

Do similar rules apply to chromatic patterns? It is well known that stereopsis is poor for chromatic isoluminant patterns (for review see Livingstone and Hubel, 1987; Cavanagh, 1991; Kovacs and Julesz, 1992).

Recently Kulikowski (1992) reported that colored patterns in antiphase are not only difficult to fuse, but also produce a hitherto unknown perceptual phenomenon of binocular chromatic rivalry, which means integrating the same color from both eyes and suppressing the other color.

It would be interesting to know whether stereopsis for chromatic stimuli is inferior to achromatic stereopsis when the patterns to be fused vary in an additional dimension, other than luminance, color, or disparity. In the experiments reported here, we show that stereopsis of antiphase chromatic patterns close to isoluminance is stronger when they consist of short segments forming a regular color checkerboard, referred to as *regular* chromatic texture (note that the word texture usually refers to random or pseudorandom patterns). We shall argue that the chromatic processing of color–texture can be segregated from other chromatic mechanisms.

Methods

Stimuli

In the initial experiments, space periodic patterns varying in color and spatial frequency were generated on a television monitor as described by Murray et al. (1987), Parry et al. (1988), and Kulikowski et al. (1989). This technique makes it possible to adjust independently both contrast and luminance of the two colored components in order to test either red–green or blue–yellow color-opponent mechanisms. In the extreme conditions the patterns could be luminance modulated (e.g., dark/light as in figure 3.1, top, or monochromatic: either purely red, or purely green). The desired state for testing color-opponent mechanisms is equal luminance, i.e., isoluminance of the two colors. In the experiments with TV monitors isoluminance of red–green components was achieved by using heterochromatic flicker photometry: for 12.5 Hz red–green pattern reversal, the luminance ratio of red and green was varied until flicker was minimal. (The individual subjects were tested in this way since the isoluminance ratio varies slightly for different subjects.) The same technique could be used for blue–yellow mechanism, but in this case at least two additional conditions must be fulfilled:

1. The colors have to be chosen to correspond to the tritanopic confusion line (that is, any modulation must be invisible to the red-green mechanism).

2. Chromatic aberration must be carefully monitored since the errors are greater than for the red–green pattern. In theory this is not achievable using colors on a plane (McKeefry and Kulikowski, 1994), but in practice a blue–yellow pair is not strongly affected by chromatic aberration. Besides, our results showed that precise isoluminance is not necessary to perceive the effects described below.

For simplicity, this chapter deals only with patterns consisting of two vertical colored stripes forming a spatial cycle. The colored stripes were on a white background and surrounded by a black outline with markers to facilitate fusion. Since it is difficult to reproduce colors, we first use a black–white pattern (figure 3.1, top) in order to introduce the readers and subjects to the problem.

In most experiments, which will be published separately, we used red-green pairs of paper stripes of variable saturation, some of which were made of standard Munsell papers, for example, red: 2.5R 5/12 and green: 5G 5/8. Each stripe in a pair was four times longer than its width. In subsequent experiments the colored patches were made shorter, that is, length-to-width ratio of each color patch was modified; ultimately a chromatic checkerboard was formed. The two pairs were viewed binocularly by each eye viewing one pair; the pairs were always presented in spatial antiphase, that is, an orange (or red)

patch in one eye corresponded to green in the other eye and vice versa (figure 3.1).

In these experiments free viewing is sufficient for most subjects to fuse the patterns. However, it is helpful for naive observers to use a device called the Maddox wing, in which fields of view of both eyes are separated by a septum (each eye looks at the field on the same side). Experienced observers may also try to fuse patterns by crossing their eyes.

Subjects

Observers who were used in this study had normal color vision and stereopsis (binocular vision). The readers who want to check these percepts (figure 3.1) must fulfill these requirements.

Results and Comments

Long Bars

When pairs of light and dark stripes are presented binocularly in spatial antiphase and the fixation markers fused, one bar is seen either in front of, or behind the remaining bars (figure 3.1A).

With colored stripes (if figure 3.1B is in color) stereopsis is rarely achieved (see Kulikowski, 1992). In other words, it is rare to see one colored bar in the mid-line to be at a different depth than the flanks (cf. Kulikowski, 1992). The closer to isoluminance both stripes are, the more difficult is depth perception. Many normal subjects simply do not perceive it at all. Quite often one eye may dominate the percept, but such cases are already well documented.

More importantly, however, very unstable sensations are observed, among which the most prominent is seeing an almost uniformly colored patch, either red or green, as though these colors were integrated from different visual fields of two eyes. This is binocular chromatic rivalry since one color is not seen continuously in time, but after few seconds is replaced by the other color. Often alternations of the integrated component colors (with only brief transitions) are produced: the whole fused area is seen as uniform red, then uniform green, then red, etc. The integrated colors have almost the same apparent saturation as seen monocularly. The transitional, intermediate percepts of figure 3.1B (if it is in color) may include seeing a narrow bar of one color with the flanks of the opposite color (Kulikowski, 1992). To experience the whole range of these percepts the readers should try fusing the colored version of figure 3.1B at various viewing distances.

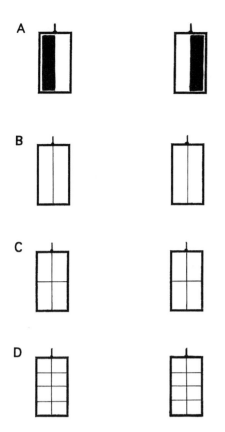

Intersected Stripes and Checkerboard Patterns

The colored patches shown in figure 3.1C have shorter segments and the colors are reversed in the middle. A further reduction in length leads to the formation of the color checkerboard pattern shown in figure 3.1D. When the patterns in figure 3.1C or D are fused, the binocular chromatic rivalry is markedly reduced in the frequency of its occurrence (as compared with figure 3.1B). "Rivalrous" chromatic integration, which still occurs, is horizontal, across the pattern. In other words, occasionally one color is seen covering the area of two elements, or two squares in the case of checkerboards. As a result of weaker chromatic rivalry, depth perception is elicited more readily and more frequently using the patterns in figure 3.1C or D, than when fusing the patterns in 3.1B. Once the elements are seen at different depths than the flanks (either in front or behind), depth perception is more stable than in figure 3.1B.

What Restores Stereopsis in Patterns with Chromatic Checks?

We can restate these observations and invoke some psychophysical explanations, for example, by saying that shorter segments can interrupt spatial integration in the color channel which is restricted to low spatial frequencies

Figure 3.1

This figure provides (*A*) luminance-modulated (dark/light) pairs of stripes for reference (*top*) and below three pairs of frames with outlines that may be turned into colored patterns (*B, C, D*). The frames should be colored as instructed (see "Preparation of the colored figures").

Viewing: The top pattern has two pairs of achromatic stripes, dark/light and light/dark. Cover the remaining figures to avoid distribution. Concentrate on the short vertical segments above the outlines and try to fixate the junctions of these segments with the outlines in order to binocularly fuse the patterns. Initially use a septum, i.e., a cardboard partition (over 30 cm long) between your eyes and the mid-line between the pair of patterns, so that the left eye looks at the left pair and right eye at the right pair (later the septum may not be needed). Try to fuse the segments, so that they are seen as a single object, then without changing the fixation point try to shift your attention to the patterns within the frames.

Observations: Four pairs of patterns shown produce different percepts. (*A*) *Top*: An achromatic pair of patterns in spatial antiphase is most commonly perceived as a single dark bar behind the frame (further details in Kulikowski, 1978). (*B*) *Second row from top*: A pair of orange-green (*left*) and green-orange (*right*) stripes most often produces chromatic rivalry—the area being totally orange, or totally green. (*C*) *Third row from top*: A pair of intersected stripes is seen ambiguously, but sometimes in depth. (*D*) *Bottom row*: A pair of "reversed" colored checkerboards often elicits depth perception.

Preparation of the colored figures: The reader may make such colored patterns by using standard orange and light-green highlighters that have roughly similar reflectance, i.e., they are nearly isoluminant (avoid red highlighters since they are usually darker than green). Standard colors of the same reflectance (e.g., the same Munsell value) are obviously better, if available. First, practice making patches of equal reflectance using orange and light-green highlighters on a piece of paper. Second, copy the master figure several times, so that you can practice making such patterns without destroying the original. Third, try to color the patches outlined as evenly as possible (they should seem equally bright). Note that the thin lines within the outlines are needed only at preliminary stages of preparation of the figures; it actually helps to make them as indistinct as possible. Patterns in rows 2–4 from the top (parts *B*–*D*) should be colored alternately. (*B*) Thus the second row has orange-green vertical stripes in the left panel and green-orange stripes in the right panel. (*C*) The patterns in both the left and the right panels are intersected; use the same sequence as in (*B*) for its upper half, i.e., orange-green and green-orange, but reverse this sequence in the lower half, i.e., from the left: green-orange and orange-green. (*D*) The bottom pattern consists of two checkerboard frames, which should be colored alternately to form colored checkerboards; colors in both checkerboards should alternate.

Illumination: Stripes of different colors shown here ought to be of equal luminance, i.e., isoluminant. This can be achieved by varying the illuminating light, most conveniently using two light sources (orange and green).

(Mullen, 1985; Parry et al., 1988), or that the shorter segments promote stereopsis based on horizontal disparity.

However, our experiments with binocular rivalry and stereopsis can also be used to probe the information flow and the structure of the neural pathways. In this sense our technique is similar to psychoanatomical studies (see Blake, this volume). It is, therefore, tempting to formulate a hypothesis in the neurophysiological terms, especially so because the comparable data on single units are available.

Color-opponent cells that process color information in the primary visual cortex (V1) are monocularly activated (De Valois, 1991; Dow, 1991) and have low spatial and low temporal resolution limits (Livingstone and Hubel, 1987; Kulikowski and Walsh, 1993). It is, therefore, not surprising that chromatic isoluminant patterns elicit either poor depth perception or none (but see Vidyasagar, 1976, for interocular transfer). However, isoluminant borders (especially between red and green) can activate most cells in the magnocellular pathway, which is considered to be the main basis for stereopsis (Cavanagh, 1991; Lee, 1991). There are also many "hypercomplex-type" cells in superficial (supragranular) layers of the macaque striate cortex, some of which are binocularly activated by chromatic texture (see below).

The simplest explanation for better depth perception in figure 3.1C and D is that a chromatic checkerboard pattern has more chromatic contours than a grating. However, only horizontal contours have been increased and those do not provide direct cues for depth perception (e.g., Bishop, 1982).

An alternative explanation is that the fusion of chromatic texture patterns involves another chromatic-sensitive channel that has binocularly responsive units and a spatiotemporal response profile, more suitable for processing color–texture information than is the color-opponent channel (Livingstone and Hubel, 1987; Ts'o and Gilbert, 1988). The obvious candidates may be the cells with concealed chromatic opponency in the interblob regions of the superficial layers of the macaque visual cortex (Dow, 1991). Many of these cells are binocularly activated, and they respond well only to short line segments. These are called end-stopped cells, the properties of which have been observed in several cortical regions (Zeki, 1978; Desimone et al., 1985). Moreover, the binocularly activated complex cells that prefer short segments of color texture, including isoluminant, are also found in cortical visual area V1. In addition, their responses to a temporally modulated checkerboard tend to peak at a higher temporal frequency (approaching 5 Hz), than do

chromatic opponent cells—around 1 Hz (Kulikowski and Walsh, 1993).

Discussion

These data demonstrate for the first time that different mechanisms operate for the fusion of chromatic stripes (gratings) and regular chromatic texture. One may expect that this process is not weakened by motion of chromatic-texture patterns and that the fusion of chromatic texture would be useful in breaking camouflage.

In recent years the properties of color-opponent channels that process color information have been carefully evaluated in psychophysical experiments: both spatial and temporal resolution of isoluminant colored gratings that are aberration free has been confirmed to be low compared with achromatic patterns (Mullen, 1985; McKeefry and Kulikowski, 1994; see also Kelly, 1989). Moreover, the spatiotemporal properties of blue-yellow mechanisms turned out to be very similar to those of the red-green channels (McKeefry and Kulikowski, 1994). In accord with these psychophysical findings, dual-opponent cells with similar response characteristics (low spatial, low temporal frequency preference) have also been found in the monkey visual cortex using stimuli similar to those in human experiments (Kulikowski and Vidyasagar, 1986; Kulikowski and Walsh, 1993).

On the other hand, some recent experiments cast doubt on the notion that the coarse and slow color channel is exclusively responsible for all chromatic processing (e.g., Papathomas et al., 1991). These and other related experiments suggest that the red-green chromatic patterns under normal conditions (in which chromatic aberration is not eliminated) may be detected with higher acuity and temporal resolution (i.e., much faster) than the blue-yellow patterns. The traditional view still persists that the red–green chromatic channel has higher resolution that the blue-yellow channel (e.g., Lennie et al., 1990, figure 7). Even the studies that distinguish between detection and identification of colors tend to overestimate resolution of the red-green channel, if chromatic aberration is not corrected (Granger and Heurtley, 1973). These observations cannot be dismissed as artifacts (e.g., due to chromatic aberration activating the achromatic system) since they produce some chromatic sensations, although not always corresponding to the original colors. In addition, chromatic sensations may even be generated by achromatic moving patterns such as the Benham disc (Kozak et al., 1989). This observation, again, would be difficult to reconcile with the color-opponent mechanism whose channels give rise to categorical color perception (Mullen and Kulikowski, 1990) and that have similar spatio-temporal properties for red-green and blue-yellow stimulation (McKeefry and Kulikowski, 1994). Our present demonstration suggests that the putative chromatic mechanism (that is different from the low-pass color mechanism, Mullen, 1985) is also capable of subserving stereopsis.

In conclusion, we propose that there is a separate chromatic-texture mechanism that is consistent with the phenomena reported here and with the properties of cells in area V1, which are binocularly activated and optimally driven by short colored line segments (Kulikowski and Walsh, 1994). These findings should also provide some data for the development of neurophysiologically plausible models for stereopsis, such as the one proposed by Tyler in this volume.

Acknowledgments

This research was supported by the Visual Sciences Fund. We thank John Simpson for very helpful technical assistance. V. W. was the former Wellcome Trust scholar.

References

Bishop, P. O. (1982). Binocular vision. In R. A. Moses (Ed.), *Adler's Physiology of the Eye* (pp. 545–649). St. Louis: C. V. Mosby.

Cavanagh, P. (1991). Vision at equiluminance. In J. J. Kulikowski, V. Walsh, and I. J. Murray (Eds.), *Limits of Vision* (pp. 234–250). London: Macmillan.

Desimone, R., Schein, S. J., Moran, J., and Ungerleider, L. G. (1985). Contour color and shape analysis beyond the striate cortex. *Vision Res. 25*, 441–452.

De Valois, R. L. (1991). Orientation and spatial frequency: Properties and modular organization. In A. Valberg and B. B. Lee (Ed.), *From Pigments to Perception* (pp. 261–267). New York: Plenum.

Dow, B. (1991). Orientation and color columns in monkey striate cortex. In A. Valberg and B. B. Lee (Eds.), *From Pigments to Perception* (pp. 269–274). New York: Plenum Press.

Fender, D., and Julesz, B. (1967). Extension of Panum's area in binocularly stabilized vision. *J. Opt. Soc. Am. 57*, 819–830.

Granger, E. M., and Heurtley, J. C. (1973). Visual chromaticity modulation transfer function. *J. Opt. Soc. Am. 63*, 1173–1174.

Hyson, B., Julesz, B., and Fender, D. H. (1983). Eye movements and neural remapping during fusion of misaligned random-dot stereograms. *J. Opt. Soc. Am. 73*, 1665–1673.

Julesz, B. (1971). *Foundations of Cyclopean Perception.* Chicago: University of Chicago Press.

Kelly, D. H. (1989). Spatial and temporal interactions in color vision. *J. Imaging Tech. 15*, 82–89.

Kozak, W. M., Reitboeck, H. J., and Meno, F. (1989). Subjective color sensations elicited by moving patterns: Effect of luminance. In J. J. Kulikowski, C. M. Dickinson, and I. J. Murray (Eds.), *Seeing Contour and Colour* (pp. 294–310). Oxford: Pergamon Press.

Kovacs, I., and Julesz, B. (1992). Depth, motion and static-flow perception at metaisoluminant color contrast. *Proc. Natl. Acad. Sci. U.S.A. 89*, 10390–10394.

Kulikowski, J. J. (1978). Limit of single vision in stereopsis depends on contour sharpness. *Nature (London) 275*, 126–127.

Kulikowski, J. J. (1992). Binocular chromatic rivalry and single vision. *Opthal. Physiol. Optics 12*, 168–170.

Kulikowski, J. J., Murray, I. J., and Parry, N. R. A. (1989). Electrophysiological correlates of chromatic-opponent and achromatic stimulation in man. In B. Drum and G. Verriest (Eds.), *Colour Vision Deficiencies IX* (pp. 145–153). Dortrecht, the Netherlands: Kluver Academic Publishers.

Kulikowski, J. J., and Vidyasagar, T. R. (1986). Space and spatial frequency: analysis and representation in macaque striate cortex. *Exp. Brain Res. 64*, 5–18.

Kulikowski, J. J., and Walsh, V. (1993). Colour vision: isolating mechanisms in overlapping streams. *Prog. Brain Res. 95*, 417–426.

Kulikowski, J. J., and Walsh, V. (1995). In preparation.

Lee, B. B. (1991). Spectral sensitivity in primate vision. In J. J. Kulikowski, V. Walsh, and I. J. Murray (Eds.), *Limits of Vision* (pp. 191–200). London: Macmillan.

Lennie, P., Trevarthen, C., van Essen, D., and Wassle, H. (1990). Parallel processing of visual information. In L. Spillmann and J. S. Werner (Eds.), *Visual Perception* (pp. 103–128). San Diego: Academic Press.

Livingstone, M. S., and Hubel, D. H. (1987). Psychophysical evidence for separate channels for the perception of form, color, movement and depth. *J. Neurosci. 7*, 3416–3468.

McKeefry, D., and Kulikowski, J. J. (1994). Psychophysical and occipital responses to aberration-free blue/yellow and red/green gratings. *Colour Vision Defic. XII.* Drum, B. (Ed.), Dortrecht, the Netherlands: Kluver Academic Publishers (in press).

Mullen, K. T. (1985). The contrast sensitivity of human colour vision to red-green and blue-yellow chromatic gratings. *J. Physiol. 359*, 381–400.

Mullen, K. T., and Kulikowski, J. J. (1990). Wavelength discrimination at detection threshold. *J. Opt. Soc. Am. A 7*, 733–742.

Murray, I. J., Parry, N. R. A., Carden, D., and Kulikowski, J. J. (1987). Human visual evoked potentials to chromatic and achromatic gratings. *Clin. Vision Sci. 1*, 231–244.

Ogle, K. N. (1950). *Researches in Binocular Vision.* Philadelphia: W. B. Saunders.

Papathomas, T. V., Gorea, A., and Julesz, B. (1991). Two carriers for motion perception: Color and luminance. *Vision Res. 31*, 1883–1892.

Parry, N. R. A., Kulikowski, J. J., Murray, I. J., Kranda, K., and Ott, H. (1988). Visual evoked potentials and reaction times to chromatic and achromatic stimulation: Psychopharmacological applications. In

I. Hindmarch, B. Aufdembrinke, and H. Ott (Eds.), *Psychopharmacology and Reaction Time*. New York: John Wiley.

Regan, D. (1991). *Binocular Vision*. London: Macmillan.

Ts'o, D. Y., and Gilbert, C. D. (1988). The organization of chromatic and spatial interactions in the primate striate cortex. *J. Neurosci. 8,* 1712–1727.

Vidyasagar, T. R. (1976). Orientation-specific contour adaptation at a binocular site. *Nature (London) 261,* 39–40.

Zeki, S. (1978). Uniformity and diversity of structure and function in rhesus monkey prestriate visual cortex. *J. Physiol. 277,* 273–290.

4

Review of Computational Models of Stereopsis

Daphna Weinshall and Jitendra Malik

Binocular stereopsis is based on the cue of *disparity*—the two eyes receive slightly different views of the three-dimensional world. This disparity cue, which includes differences in position, both horizontal and vertical, as well as differences in orientation or spacing of corresponding features in the two images, can be used to extract the three-dimensional structure of the scene. The extraction of three-dimensional information is usually composed of two stages, correspondence and geometric interpretation. We start with a discussion of models for the measurement of retinal disparity and then we discuss the geometric interpretation of the disparity field: what can be inferred from it about the three-dimensional structure of the world?

The Estimation of the Disparity Field

Estimation of the positional disparity field requires a solution of the correspondence problem—one needs to determine which feature in the left eye's retinal image corresponds to which feature in the right eye's retinal image. Julesz's development of the random-dot stereogram demonstrated the amazing ability of the human visual system to solve the correspondence problem as part of early vision (Julesz, 1960, 1971). He pioneered two stereopsis models (Julesz, 1962, 1971). In this section we discuss the basic computational constraints typically used by correspondence algorithms, and the circumstances in which these constraints fail. We then review relevant psychophysical data and a few matching algorithms.

Basic Computational Constraints

To match two images, depicting the same scene but from different points of view, it is necessary and helpful to exploit some constraints. The constraints range from some that are based on physical understanding of the imaging process, to heuristic constraints that are expected to be "usually" true and that simplify the computation.

Similarity

The similarity constraint prefers the matching of similar (or identical) elements in the two images. This constraint is more powerful when the matched elements are complex and distinctive, such as windowed patches or multiple filter outputs. If the elements being matched are just black or white dots in a random-dot stereogram, there are plenty of these and similarity does not constrain the possible choices by very much. Similar remarks apply to the use of simple edge elements (like zero-crossings). It should also be noted that in general we can expect the elements that are used in correspondence to be only similar between the two images, not identical. For example, the gray levels change between the two images just because each camera is oriented differently with respect to the light sources, and edge elements will have slightly different orientations in the two eyes.

Uniqueness

Assuming that the elements in the scene come from objects in the real world, it makes sense to require that an element in one image should be matched to at most a single element in the other image. This assumption is often true; it fails when an object, say a nail, is occluded by another nail with respect to one camera, say the left one. In this case the two nails are projected to one nail in the left image and two nails in the right image. This is Panum's limiting case. In this limiting case, the single nail in the left image should be matched to both nails in the right image.

Epipolar Geometry

By virtue of the basic geometry involved in a pair of eyes (or cameras) viewing a three-dimensional scene, corresponding points must always lie along epipolar lines in the images. These lines correspond to the intersections of an epipolar plane (the plane through a point in the scene and the nodal points of the two eyes) with the left and right image planes. Exploiting this epipolar constraint reduces an initially two-dimensional search to a one-dimensional one. Obviously determination of the epipolar lines requires a knowledge of the viewing geometry. The difficulty here is to compute the epipolar geometry in the case of variable camera geometry (e.g., Longuet-Higgins, 1981; see the next section on geometry for possible ways this could be done).

Ordering Constraint

When two elements are positioned one beside the other in one image, and one of them (say the left one) is matched to another element in the second image, the ordering constraint would instruct the algorithm to look for a match for the right element to the right of the match of the left element in the second image (Yuille and Poggio, 1984). This matching preserves the order of the elements in both images. This constraint is heuristic and is violated in physical situations (see, e.g., figure 4.1). Nevertheless, it is true most of the time, such as when the two elements lie on a connected visible part of a single smooth surface. In computer vision, this constraint is often used because it permits the use of dynamic programming.

Piecewise Smoothness

Assuming that the scene consists of piecewise smooth opaque surfaces, the disparity field is going to be piecewise smooth. This suggests that the disparities of nearby elements in the image should not be too different—the continuity constraint of Marr (1982). Therefore if we match an element to another element in the second image, we should look for matches to neighboring elements only around, and not far from, its match in the second image. Of course, this is not true at object boundaries.

In stereograms of transparent surfaces, where each surface is defined by a group of random dots at a certain disparity, neighboring dots may have very different disparities if they belong to different transparent surfaces. People have no difficulty seeing transparent planes in such stereograms, but algorithms that strictly impose the continuity constraint usually encounter difficulties.

One way to implement this constraint is via the disparity gradient concept (Burt and Julesz, 1980). The disparity gradient is defined for two elements in one image, each assigned a specific disparity: it is the disparity difference between the two elements divided by the positional difference between the elements (averaged over both images). Elements on a smooth surface, say a tilted plane, might be correctly assigned very different disparities if they are located on two different ends of the plane, but the disparity gradient between any two elements will always be small. For example, if the elements are located on two different ends of the plane, the disparity gradient is small since the large disparity difference is divided by another large number, the positional difference between the elements. The disparity gradient constraint is related to the ordering constraint (Pollard, Mayhew, and Frisby, 1985).

Choice of Matching Primitives

Different approaches to the correspondence problem exploit the constraints described above in different ways. The two best studied approaches are area correlation (Hannah, 1974; Nishihara, 1984) and edge matching

(Marr and Poggio, 1979; Grimson, 1981; Baker and Binford, 1981; Pollard, Mayhew, and Frisby, 1985).

A simple idea, which appeared in earlier works of photogrammetry and image processing, is the correlation maximization rule (see also Nishihara, 1984). The basic idea is to correlate image patches with each other, where the gray-level correlation function can be defined as follows:

$$\text{correlation}(D_x, D_y) = \sum_i^W \sum_j^W I(x_i^r, y_j^r) I(x_i^l + D_x, y_j^l + D_y)$$

Here $I(x_i, y_j)$ denotes the image intensity at location (x_i, y_j) of the right (superscript r) or left (superscript l) image, W denotes the size of the window, and (D_x, D_y) denotes the disparity of the element in the left image with respect to the right image. A correlation maximization algorithm will choose the disparity pair (D_x, D_y) that maximizes the correlation function. This idea can be generalized to the use of cross-correlation operators, operating on filtered images filtered by any of the filters described below.

The difficulties with approaches based on area correlation are well known. Because of the difference in viewpoints, the effects of shading can give rise to differences in brightness for nonlambertian surfaces. A more serious difficulty arises from the effects of differing amounts of foreshortening in the two views whenever a surface is not strictly frontoparallel. Still another difficulty arises at surface boundaries, where a depth discontinuity may run through the region of the image being used for correlation. Finally, one of the problems of naively implemented correlation algorithms is the way the smoothness constraint is implemented: instead of enforcing smoothness, it enforces frontoparallelism, by attempting to assign the same disparity to neighboring image locations.

In typical edge-based stereo algorithms, edges are deemed compatible if they are near enough in orientation and have the same sign of contrast across the edge. To cope with the enormous number of false matches, a coarse-to-fine strategy may be adopted (Marr and Poggio, 1979; Grimson, 1981). In some instances, additional limits can be imposed, such as a limit on the rate at which disparity is allowed to change across the image (Pollard, Mayhew, and Frisby, 1985). Although not always true, assuming that corresponding edges must obey a left-to-right ordering in both images, ordering can also be used to restrict the number of possible matches and lends itself to efficient dynamic programming methods (Baker and Binford, 1981). With any edge-based approach, however, the resulting depth information is sparse, available only at edge locations. Thus a further step is needed to interpolate depth across surfaces in the scene.

A third approach is based on the idea of first convolving the left and right images with a bank of linear filters tuned to a number of different orientations and scales (Kass, 1993; Jones and Malik, 1992). The choice of filters is loosely modeled after receptive fields of cells in V1. The responses of these filters at a given point constitute a vector that characterizes the local structure of the image patch. The correspondence problem can be solved by seeking points in the other eye's view where this vector is maximally similar. The primary goal in using a large number of spatial filters, at various orientations, phases, and scales is to obtain rich and highly specific image features suitable for stereo matching, with little chance of encountering false matches.

It is interesting to note that, when approached as a problem of determining which black dot in one view corresponds with which black dot in the other, the correspondence problem seems quite difficult for Julesz random-dot stereograms. However using a different primitive, such as in area correlation or the approach based on spatial filters, random-dot stereograms are among the richest stimuli—containing information at all orientations and scales, making stereo-matching quite straightforward and unambiguous.

Psychophysical Evidence

It is not clear how many of the "hacks" and computational constraints described above are used in biological systems; much psychophysics is still needed. Below we describe some relevant psychophysical evidence for the use of these constraints.

Uniqueness and Smoothness

Krol and van de Grind (1980) described a psychophysical experiment where subjects were shown two nails one behind the other. The projection of the nails onto the retinas is illustrated in figure 4.1. The correct matching of the nails is not order preserving; using the notations of figure 4.1, L_1 should be matched to R_2 and L_2 should be matched to R_1. However, humans choose the other solution, the matching of L_1 to R_1 and L_2 to R_2, which is both continuous and order preserving, *but false*. This false matching leads to the double nail illusion, the illusory percept of two nails one beside the other (rather than one behind the other). This illusion seems to confirm the relevance of some of the above computational constraints to the explanation of human vision.

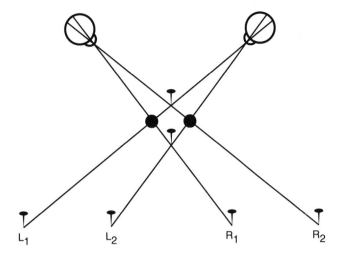

Figure 4.1
The double nail illusion: the subject views two nails, one approximately behind the other, which are projected to two nails in each of the left and right retinas. The subject falsely perceives two nails one next to the other, located in the space locations marked above by filled circles.

Uniqueness

The uniqueness constraint is violated in a case like Panum's limiting case. Braddick (cited in Marr, 1982) described random-dot stereograms, where each dot appeared once in the left image and twice in the right image (i.e., the right image had two copies of the random dot pattern, like a badly received television picture having "shadows"). People see two transparent surfaces in such stereograms, as if they match each dot in the left image simultaneously with its two corresponding dots in the right image. However, Grimson argued that this does not rule out the uniqueness constraint, since uniqueness is preserved when matching is done from the right image to the left (Grimson, 1981).

A generalization of this case is described in Weinshall (1989), where experiments with similar random-dot stereograms are reported, only that the random-dot pattern is copied twice *both* in the left and the right images. The distance between the two copies in the left image was typically different from the distance between the two copies in the right image. Therefore each copy of the random-dot pattern could be matched to one copy of the random-dot pattern in the other image. The situation is similar to the case depicted in figure 4.1, where L_1 symbolizes one copy of the random-dot pattern in the left image, L_2 is the second copy of the random-dot pattern in the left image, and similarly for R_1, R_2 in the right image.

People see in these stereograms four transparent layers, whose disparities correspond to matching L_1 both to R_1

and R_2, and L_2 both to R_1 and R_2. This perception therefore corresponds to multiple matching of the whole random-dot pattern. However, this perception can be simulated by an algorithm that enforces locally the unique matching constraint, where some dots from L_1 (or L_2) are matched to dots in R_1, and other dots in L_1 (or L_2) are matched to dots in R_2. This is discussed in Weinshall (1991), showing only weak evidence of the violation of the uniqueness constraint at the individual element level in human stereo vision.

Piecewise Smoothness

Since the scene is assumed to consist of piecewise smooth surfaces, the disparity map is piecewise smooth. Exploiting this constraint requires some subtlety so that we do not smooth away the disparity discontinuities associated with surface boundaries in the scene. There is good psychophysical evidence supporting disparity interpolation and segmentation in humans (Mitchison, 1988).

Occlusion

We must also deal correctly with regions that are only monocularly visible. Whenever there is a surface depth discontinuity that is not purely horizontal, distant surfaces are occluded to different extents in the two eyes, leading to the existence of unpaired image points that are seen in one eye only. The realization of this goes back to Leonardo Da Vinci. Recent psychophysical work has convincingly established that the human visual system can exploit this cue for depth in a manner consistent with the geometry of the situation (Nakayama and Shimojo, 1990; Anderson and Nakayama, 1994).

Algorithms for Solving the Correspondence Problem

The computational literature is full of descriptions of many algorithms and elaborate systems for solving the correspondence problem in stereopsis. We have come a long way from simple algorithms such as the cooperative matching algorithm of Marr and Poggio (1976). The different algorithms make different choices of matching primitives (areas, edges, or filter outputs) and exploit the constraints from the section on "Basic Computational Constraints" in various ways.

We will just mention one of these approaches here. Prazdny (1985) described a matching algorithm where a list is maintained at each element in the image, keeping an entry for each disparity that corresponds to a feasible match. Each such disparity receives decreasing support from its neighboring elements (within a certain neighborhood) with increasing disparity gradient (see definition in the section on "Basic Computational Constraints"). The most supported disparity is selected at each feature. Thus, since the algorithm uses the disparity gradient to evaluate the quality of a particular match, larger differences in disparity are tolerated for features that are further apart. This algorithm can handle smooth surfaces that are not fronto-parallel (such as tilted planes), and it can handle transparent objects. A similar algorithm, which later evolved into a complex system, is described in Pollard et al. (1985).

The voluminous literature mentioned is aimed at explicitly solving the correspondence problem. An interesting alternative, where the correspondence problem is solved only implicitly, is the use of phase based approaches (Fleet, Jepson, and Jenkin, 1991, for example). The disparity is expressed in terms of phase differences in the outputs of local, bandpass filters applied to the left and right views. Examples of such filters would be sine and cosine Gabor filters. One advantage is that subpixel accuracy is automatic. A disadvantage is that the disparity range is limited to a fraction of the period of the bandpass signal. Recently Ohzawa et al. (1991) identified cortical neurons in cat with Gabor receptive fields that seem to respond to phase disparity. A weakness seems to be the limited disparity range $\lambda/2$ of these mechanisms that would fall short of the empirical measurements of Schor and Wood (1983), who observed that the upper disparity limit for stereopsis could be over 10 times the spatial period of the stimulus at high spatial frequencies (> 2 cpd). See Tyler's chapter for further details on this issue (figure 1.4).

The Geometric Interpretation of the Disparity Field

In the previous section we discussed how to compute the disparity field. But assuming this is given, what should be done with it? What is (or should be) computed from the disparity field? Possibly, depth at each point should be recovered, or rather some (more qualitative) measure of depth.

Disparity Interpretation: Computational Angle

The study of the relationship between disparity and scene geometry has a long history including most notably the work of Helmholtz (1925) and Ogle (1950) (see also figure 1.2 in Tyler's chapter). More recently, Koenderink and van Doorn (1976) presented a fairly complete analysis of the binocular disparity field, allowing for asymmetric fixation and associated cyclotorsion. A key observation is that the mapping between disparity and scene geometry depends on the viewing parameters: in particular, it depends on the direction and distance of the point of binocular fixation. Let us examine this under the "small baseline" approximation, i.e., assuming that the interocular distance b is small compared to the fixation distance d, and that the fixation point is in the equatorial plane. The gaze angle γ is defined to be the angle between the cyclopean visual axis and the primary direction. One can show (e.g., Gårding et al., 1993b) that the horizontal and vertical components of the disparity $[h, v]$ of the point at depth $d + \delta$ (δ is the relative depth) with cyclopean image coordinates (x, y) are given by the formulas

$$h = \frac{b \cos \gamma}{d}\left(\frac{\delta}{d + \delta} + \frac{d \tan \gamma}{d + \delta}x + x^2 \right) \tag{4.1}$$

$$v = \frac{b \cos \gamma}{d}\left(\frac{d \tan \gamma}{d + \delta}y + xy \right) \tag{4.2}$$

Given the horizontal disparity h, the relative depth δ can be estimated only if the fixation distance d and gaze angle γ are known. The disparity interpretation problem has been to figure out if, and how, the human visual system accomplishes this. Some of the proposed mechanisms have been based on using the vertical disparity field. It can be seen from the equations that typically the vertical disparities are much smaller than the horizontal disparities. Due to this, it has been a long-standing debate whether humans are able to detect and use vertical disparities.

There are three approaches to the interpretation problem:

1. Finding shape modulo some transformation. One can find shape up to a relief transformation rather easily without a full determination of viewing parameters (Helmholtz, 1925; Gårding et al., 1993b). We are settling here for less than the full shape, for the sake of robustness and less demanding computations. Two models were proposed, both of which are gaze invariant (namely, three-dimensional information is computed without recovering the camera calibration, or the angle of gaze). The polar disparities model (Weinshall, 1990; Liu, Stevenson, and Schor, 1994) uses the difference between the polar angles of matched points in the two images, or the polar disparity, to approximate depth up to a scaling factor, which in turn depends on the angle of gaze of the eyes. It is shown that the slant and tilt of surfaces depend only on the polar disparities up to a scaling factor. The deformation model (Koenderink and van Doorn, 1976) analyzes the behavior of the gradient of the disparity field. It shows that the deformation component of the disparity field carries all the information concerning the slant of a surface element.

2. Using vertical disparity to calibrate the system fully. The core ideas behind the algorithms to determine viewing geometry date back to work in the photogrammetry community in the beginning of this century and have been rediscovered and developed in the work on structure from motion in the computational vision community. Given a sufficient number of corresponding pairs of points in two frames (at least five), one can recover the rigid-body transformation that relates the two camera positions except for some degenerate configurations. In the context of stereopsis, Mayhew and Longuet-Higgins (1982) and Gillam and Lawergren (1983) were the first to point out that the viewing geometry could be recovered purely from information present in the two images obtained from binocular viewing.

3. Using extraretinal information about eye position. The oculomotor system does have access to the information about the angle of gaze, vergence, etc., that is needed for calibration of the relationship between depth and disparity, so in principle that could be "communicated" to the visual system. We need to distinguish between the static case and the dynamic case (during eye movements). The interaction between the oculomotor system and the stereopsis system during eye movements merits further study. Some interesting observations may be found in Steinman et al. (1985) and in Enright (1991), who notes that the ability to discriminate the depths of two targets is largely unaffected by eye movements from one target to another. Computationally, depth ordering expressions, which are computable from image measurements, are described in Weinshall (1990).

These models, while logically distinct, are not mutually exclusive. For example, the calibration of the relationship between depth and disparity could be done using a combination of vertical disparity as well as extraretinal information about eye position—indeed under natural viewing conditions the two are expected to provide information that could yield more robust estimates than from either cue alone. On the other hand, finding shape up to a relief transformation can be the first step of an algorithm that later uses extraretinal information to compute precise shape (Gårding et al., 1993b).

In the next section we discuss a number of psychophysical experiments that could try to discriminate among these models.

Psychophysics of Disparity Interpretation

The induced effect was first reported by Ogle (1950). In this experiment, subjects view a frontoparallel plane. On one eye (say the right eye, see figure 4.2) they put a

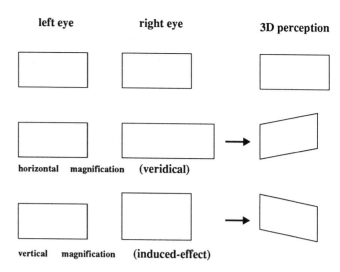

Figure 4.2
The induced-size effect (see text).

distorting lens, magnifying either the horizontal or the vertical dimension. When the horizontal dimension is magnified (second row in figure 4.2), the plane is perceived to be tilted to the right. This is the veridical geometric interpretation of the stimulus. However, when the vertical dimension is magnified (third row in figure 4.2), the plane is perceived to be tilted to the left. This interpretation is *false*, namely, a plane tilted to the left would not create such a stereo pair.

This illusion was called the "induced-size effect" by Ogle. His explanation was that initially humans see the vertical magnification as large vertical disparities. Knowing that vertical disparities should normally be small, they compensate for the unnaturally large vertical disparties by isotropically shrinking the right image until the vertical disparities disappear. This leads to a situation where the left image is horizontally magnified with respect to the right image, which can be correctly interpreted as a leftward tilting plane. This explanation is hardly computational, but it does argue that people perceive vertical disparities and use them to interpret the scene.

Koenderink and van Doorn's def model (1976) relates the perceived slant of a plane to the deformation component of the derivative of the disparity field; this component is equally affected by a horizontal expansion of the left eye's image as a vertical expansion of the right eye's image by the same amount. This provides a correct quantitative explanation of the induced effect.

Another (local) explanation for the induced effect does not use the vertical disparities directly, but rather the polar disparities (Weinshall, 1990). Here a one-dimensional disparity field is used, but rather than taking the horizontal disparities, which is an unnatural choice in a system whose lenses are spherical, it is the polar disparities which are used. The disparity field at each image element is the difference between the position of the element in one image, and the position of the matched element in the other image. When we use Cartesian coordinates, this field has two components: vertical and horizontal. When we use polar coordinates, this field has two components also: polar and radial. It is shown in Weinshall (1990) that the tilt of a plane can be computed from the polar disparity field only, and that the induced effect is a side effect of this computation, when one image is vertically magnified with respect to the other.

The induced effect can be explained by Mayhew and Longuet-Higgins's (MLH) model (1982). In this scheme the vertical disparities are used to compute the angle of gaze of the cameras. When the vertically magnified image pair is used, the angle of gaze is computed to be sideways (although the subject is looking forward), and this error leads to the false perception of a plane titled leftward.

How does one discriminate among these explanations? The MLH explanation is global: the angle of gaze should be computed once for the whole image, and therefore there can be only a single distortion of the induced-size type in the image. Koenderink and van Doorn's and Weinshall's explanations are local. There seems to be some evidence that the induced-size effect is a local phenomenon, that can take different values in different locations in the image (Rogers and Koenderink, 1986). Clearly, more psychophysics is necessary.

Still, does the induced effect prove that vertical disparities are detected and used by the visual system? Arditi, Kaufman, and Movshon (1981) argued that it is possible to explain the induced effect using horizontal disparities only. However, their explanation does not explain the induced effect in stimuli such as the inverted V pattern used by Westheimer (1984). A few studies, such as Cumming, Johnston, and Parker (1991) concluded that vertical disparities are not used by the human visual system, but reinterpretation using the polar disparities model and additional experiments (Gårding et al., 1993a; Liu, Stevenson, and Schor, 1994, seem to suggest that humans see and use more than just the horizontal disparity field (possibly they use polar disparities, or vertical disparities).

The induced effect provides a rather indirect test of the disparity scaling mechanism. Some studies have tried to address directly the question of whether vertical disparities are utilized to calibrate the system to provide metric depth measurements. Cumming et al. (1991) used a task where the observers were asked to judge which of a series of stereograms portraying elliptic cylinders appeared circular. The axis of the cylinder is aligned horizontally in the frontoparallel plane. The vertical disparities are manipulated so that they correspond to different fixation distances. Cummings et al. (1991) found that manipulating vertical disparities had no measurable effect, while changing the vergence angle had a measurable effect in the direction corresponding to its affect on the perceived fixation distance.

In Cumming et al.'s study (1991), the angular extent of the stereoscopic surface was small (8–11°). Rogers and Bradshaw (1993) used large field displays (up to 80 × 70°) where observers were asked to make judgments about the amount of perceived peak-to-trough depth of sinusoidal corrugations. Again, they manipulated both the vergence and vertical disparities. They found that, for small fields of view, vergence manipulations account for the variations in perceived depth; for large fields of view, the manipulation of vertical disparity accounted for most of the variations in perceived depth with vergence playing a smaller role. So this study argues that the visual system is using a combination of the approaches suggested earlier in this section. Independent of the debate on how vertical disparity is utilized by the visual system, one may also note the psychophysical work of Westheimer and Pettet (1992), which demonstrates the existence of mechanisms sensitive to vertical disparity using very simple stimuli, composed of just a few dots.

Finally, it should be noted that corresponding elements in the left and right eyes do not differ only in positional disparity (horizontal or vertical), but also in orientation and spacing (or spatial frequency). This was initially proposed by Blakemore, Fiorentini, and Maffei (1972) and several attempts have been made to establish that orientation and spatial frequency disparity mechanisms exist independently of the positional disparity mechanisms (see, e.g., Rogers, 1992). A possible advantage of such mechanisms is that they could code directly for stereoscopic slant and tilt of surfaces instead of estimating these by differentiating an estimated depth. For a possible computational model, see Jones and Malik (1992b).

Discussion

Which is the correct way to explain human perception? On the one hand, it seems that humans do not have access to the complete reconstruction of the scene: they do not seem to have precise depth map descriptions of objects, and they do not really know quantitatively the exact configuration of their eyes. This does not rule out the possibility that these quantities are computed, but cannot be directly accessed. In addition, the parameters of the viewing system such as gaze and fixation distance are important for the computation of the epipolar geometry of the stereo pair, which is needed by many algorithms to compute image matching efficiently. This question is the subject of on-going research.

References

Anderson, B. L., and Nakayama, K. (1994). Towards a general theory of stereopsis: Binocular matching, occluding contours, and fusion. *Psychol. Rev. 101*, 414–445.

Arditi, A., Kaufman, L., and Movshon, J. A. (1981). A simple explanation of the induced size effect. *Vision Res. 21*, 755–764.

Blakemore, C., Fiorentini, A., and Maffei, L. (1972). A second neural mechanism of binocular depth discrimination. *J. Physiol. (London) 226*, 725–749.

Baker, H. H., and Binford, T. O. (1981). Depth from edge- and intensity-based stereo. *Proc. Seventh IJCAI*, Vancouver, BC, pp. 631–636.

Burt, P., and Julesz, B. (1980). A disparity gradient limit for binocular fusion. *Science 208*(9), 615–617.

Cumming, B. G., Johnston, E. B., and Parker, A. J. (1991). Vertical disparities and perception of three dimensional shape. *Nature (London) 349*, 411–413.

Enright, J. T. (1991). Exploring the third dimension with eye movements: Better than stereopsis. *Vision Res. 31*(9), 1549–1562.

Fleet, D. J., Jepson, A. D., and Jenkin, M. R. M. (1991). Phase-based disparity measurement. *CVGIP: Image Understand. 53*(2), 198–210.

Gårding, J., Porrill, J., Frisby, J. P., and Mayhew, J. E. W. (1993a). Gaze-invariant binocular depth perception and vertical disparity. Unpublished Draft, Royal Institute of Technology, Stockholm, Sweden.

Gårding, J., Porrill, J., Frisby, J. P., and Mayhew, J. E. W. (1993b). Binocular stereopsis, vertical disparity and relief transformations. Unpublished Draft, Royal Institute of Technology, Stockholm, Sweden.

Gillam, B., and Lawergren, B. (1983). The induced effect, vertical disparity, and stereoscopic theory. *Percept. Psychophys. 34*(2), 121–130.

Grimson, W. E. L. (1981). *From Images to Surfaces*. Cambridge, MA: MIT Press.

Hannah, M. J. (1974). Computer matching of areas in images. Technical Report AIM-239, Artificial Intelligence Laboratory, Stanford University.

Helmholtz, H. von (1925). In J. P. C. Southhall (trans.), *Treatise on Physiological Optics* (Vol. 3). New York: Dover.

Jones, D. G., and Malik, J. (1992a). Computational framework for determining stereo correspondence from a set of linear spatial filters. *Image Vision Comp. 10*, 699–708.

Jones, D. G., and Malik, J. (1992b). Determining three-dimensional shape from orientation and spatial frequency disparities. In G. Sandini (Ed.), *Lecture Notes in Computer Science 588* (pp. 661–669). Berlin: Springer-Verlag.

Julesz, B. (1960). Binocular depth perception of computer-generated patterns. *Bell Syst. Tech. J. 39*, 1125–1162.

Julesz, B. (1962). Towards the automation of binocular depth perception (AUTOMAP). *Proc. IFIPS Cong.*, Munich.

Julesz, B. (1971). *Foundations of Cyclopean Perception* (pp. 439–444). Chicago: University of Chicago Press.

Kass, M. (1983). Computing visual correspondence. *Proc. DARPA Image Understanding Workshop*, pp. 54–60.

Koenderink, J. J., and van Doorn, A. J. (1976). Geometry of binocular vision and a model for stereopsis. *Biol. Cybern. 21*, 29–35.

Krol, J. D., and van de Grind, W. A. (1980). The double nail illusion: Experiments on binocular vision with nails, needles, and pins. *Perception 9*, 651–669.

Liu, L., Stevenson, S. B., and Schor, C. M. (1994). A polar coordinate system for describing binocular disparity. *Vision Res. 34*, 1205–1222.

Longuet-Higgins, H. C. (1981). A computer algorithm for reconstructing a scene from two projections. *Nature (London) 293*, 133–135.

Marr, D. (1982). *Vision*. San Francisco: W. H. Freeman.

Marr, D., and Poggio, T. (1976). Cooperative computation of stereo disparity. *Science 194*, 283–287.

Marr, D., and Poggio, T. (1979). A computational theory of human stereo vision. *Proc. R. Soc. London B 204*, 301–328.

Mayhew, J. E. W., and Longuet-Higgins, H. C. (1982). A computational model of binocular depth perception. *Nature (London) 297*, 376–378.

Mitchison, G. (1988). Planarity and segmentation in stereoscopic matching. *Perception 17*, 753–782.

Nakayama, K., and Shimojo, S. (1990). DaVinci stereopsis: Depth and subjective occluding contours from unpaired image points. *Vision Res. 30*(11), 1811–1825.

Nishihara, H. K. (1984). Practical real-time imaging stereo matcher. *Opt. Engi. 23*(5), 536–545.

Ogle, K. N. (1950). *Researches in Binocular Vision*. Philadelphia: Saunders.

Ohzawa, I., DeAngelis, G. C., and Freeman, R. D. (1991). Stereoscopic depth discrimination in the visual cortex—neurons ideally suited as disparity detectors. *Science 249*(4972), 1037–1041.

Pollard, S. B., Mayhew, J. E. W., and Frisby, J. P. (1985). A stereo correspondence algorithm using a disparity gradient limit. *Perception 14*, 449–470.

Prazdny, K. (1985). Detection of binocular disparities. *Biol. Cybern. 52*, 93–99.

Rogers, B., and Koenderink, J. (1986). Monocular aniseikonia: A motion parallax analogue of the disparity-induced effect. *Nature (London) 322*, 62–63.

Rogers, B. J. (1992). The perception and representation of depth and slant in stereoscopic surfaces. In G. Orban and H. H. Nagel (Eds.), *Artificial and Biological Vision Systems* (pp. 241–266). ESPRIT Basic Research Series. Berlin: Springer-Verlag.

Rogers, B. J., and Bradshaw, M. F. (1993). Vertical disparities, differential perspective and binocular stereopsis. *Nature (London) 361*, 253–255.

Schor, C. M., and Wood, I. (1983). Disparity range for local stereopsis as a function of luminance spatial frequency. *Vision Res. 23*(12), 1649–1654.

Steinman, R. M., Levinson, J. Z., Collewijn, H., and van der Steen, J. (1985). Vision in the presence of known natural retinal image motion. *J. Opt. Soc. Am. A 2,* 226–233.

Weinshall, D. (1989). Perception of multiple transparent planes in stereo vision. *Nature (London) 341,* 737–739.

Weinshall, D. (1990). Qualitative depth from stereo, with applications. *Comp. Vision, Graphics, Image Process. 49,* 222–241.

Weinshall, D. (1991). Seeing 'ghost' planes in stereo vision. *Vision Res. 31*(10), 1731–1748.

Westheimer, G. (1984). Sensitivity for vertical retinal image differences. *Nature (London) 307,* 632–634.

Westheimer, G., and Pettet, M. W. (1992). Detection and processing of vertical disparity by the human observer. *Proc. R. Soc. London B 250,* 243–247.

Yuille, A. L., and Poggio, T. (1984). A generalized ordering constraint for stereo correspondence. Technical Report AIM-777, Artificial Intelligence Laboratory, Massachusetts Institute of Technology.

5

Stereoscopic Processing in Monkey Visual Cortex: A Review

Gian F. Poggio

Stereoscopic depth perception rests on the brain's ability to measure differences between the images in the two eyes. In binocular vision, the two monocular fields of view are largely superimposed; separate images of the visual world are present in left and right eyes, and a single three-dimensional (3D) representation of that world is constructed in the visual brain. The paired images of a single object in space are essentially identical, but, as dictated by the geometry of binocular vision, do not necessarily occupy the same positions on the two retinas. Indeed, the images are topographically in register (*correspondence*) only for a small set of objects, those objects located at or close to the distance of convergent fixation. The images of all other objects occupy horizontally shifted retinal positions (*disparity*): left and right images of objects beyond the point of fixation are closer to each other, those of nearer objects are farther apart. It has been recognized since Wheatstone's demonstration with the stereoscope (1838), and conclusively proven by Julesz's studies (1960, 1971) with random-dot stereograms, that horizontal retinal disparity is the most important and accurate source of information for judgments of relative depth (stereopsis).

The discovery by Hubel and Wiesel (1959) that single neurons in the primary visual cortex (V1) of the cat respond to stimulation of either eye provided the first physiological evidence for the neural combination of left and right retinal images, and opened the path for the experimental investigation of the neurophysiology of binocular vision. In primates, the central visual projections originating from the ganglion cells in left and right retinas remain essentially separate up to the input to visual area V1 (layer 4). Beyond that, neurons in visual cortex, from the other neurons in V1, to those in areas V2 through V5 and beyond, receive inputs from both eyes.

A neuron in the visual cortex of the brain "sees" the world through a pair of *receptive fields*, one in each eye, and its pattern of activity reflects at all times the interaction of inputs from the two eyes. Neurophysiological studies have revealed that the response of a large proportion of visual cortical neurons depends critically upon the relative horizontal position of the pair of corresponding image features in the two eyes, an effect called *disparity selectivity*. Disparity-selective neurons were discovered by Barlow, Blakemore, and Pettigrew (1967) and Nikara, Bishop, and Pettigrew (1968) in the primary visual cortex of the cat. The properties of these cells were analyzed in some detail by Bishop and his collaborators (Pettigrew, Nikara, and Bishop, 1968; Joshua and Bishop, 1970; Bishop and Henry, 1971; Bishop, Henry, and Smith, 1971; Maske, Yamane, and Bishop, 1986), as well as in other laboratories (Hubel and Wiesel, 1973; von der Heydt et al., 1978; Fischer and Krueger, 1979; Ferster, 1981). In the macaque monkey, disparity-selective neurons have been identified in the striate cortex (V1) and in all prestriate visual areas from V2 to V5 (Hubel and Wiesel, 1970; Poggio and Fischer, 1977; Poggio and Talbot, 1981; Maunsell and Van Essen, 1983; Poggio, 1984, 1990; Poggio et al., 1985, 1988; Burkhalter and Van Essen, 1986; Felleman and Van Essen, 1987; Hubel and Livingstone, 1987; Roy, Komatsu, and Wurtz, 1992).

The binocular pair of receptive fields of a disparity-selective neuron must have a structural organization such as to detect binocular image disparity. The analysis of the organization of the receptive field, conducted mainly in the cat, has shown that the field is in general not spatially uniform, and that excitatory and inhibitory subregions may be recognized within it. The subregions may be completely distinct, or may overlap to various degrees. The pair of associated fields in the two eyes usually have a similar structure, but not necessarily the same spatial arrangement (Hubel and Wiesel, 1962, 1968; Schiller, Finlay and Volman, 1976a,b; Movshon, Thompson, and Tolhurst, 1978; Dean and Tolhurst, 1983; Mullikin, Jones, and Palmer, 1984a,b; Skottun and Freeman, 1984; Camarda, Peterhans, and Bishop, 1985; Maske, Yamane, and Bishop, 1984, 1986; Ohzawa and Freeman, 1986a,b; Emerson et al., 1987; Szulborski and Palmer, 1990; Ohzawa, DeAngelis, and Freeman, 1990). Optimal binocular responses are evoked when left and right RFs are *functionally* superimposed, that is, when corresponding components (subfields) of the two fields are in register, and receive images of essentially the same configuration.

Horizontal disparity sensitivity is obtained because left and right RFs of the cortical neuron are not spatially matched (*receptive field disparity*), either because of a positional incongruity of two fields of identical internal structure, or because of a lateral spatial misalignment of synergistic subfields within the left and the right fields, which are as a whole coextensive over corresponding retinal regions (Barlow, Blakemore, and Pettigrew, 1967; Nikara, Bishop, and Pettigrew, 1968; Poggio and Fischer, 1977; Poggio, Gonzalez, and Krause, 1988; Ohzawa, De-

Angelis, and Freeman, 1990; Freeman and Ohzawa, 1990; DeAngelis, Ohzawa, and Freeman, 1991). The phenomenon of receptive field disparity is thought to play a basic role in stereopsis because under conditions of binocular convergent fixation, different groups of cortical neurons would be selectively activated by objects at different relative depth (Joshua and Bishop, 1970; Bishop and Henry, 1971). Cortical visual neurons may also be sensitive to other forms of binocular disparity, for example, orientation disparity (Haenny et al., 1980) or temporal disparity (Gardner, Douglas, and Cynader, 1985), and a small number of cells has been observed that specifically signal motion in depth (Zeki, 1974; Cynader and Regan, 1978; Poggio and Talbot, 1981). Neurons that respond to uniquely binocular stimulation may be collectively regarded as "stereoscopic neurons" on the conjecture that their response reflects the basic cortical processing that leads to binocular depth perception.

This chapter summarizes the observations that my colleagues and I have made, over the past several years, on the response evoked by stereoscopic patterns in single neurons in the striate (V1), and prestriate (V2, V3–V3A) visual cortical areas of the alert rhesus monkey. In particular, I want to outline the functional properties of disparity selective neurons, and to evaluate how these properties may be reflected in the behavioral and psychophysical aspects of binocular vision.

Experimental Preparation

The experiments were conducted on visually attentive and behaving male rhesus macaques (3–5 kg body weight) without the use of anesthetics or other drugs. The monkeys were trained to maintain steady eye fixation for several seconds, while visual patterns were displayed on high-resolution monitors, separately for each eye, and the neuron's impulse activity concurrently recorded with platinum/iridium microelectrodes. The position of the eyes was monitored with an infrared optoelectronic system that detected the corneal light reflex (Poggio and Talbot, 1981; Motter and Poggio, 1984) or, more recently, with a close-circuit television system. Luminous bars (slits) were used to locate the "minimum-response field" (Barlow et al., 1967) and to define the basic 2D properties of each neuron studied. The size, orientation, and speed of the bar were adjusted to evoke optimal binocular responses, as the bar was made to move back and forth across the neuron's receptive field (1°/sec to 4°/sec), or it was held stationary over it, and flashed on and off. Binocular disparity selectivity was analyzed with stereoscopic stimuli positioned over the receptive fields of the neuron under study. Three types of stereopatterns were employed: solid-figure stereograms (SFS), "cyclopean" (CYC) dynamic random-dot stereograms, and dynamic random-dot correlograms (UNC) (see below). Monocular responses to all types of stimuli were also recorded. Macaque monkeys are believed to see depth in random-dot stereograms (Bough, 1970; Cowey, Parkinson, and Warnick, 1975). In our experiments, however, the animal was not required to, and most likely did not direct its attention to the stereoscopic stimulus, a stimulus that had no relevance for the behavioral task the monkey was performing. The behavioral paradigm, stimulus generation, and data collection were controlled on-line with a digital computer (PDP11/34, or PC286). Details of the experimental setup, visual stimulation, and data analysis have been described previously (Poggio, Doty, and Talbot, 1977; Poggio and Fischer, 1977; Poggio and Talbot, 1981; Poggio, 1984; Poggio, Gonzalez, and Krause, 1988; Poggio, 1990).

Experimental Observations in the Alert Monkey

Binocular positional disparity may be defined by its two orthogonal components: horizontal disparity (HD) and vertical disparity (VD). Horizontal disparity gives rise to stereopsis; vertical disparity does not. Indeed, psychophysical evidence indicates that even small amounts of VD interfere with binocular fusion and depth discrimination (Fender and Julesz, 1967; Nielsen and Poggio, 1984). Therefore, we have analyzed the responses of cortical neurons to HD while keeping VD = 0. The results are described below under "Horizontal Disparity." A brief account of our preliminary observations (unpublished) on the effect of VD/HD interaction on neural activity is given below under "Vertical Disparity."

Horizontal Disparity (HD)

The analysis of binocular interaction under conditions of normal binocular vision in the alert, behaviorally trained macaque has shown that a substantial proportion of neurons in striate cortex V1, as well as in prestriate areas V2 and V3−V3A, give differential responses to horizontal binocular disparity (Poggio and Fischer, 1977; Poggio and Talbot, 1981; Poggio, Gonzalez, and Krause, 1988; Poggio, 1990). The amplitude and nature of the response vary along the disparity dimension, and determine the *disparity selectivity profile* of the neuron. It may be assumed that maximal responses are obtained when the retinal sep-

aration between left and right components of the disparate stimulus corresponds to the horizontal misalignment between the synergistic components of the binocularly matched receptive fields. The stereoscopic properties of cortical neurons were analyzed with isolated bar patterns (solid figure stereograms), and with dynamic random-dot stereopatterns (cyclopean stereograms and correlograms), which provided complementary information results leading to an insight of the operational properties of stereoscopic neurons in visual cortex. The characteristics of the stimulating patterns and the response they evoked are described in what follows.

Solid Figure Stereograms (SFS)

Simple bar stereograms were constructed using the bright narrow bar of the spatiotemporal configuration previously defined as optimal for the neuron under study. Left and right bar patterns were presented simultaneously to each eye, moving or flashing, at a series of horizontal disparities, uncrossed, zero, and crossed, with smallest increment of $0.05°$. They were displayed either against a dynamic random-dot background or against a featureless dark field, depending on the one with which the larger response was obtained (Squatrito, Trotter, and Poggio, 1990). The length of the solid bar ranged for different cells between $0.5°$ and $2.0°$, and its width was usually narrow, $0.05°$ or $0.30°$.

On the basis of the response profiles obtained with SFSs, two types of disparity-selective neurons were recognized: "tuned" neurons (excitatory and inhibitory) and "reciprocal" neurons (near and far). The term "flat" was given to those binocular neurons that are not sensitive to horizontal disparity (Poggio and Fischer, 1977; Poggio, Gonzalez, and Krause, 1988). Similar types of disparity-selectivity have been observed in anesthetized and paralyzed cats (Fischer and Krueger, 1979; Ferster, 1981; LeVay and Voigt, 1988) and monkeys (areas V1 and V2: Hubel and Livingstone, 1987; areas V2 and V3: Felleman and Van Essen, 1987; area MT: Maunsell and Van Essen, 1983; Roy, Komatsu, and Wurtz, 1992). Outlines of representative disparity response profiles are shown in figure 5.1.

Tuned neurons respond with excitation or inhibition within a narrow range of disparities and may give the opposite response to disparate images outside this range. "Tuned excitatory" neurons that respond maximally to binocular images with zero or near-zero horizontal disparity ($\pm 0.05°$) are termed *tuned zero* (T0), and tuned neurons with peak response facilitation at larger disparities, crossed or uncrossed, are labeled *tuned near* (TN) and

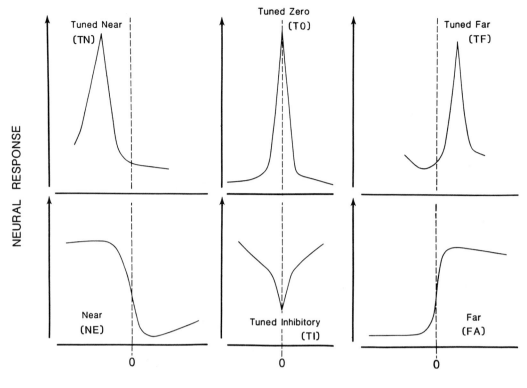

HORIZONTAL DISPARITY

Figure 5.1

Disparity selectivity profiles for neurons in areas V1, V2, and V3–V3A of monkey visual cortex. The curves were drawn by hand through plots of the neural responses (impulses/second) evoked by luminous bars of optimal configuration, and moving in the preferred direction across the neuron's receptive field, at a series of horizontal binocular disparities, crossed (−), zero (0), and uncrossed (+) (solid figure stereograms, SFS). The selectivity profiles that are obtained with dynamic random-dot stereograms (CYC) are not qualitatively differ- ent. The curves outlined in the figure are representative of the types of disparity selectivity we have observed. For T0 and TI neurons, peak response amplitude was evoked by stereopairs of zero disparity ($\pm 0.05°$). TN and TF neurons had peak responses to larger disparities, crossed and uncrossed, respectively. NE and FA neurons are character- ized by response profiles with a smooth transition from maximal exci- tation to maximal inhibition, with the midpoint level of activity at or very close to zero disparity.

tuned far (TF), respectively.[1] T0 neurons have narrow and symmetric excitatory response profiles, with inhibitory sides extending to larger disparities. They typically give very similar responses (often responding minimally, or not at all), to monocular stimulation of either eye (ocular balance). Many of these neurons are directionally selec- tive, often strictly unidirectional. TN and TF neurons, on the other hand, have broader excitatory tuning curves, usually with a clear inhibitory component tailing toward the zero disparity, give different responses to monocular stimulation of left and right eyes (ocular unbalance), and are less frequently directionally sensitive. Moreover, ma- jor differences exist between the responses of T0 neurons

and of TN/TF neurons to binocular image correlation (Poggio et al., 1988), as described later on.

"Tuned inhibitory" neurons (TI) have disparity re- sponse profiles opposite to those of the T0 neurons: their binocular responses are suppressed within the same nar- row range of disparities over which the T0 neurons are binocularly facilitated. Peak suppression occurs within $\pm 0.05°$ of disparity and response facilitation at larger disparities is commonly observed.

Reciprocal neurons either give binocular excitatory re- sponses to bars with crossed disparities, and are inhibited by bars with uncrossed disparities, *near neurons* (NE), or display the opposite behavior: excitatory responses to

---

1. The initial observations by Poggio and Fischer (1977) were made mainly in regions of area V1 and V2 subserving central vision (1°–2° of eccentricity), and predictably the vast majority of tuned excitatory neurons studied (90%) had preferred disparities within $\pm 0.10°$, with half of them tuned to zero-disparity. They were labeled TE. In later experiments (Poggio, Gonzalez, and Krause, 1988) cortical areas V2 and V3–V3A, and more peripheral regions of visual field representation, were also explored (to 8° of eccentricity). Tuned neurons with peaks at large disparities were commonly found, up to 0.6°, and were labeled tuned near (TN) and tuned far (TF) for descriptive purposes. Neurons with tuned properties as those originally described as TE were labeled T0.

uncrossed disparities, and inhibitory responses to crossed ones, *far neurons* (FA). The excitatory peaks and inhibitory troughs are frequently around 0.2° of disparity. For some of these neurons, horizontal disparity sensitivity may extend over a range of $\pm 1°$; other neurons have a narrower, S-shaped response profile. A characteristic feature of the disparity sensitivity of the far and near neurons is a smooth response gradient from maximal excitation to maximal inhibition with the mid-point of response activity at, or close to, zero disparity (see figure 5.1).

All types of stereoscopic neurons described above were observed in all regions of visual cortex we explored. Tuned excitatory neurons (T0, TN, TF) were, on average, twice as numerous as reciprocal neurons (NE/FA). The incidence of disparity selectivity increases from striate to prestriate cortex: the observed ratios of disparity-selective to disparity-insensitive, flat neurons are 1:1 for V1, 2:1 for V2, and 4:1 for V3–V3A. In area V1, tuned excitatory neurons at small disparities (T0) are found most frequently in layers 4c-alpha and 4b, but stereoscopic neurons are encountered also in all other layers (Poggio, 1984). In area V2, disparity-selective neurons are found segregated in zones interleaved with regions with no stereo neurons. Hubel and Livingstone (1987) have shown that the disparity neurons in V2 of the monkey are located in the cytochrome oxidase stained "thick" stripes, and not in the "thin" or in the "pale" stripes. Stereoscopic neurons in areas V3–V3A tend to occur in clusters (Poggio, Gonzalez, and Krause, 1988). Disparity selectivity for isolated bar stereograms is found in the same proportion among neurons with *simple* and with *complex* receptive fields (Hubel and Wiesel, 1962, 1968; Schiller, Finlay, and Volman, 1976a), and there is no evidence of any correlation between the simple/complex properties and the tuned/reciprocal disparity types.

Dynamic Random-Dot Stereograms or Cyclopean Stereograms (CYC)

These were constructed as described by Julesz (1960, 1971). Binocular "figures" (squares) of identical random-dot patterns were displayed centered in a random-dot "background" field (5° or 10°) at a series of disparities including zero. Figure and background had the same dot density (10–50%), luminous intensity, and interdot separation; only a positional disparity between left and right figures would differentiate these otherwise identical stereopatterns of randomly distributed dots.

Uncorrelated Stereograms or Correlograms (UNC)

These stereograms were constructed as those described above, with the important differences that the dot patterns within the outline of left and right "figures" were not the same, but were randomly different from each other (uncorrelation), their patterns changing from frame to frame of the display at 67 or 100/sec (Tyler and Julesz, 1978; Poggio, Gonzalez, and Krause, 1988).

A proportion of neurons in areas V1, V2, and V3–V3A of the alert macaque responds readily and strongly to dynamic random-dot stereograms; we refer to these neurons as "cyclopean" neurons. All types of disparity selectivity to SFS (tuned, reciprocal, and flat) were also observed with CYC stereograms. For any one neuron, however, the response profiles that were obtained with isolated bars and with random-dot stereopatterns are qualitatively the same, but the magnitude of the response and the range of effective disparities may be different. All types of disparity selectivity were found in all monkeys and in all cortical areas examined (Poggio, 1980, 1990; Poggio et al., 1985, 1988).

Cortical visual neurons, so often sensitive to the spatio-temporal configuration of contour patterns (e.g., size, orientation, contrast, velocity, and direction of motion), appear to have less strict requirements for random-dot patterns. For any one cell, cyclopean figures larger than the size of the "optimal" solid bar figure commonly evoked stronger responses and sometimes were needed to elicit any response at all (Poggio et al., 1985). The response to RDS of stationary large figures may often be as strong as or stronger than the response evoked by SFS; the reverse was usually true with moving random-dot figures of the size and orientation of the isolated bar.

The number of neurons responding to RDS increased from the striate to the prestriate areas, from about 30% in V1 to 60% in V2 and to 70% in V3–V3A. This increase was due mainly to neurons with tuned-near or tuned-far disparity selectivity (TN, TF), which represented nearly one-half of the disparity neurons in V2 and V3–V3A, and which were the most frequently sensitive to CYC stimulation (72%). Of all the neurons with other disparity selectivity profiles for solid bars, about 30% responded to random-dot stereograms. The 2D and 3D properties of cortical cells appear to be largely independent of each other, and orientation and directional selectivity may coexist with all types of stereo properties. Remarkably, however, the vast majority of neurons (90%) that responded to dynamic CYC stereograms had *complex* receptive field properties, whereas in their response to solid bar stereograms neurons were evenly split between simple and complex (Poggio et al., 1985, 1988; Poggio, 1990).

Stimulation with random-dot stereopatterns has shown that disparity selectivity is not the only cyclopean property of cortical visual neurons. A substantial proportion of cells is sensitive to binocular image correlation, and an

Poggio: Stereoscopic Processing in Monkey Visual Cortex

operational association exists between disparity selectivity and correlation sensitivity (see below).

Vertical Disparity (VD)

We have used dynamic random-dot stereograms (CYC) and correlograms (UNC) to assess the effect of vertical misalignment of the "figure" on the response of cortical visual neurons (more frequently in areas V3–V3A). Both binocular vertical relations were tested: left eye image higher ($+$) or lower ($-$) than right eye image. The majority of our observations were made on neurons that displayed HD selectivity. In these cells, vertical disparity consistently affected the neuron's response to HD: Vertical misalignments as small as $\pm 0.1°$ introduced between left and right "figures" of random-dot stereograms positioned over the neuron's receptive field consistently reduced the response evoked by a simultaneously present horizontal disparity. The effect was particularly evident at the horizontal disparity that evoked the largest response from the neuron in the absence of vertical disparity (VD = 0). As described above, the HD selectivity profiles of cortical neurons commonly include both excitatory and inhibitory components. The effect of VD is simply that of reducing the response evoked by HD, a reduction that affects both the excitatory and the inhibitory response, and that occasionally may cancel the response and bring the neuron's ongoing activity to the "spontaneous" level. In a small group of HD-insensitive neurons (flat), the vertically disparate stereopatterns did not modify the response other than at HD = 0, where it had an excitatory effect that was most likely the result of binocular image uncorrelation (see below). Outside the range of effective horizontal disparities, no evident changes on neural activity were observed that could be ascribed to vertical disparity. Our observations are too limited to rule out the existence of neurons with response selectivity for vertical disparity, but we have found none with RDS stimulation.

These physiological findings are consonant with the psychophysical observations of Nielsen and Poggio (1984), who showed that in random-dot stereograms, only a small amount (3.5 arcmin) of VD can be tolerated before depth discrimination (front/behind) reduces to chance level. Both the single-unit results and the psychophysical ones suggest that the binocular stereo matching is based on a 1D analysis, which is considerably simpler than the 2D analysis required if both disparities were to be processed.

Disparity Selectivity and Binocular Correlation

The results of our studies have shown that a large proportion of neurons in the visual cortex of the macaque signal horizontal binocular disparity. Moreover, the analysis of the responses to dynamic random-dot stereopatterns has revealed that neurons tuned to zero and near-zero disparities, and neurons tuned to larger disparities give very different responses to binocular image correlation (Poggio, Gonzalez, and Krause, 1988). Accordingly, separate "systems" of disparity-selective neurons were defined (Poggio, 1990): (1) the zero-disparity systems, including T0 and TI cells, and (2) two systems with the same correlation properties but mirror ranges of disparity selectivity, the near-disparity system (TN and NE) and the far-disparity system (TF and FA).

Zero-Disparity System or Correspondence System

It is composed of neurons narrowly tuned to stereopatterns of zero or near-zero disparities (T0, TI). T0 neurons give sustained excitatory responses to RDS of zero and near-zero disparities, and inhibitory responses to RDS of larger disparities, both crossed and uncrossed. Excitation results from the concurrent stimulation of topographically corresponding receptive fields in left and right eyes by identical random-dot patterns (binocular correlation). Inhibition obtains from stimulation with stereopairs at disparities larger than the excitatory ones, the results of the different dot pattern/receptive field relations in the two eyes (binocular uncorrelation). This is confirmed by the suppression of activity that occurs when left and right fields are covered with topographically corresponding but texturally different binocular patterns (UNC). TI neurons give responses opposite to those of the tuned excitatory: suppression by RDS of zero disparity (correlation), and activation by disparate patterns (uncorrelation).

It may be suggested that during binocular vision, the T0 population is activated, and the TI suppressed by objects at or close to the plane of fixation, and, reversing their response, respectively inhibited and excited by nearer or farther objects. The ongoing activity of these two functional sets of neurons may operate in binocular vision by defining the reference plane of fixation, and may represent the essential neural substrate for binocular single vision, carrying information for fusional mechanisms. Moreover, neurons of this system, finely tuned to signal small disparities, could represent the neural substrate for fine stereoscopic discrimination.

Near-Disparity System and Far-Disparity System

They include (1) neurons tuned to non-zero disparities (tuned near and tuned far), and (2) neurons giving extended and reciprocal responses to crossed and uncrossed disparities (near and far). (1) Tuned excitatory neurons with peak binocular facilitation at disparities larger than about $\pm 0.1°$ (TN, TF) give similar peak excitatory responses to SFS and to RDS, but the shape of the tuning curves is frequently not the same. Neurons of this type respond to RDS more frequently than any other stereoscopic type (70%). At variance with the T0 neurons, however, TN and TF neurons respond to binocularly uncorrelated patterns (UNC) with activation and never with suppression. These responses are usually smaller, and never larger, than the responses at the preferred disparity, suggesting that they are evoked by those elements of the uncorrelated stereopair that occur with the correct excitatory disparity for the neuron. The depth response profile of these cells appears to be determined chiefly by positional disparity sensitivity, with image contrast correlation playing a lesser role in their stereo selectivity. (2) Only about 30% of the neurons that display reciprocal disparity selectivity to SFS respond also to RDS. Whereas the excitatory response to crossed (NE) or uncrossed (FA) disparities is always evident (even though usually over a range narrower than the range that obtains with isolated contrast bars), the inhibitory response to the reciprocal disparities may be limited in amplitude or/and extent, or it may not be present at all. The response properties of the TN/TF neurons and the characteristics of binocular interaction are similar to those of the NE/FA cells, and it may well be that there exists disparity selectivity profiles intermediate between the two.

The proposition may be advanced that during binocular vision, neurons of the near- and far-disparity systems signal the horizontal disparity of objects whose nearly identical images project upon the neuron's receptive fields in the two eyes. These neurons would discharge at a maintained level in response to the uncorrelated images of different objects in the two eyes, and increase or decrease their activity in the presence of objects at the "correct" depth, that is, within the region of space of their receptive field superposition. Moreover, the populations of NE and FA neurons could also contribute to stereoacuity by signaling small disparity changes through their finely graded response transition from suppression to facilitation about the zero disparity, perhaps via the rapid and opposite change in the activity of the two reciprocal types of neurons.

The transition from the zero-system to the near- or to the far-disparity systems is not abrupt, and in the range from $\pm 0.05°$ and up to $\pm 0.2°$ of disparity, neurons with the same disparity selectivity may have different correlation properties: about one-half of the tuned neurons in this range are activated by uncorrelation, like other TN/TF neurons, whereas the other half is suppressed, as typical of the T0 neurons (Poggio, Gonzalez, and Krause, 1988).

Disparity-Insensitive Neurons

Some cortical neurons, more frequently observed in striate than in prestriate cortex, give similar excitatory responses to SFS stereograms at all disparities, including zero (flat neurons, FL). About one-third of these neurons respond also, and in a similar way, to cyclopean patterns (CYC), except, of course, to those of zero disparity in which the dot patterns in left and right eyes are identical. The response profile of the FL neuron to CYC is therefore very similar to that of the tuned inhibitory neuron (TI). When the textural correlation between left and right stereopairs is removed (UNC), the FL neurons respond equally well at all disparities including zero, their response profile now being the same as that which obtains with SFS. This response behavior suggests that the FL neurons, like the T0 and TI neurons, are sensitive to binocular correlation. The lack of responses to stereograms of zero disparity and their occurrence with disparate stereograms also suggest that the receptive fields of these neurons are in retinal correspondence. The role of the FL neurons in depth perception, if any, is as yet unknown.

Comments

The most direct evidence for the disparity selectivity property of single striate and prestriate neurons comes from studies that have shown that many of these cells respond readily and consistently to dynamic random-dot stereograms of monocularly invisible figures, in which depth emerges strictly from the interaction of the inputs from the two eyes. These findings suggest a neural substrate for one major operation that the nervous system must carry on in the reconstruction of the third dimension, that is matching the corresponding elements in the left and right retinal images. Correct matching is particularly difficult under the highly ambiguous disparity conditions of the random-dot stereograms in which all the dots have the same size and contrast, and any dot in one image could be matched with any one of a large number of dots in the other image. The results of psychophysical experiments suggest that stereoscopic matching occurs at an early stage of visual processing (Julesz, 1971). The neurophysiological findings support this notion by revealing that a substantial proportion of binocular cortical neurons, typically "complex" neurons, in the striate and prestriate cortex of the macaque monkey respond strongly to dynamic random-dot stereograms. It may be suggested that this capacity results from the spatial arrangements of the neuron's receptive fields in the two eyes, seen as being composed of numerous receptive sites, or subfields, with the subfields in one eye functionally linked with synergistic subfields of the appropriate positional disparity in the other eye. The size of the subfields should be of the order of the size of the associated monocular receptive fields at the cortical input (layer 4c) (Poggio and Poggio, 1984; Poggio, Gonzalez, and Krause, 1988). The orderly and finely organized retinotopic maps in layer 4 of the striate cortex (Blasdel and Fitzpatrick, 1984), the layer of termination of geniculate axons, could provide the arrangement for the precise matching of the binocular inputs. This anatomical substrate may set the conditions for the high resolving power of stereopsis based on a computational interpolation process similar and subsequent to that postulated to occur in layer 4C-beta for monocular hyperacuity (Barlow, 1979; Crick, Marr, and Poggio, 1981). It may be relevant to this hypothesis that T0 neurons in V1 are more frequently observed in layer 4B and 4C-alpha (Poggio, 1984).

Not all cortical visual neurons have the same repertoire of binocular properties; in particular, only a subset of the neurons with complex receptive field properties appears to have the capacity of signaling depth correctly under highly ambiguous disparity conditions. Many other cells, complex and simple alike, even though sensitive to retinal disparity of contours, do not respond to textured stereopatterns. It must be that for stereoscopic vision to be achieved, there exist in the brain not only processing mechanisms that ignore incorrect binocular matches and detect correct ones, but also mechanisms for controlling the activity of those neurons that are themselves sensitive to disparity but unable to filter out ambiguities (Poggio, 1984).

Disparity-selective neurons may also provide signals for the control of the disjunctive eye movements of convergence and divergence; because of their relatively wide range of disparity sensitivity the TN,TF and NE,FA neurons may participate in the initiation of vergence movements, whereas the T0 and TI neurons have properties that are appropriate for guiding the completion of vergence and the maintenance of binocular fixation (Poggio and Fischer, 1977).

Stereoscopic neurons typically signal disparity with little response uncertainty. Even a sharply tuned excitatory cell is securely selective for its optimal disparity, never failing to respond to stereopatterns of that disparity, and never responding as well to stimuli with disparities that differ by only a few minutes of arc. This neural property is remarkable indeed, because the jitter in the position of the eyes during fixation (Motter and Poggio, 1984) should preclude a correct binocular image superposition, especially for foveal striate neurons with small receptive

fields. Yet neurons respond as though they were insensitive to small changes in the relative positions of their receptive fields in the two eyes. This suggests that the mechanisms of binocular interaction are remarkably robust and capable of compensating dynamically for the continuous and random shifts in eye position during fixation (Motter and Poggio, 1990).

Richards (1970, 1971) investigated the human ability to discriminate large crossed and uncrossed disparities. He found that a substantial proportion of subjects could not discriminate "near" disparate stimuli from monocular stimuli, while others were unable to process "far" disparities. The defect was selective, could extend to smaller disparities (e.g., to 0.05°, Richards and Kaye, 1974), and coexist with normal fine stereopsis and good stereoacuity of less than one minute of arc (Jones, 1977). These findings led Richards (1971) to hypothesize a pooling of the activity of the disparity detectors that samples three disparity ranges: crossed, near-zero, and uncrossed. In a carefully designed study, Cormack, Stevenson, and Schor (1993) derived tuning functions in human subjects within $\pm 0.5°$ of disparity, using a subthreshold summation technique. These functions are quite similar to those that the same investigators had obtained previously with a method of adaptation (Stevenson et al., 1992). Cormack et al. (1993) conclude that "disparity processing is accomplished via a continuum of disparity-tuned channels," and refute the three "pools" hypothesis of Richards. LeVay and Voigt (1988) analyzed the disparity coding in the visual cortex of the anesthetized cat, recognized selectivity profiles similar to those observed in the alert monkey, and concluded that the various profiles belong to a continuum. Models have been constructed that show the importance of overlapping tuned channels for stereoacuity (Lehky and Sejnowski, 1990).

Our findings in the visually alert rhesus monkey indicate that a substantial proportion of neurons in striate and prestriate cortex give differential responses to horizontal retinal disparity. The majority of these neurons display *tuned* disparity selectivity spanning the range of physiological disparities through the zero disparity. The sharpness of tuning, and its symmetry, appear to be maximum for neurons tuned to the zero or near-zero disparities (T0, TI), the profile becoming wider and asymmetric for neurons tuned at larger disparities (TN, TF). The typical response profiles of these neurons (figure 5.1) are remarkably similar to the tuning functions psychophysically derived by Cormack et al. (1993). A smaller population of neurons, about one-half the tuned cells, has extended and *reciprocal* disparity selectivity (NE, FA), for which no psychophysical tuning functions have been described. Neu-

rons may also exist whose disparity selectivity profiles is intermediate between TN/TF and NE/FA.

It seems reasonable to suppose that the activity of neurons that respond selectively to horizontal retinal disparity represents the early stages of stereo processing, the output of which the brain will further elaborate and integrate with other visual (and nonvisual) signals to construct dynamically the representation of depth. On the basis of the tuned profile characteristics, ocularity, and the sensitivity to binocular image correlation, we have proposed the existence of three operational stereo systems of neurons, the zero-system (T0, TI), the near- (TN, NE) and the far-disparity (FA, TF) systems, and have suggested that qualitative estimates of depth and vergence response to large disparities are served by neurons with broad tuned properties (TN, TF), as well as by neurons with reciprocal disparity selectivity (NE, FA), whereas narrowly tuned neurons (T0, TI) operate in fine depth discrimination with the obligatory singleness of vision, and maintenance of vergence on the fixation plane. The functional boundaries between systems are not sharp, and likely to shift under different conditions of binocular vision.

On these assumptions, the deficits of stereoscopic vision selectively for the "near" or for the "far" disparity ranges described by Richards (1971) may be regarded as the result of dysfunction or defect of the set of neurons whose binocular organization—from receptive fields position and structure, to intracortical input interaction—is such as to determine the neuron's selectivity either for the crossed or for the uncrossed disparities. Neural network models on the development of binocular disparity selectivity (see Berns, Dayan, and Sejnowski, 1993) may suggest possible mechanisms for this phenomenon.

References

Barlow, H. (1979). Reconstructing the visual image in space and time. *Nature (London)* 279, 189–190.

Barlow, H., Blakemore, C., and Pettigrew, J. D. (1967). The neural mechanism of binocular depth discrimination. *J. Physiol.* 193, 327–342.

Berns, G. S., Dayan, P., and Sejnowski, T. J. (1993). A correlational model for the development of disparity selectivity in visual cortex that depends on prenatal and postnatal phases. *Proc. Natl. Acad. Sci. U.S.A.* 90, 8277–8281.

Bishop, P. O., and Henry, G. H. (1971). Spatial vision. *Annu. Rev. Psychol.* 22, 119–161.

Bishop, P. O., and Henry, G. H., and Smith, C. J. (1971). Binocular interaction fields of single units in the cat striate cortex. *J. Physiol.* 216, 39–68.

Blasdel, G. G., and Fitzpatrick, D. (1984). Physiological organization of layer 4 in macaque striate cortex. *J. Neurosci.* 4, 880–895.

Bough, E. W. (1970). Stereoscopic vision in the macaque monkey: a behavioral demonstration. *Nature (London)* 225, 42–44.

Burkhalter, A., and Van Essen, D. C. (1986). Processing of color, form and disparity information in visual areas VP and V2 of ventral extrastriate cortex in the macaque monkey. *J. Neurosci.* 6, 2327–2351.

Camarda, R. M., Peterhans, E., and Bishop, P. O. (1985). Spatial organizations of subregions in receptive fields of simple cells in cat striate cortex as revealed by stationary flashing bars and moving edges. *Exp. Brain Res.* 60, 136–150.

Cormack, L. K., Stevenson, S. B., and Schor, C. M. (1993). Disparity-tuned channels of the human visual system. *Visual Neurosci.* 10, 585–596.

Cowey, A., Parkinson, A. M., and Warnick, L. (1975). Global stereopsis in rhesus monkeys. *Q. J. Exp. Psychol.* 27, 93–109.

Crick, F., Marr, D., and Poggio, T. (1981). An information-processing approach to understanding the visual cortex. In F. O. Schmitt, F. G. Worden, G. M. Edelman, and S. G. Dennis (Eds.), *The Organization of the Cerebral Cortex* (pp. 505–533). Cambridge: MIT Press.

Cynader, M., and Regan, D. (1978). Neurons in cat parastriate cortex sensitive to the direction of motion in three-dimensional space. *J. Physiol.* 274, 549–569.

Dean, A. F., and Tolhurst, D. J. (1983). On the distinctness of simple and complex cells in the visual cortex of the cat. *J. Physiol.* 344, 305–325.

DeAngelis, G. C., Ohzawa, I., and Freeman, R. F. (1991). Depth is encoded in the visual cortex by a specialized receptive field structure. *Nature (London)* 352, 156–159.

Emerson, R. C., Citron, M. C., Vaughn, W. J., and Klein, S. A. (1987). Nonlinear directionally selective subunits in complex cells of cat striate cortex. *J. Neurophysiol.* 58, 33–65.

Felleman, D. J., and Van Essen, D. C. (1987). Receptive field properties of neurons in area V3 of macaque monkey extrastriate cortex. *J. Neurophysiol.* 57, 889–920.

Fender, D., and Julesz, B. (1967). Extension of Panum's fusional area in binocularly stabilized vision. *J. Opt. Soc. Am.* 57, 819–830.

Ferster, D. (1981). A comparison of binocular depth mechanisms in area 17 and 18 of the cat visual cortex. *J. Physiol.* 311, 623–655.

Fischer, B., and Krueger, J. (1979). Disparity tuning and binocularity of single neurons in the cat visual cortex. *Exp. Brain Res.* 35, 1–8.

Freeman, R. D., and Ohzawa, I. (1990). On the neurophysiological organization of binocular vision. *Vision Res.* 30, 1661–1676.

Gardner, J. C., Douglas, R. M., and Cynader, M. S. (1985). A time-based stereoscopic depth mechanism in the visual cortex. *Brain Res.* 328, 154–157.

Haenny, P., von der Heydt, R., and Poggio, G. F. (1980). Binocular neuron responses to tilt in depth in the monkey visual cortex. Evidence for orientation disparity processing. *Exp. Brain Res.* 41, A26.

Hubel, D. H., and Livingstone, M. S. (1987). Segregation of form, color and stereopsis in primate area 18. *J. Neurosci.* 7, 3378–3415.

Hubel, D. H., and Wiesel, T. N. (1959). Receptive fields of single neurones in the cat's striate cortex. *J. Physiol. 148*, 574–591.

Hubel, D. H., and Wiesel, T. N. (1962). Receptive fields, binocular interaction and functional architecture in the cat's visual cortex. *J. Physiol. 160*, 106–154.

Hubel, D. H., and Wiesel, T. N. (1968). Receptive fields and functional architecture of monkey striate cortex. *J. Physiol. 195*, 215–243.

Hubel, D. H., and Wiesel, T. N. (1970). Cells sensitive to binocular depth in area 18 of the macaque monkey cortex. *Nature (London) 225*, 41–42.

Hubel, D. H., and Wiesel, T. N. (1973). A re-examination of stereoscopic mechanisms in the cat. *J. Physiol. 232*, 29–30P.

Jones, R. (1977). Anomalies of disparity detection in the human visual system. *J. Physiol. 264*, 621–640.

Joshua, D. E., and Bishop, P. O. (1970). Binocular single vision and depth discrimination. Receptive field disparities for central and peripheral vision and binocular interaction on peripheral single units in cat striate cortex. *Exp. Brain Res. 10*, 389–416.

Julesz, B. (1960). Binocular depth perception of computer-generated patterns. *Bell Syst. Tech. J. 39*, 1125–1162.

Julesz, B. (1971). *Foundations of Cyclopean Perception.* Chicago: University of Chicago Press.

Lehky, S. R., and Sejnowski, T. J. (1990). Neural model of stereoacuity and depth interpolation based on a distributed representation of stereo disparity. *J. Neurosci. 10*, 2281–2299.

LeVay, S., and Voigt, T. (1988). Ocular dominance and disparity coding in cat visual cortex. *Visual Neurosci. 1*, 395–414.

Maske, R., Yamane, S., and Bishop, P. O. (1984). Binocular simple cells for local stereopsis: Comparison of the receptive field organization for the two eyes. *Vision Res. 24*, 1921–1929.

Maske, R., Yamane, S., and Bishop, P. O. (1986). Stereoscopic mechanisms: Binocular responses of the striate cells of cats to moving light and dark bars. *Proc. R. Soc. London B 229*, 227–256.

Maunsell, J. H. R., and Van Essen, D. C. (1983). Functional properties of neurons in middle temporal visual area of the macaque monkey. II. Binocular interaction and sensitivity to binocular disparity. *J. Neurophysiol. 49*, 1148–1167.

Motter, B. C., and Poggio, G. F. (1984). Binocular fixation in the rhesus monkey: Spatial and temporal characteristics. *Exp. Brain Res. 54*, 304–314.

Motter, B. C., and Poggio, G. F. (1990). Dynamic stabilization of receptive fields of cortical neurons (V1) during fixation of gaze in the macaque. *Exp. Brain Res. 83*, 37–43.

Movshon, J. A., Thompson, I. D., and Tolhurst, D. J. (1978). Receptive field organization of complex cells in the cat's striate cortex. *J. Physiol. 283*, 79–99.

Mullikin, W. H., Jones, J. J., Palmer, L. A. (1984a). Receptive-field properties and laminar distribution of X-like and Y-like simple cells in cat area 17. *J. Neurophysiol. 52*, 350–371.

Mullikin, W. H., Jones, J. J., and Palmer, L. A. (1984b). Periodic simple cells in cat area 17. *J. Neurophysiol. 52*, 372–387.

Nielsen, K. R. K., and Poggio, T. (1984). Vertical image registration in stereopsis. *Vision Res. 10*, 1133–1140.

Nikara, T., Bishop, P. O., and Pettigrew, J. D. (1968). Analysis of retinal correspondence by studying receptive fields of binocular single units in cat striate cortex. *Exp. Brain Res. 6*, 353–372.

Ohzawa, I., and Freeman, R. D. (1986a). The binocular organization of simple cells in the cat's visual cortex. *J. Neurophysiol. 56*, 221–242.

Ohzawa, I., and Freeman, R. D. (1986b). The binocular organization of complex cells in the cat's visual cortex. *J. Neurophysiol. 56*, 243–259.

Ohzawa, I., DeAngelis, G. C., and Freeman, R. D. (1990). Stereoscopic depth discrimination in the visual cortex: Neurons ideally suited as disparity detectors. *Science 249*, 1037–1041.

Pettigrew, J. D., Nikara, T., and Bishop, P. O. (1968). Binocular interaction on single units in cat striate cortex: Simultaneous stimulation by single moving slit with receptive fields in correspondence. *Exp. Brain Res. 6*, 391–410.

Poggio, G. F. (1980). Neurons sensitive to dynamic random-dot stereograms in areas 17 and 18 of the rhesus monkey cortex. *Soc. Neurosci. Abstr. 6*, 672.

Poggio, G. F. (1984). Processing of stereoscopic information in monkey visual cortex. In G. M. Edelman, W. E. Gall, W. M. Cowan (Eds.), *Dynamic Aspects of Neocortical Function* (pp. 613–635). New York: John Wiley.

Poggio, G. F. (1990). The cortical neural mechanisms of stereopsis studied with dynamic random-dot stereograms. In E. R. Kandel, T. J. Sejnowski, C. F. Stevens, and J. D. Watson (Eds.), *Cold Spring Harbor Symposia on Quantitative Biology: The Brain* (Vol. 55, pp. 749–758). New York: Cold Spring Harbor Press.

Poggio, G. F., and Fischer, B. (1977). Binocular interaction and depth sensitivity in striate and prestriate cortex of behaving rhesus monkeys. *J. Neurophysiol. 40*, 1392–1407.

Poggio, G. F., and Poggio, T. (1984). The analysis of stereopsis. *Annu. Rev. Neurosci. 7*, 379–412.

Poggio, G. F., and Talbot, W. H. (1981). Neural mechanisms of static and dynamic stereopsis in foveal striate cortex of rhesus monkeys. *J. Physiol. 315*, 469–492.

Poggio, G. F., Doty, R. W., Jr., and Talbot, W. H. (1977). Foveal striate cortex of behaving monkey: Single neuron responses to square-wave gratings during fixation of gaze. *J. Neurophysiol. 40*, 1369–1391.

Poggio, G. F., Gonzalez, F., Krause, F. (1988). Stereoscopic mechanisms in monkey visual cortex: Binocular correlation and disparity selectivity. *J. Neurosci. 8*, 4531–4550.

Poggio, G. F., Motter, B. C., Squatrito, S., and Trotter, Y. (1985). Responses of neurons in visual cortex (V1 and V2) of the alert macaque to dynamic random-dot stereograms. *Vision Res. 25*, 397–406.

Richards, W. (1970). Stereopsis and stereoblindness. *Exp. Brain Res. 10*, 380–388.

Richards, W. (1971). Anomalous stereoscopic depth perception. *J. Opt. Soc. Am. 61*, 410–414.

Richards, W., and Kaye, M. G. (1974). Local versus global stereopsis: Two mechanisms? *Vision Res. 14*, 1345–1347.

Roy, J. P., Komatsu, H., and Wurtz, R. H. (1992). Disparity sensitivity of neurons in monkey extrastriate area MST. *J. Neurosci. 12*, 2478–2492.

Schiller, P. H., Finlay, B. L., and Volman, S. F. (1976a). Quantitative studies of single-cell properties in monkey striate cortex. I. Spatio-temporal organization of receptive fields. *J. Neurophysiol. 39*, 1288–1319.

Schiller, P. H., Finlay, B. L., and Volman, S. F. (1976b). Quantitative studies of single-cell properties in monkey striate cortex. II. Orientation specificity and ocular dominance. *J. Neurophysiol. 39*, 1320–1333.

Skottun, B. C., and Freeman, R. D. (1984). Stimulus specificity of binocular cells in cat's visual cortex: ocular dominance and the matching of left and right eyes. *Exp. Brain Res. 56*, 206–216.

Squatrito, S., Trotter, Y., and Poggio, G. F. (1990). Influences of uniform and textured backgrounds on the impulse activity of neurons in area V1 of the alert monkey. *Brain Res. 536*, 261–270.

Stevenson, S. B., Cormack, L. K., Schor, C. M., and Tyler, C. W. (1992). Disparity tuning in mechanisms of human stereopsis. *Vision Res. 32*, 1685–1694.

Szulborski, R. G., and Palmer, L. A. (1990). The two-dimensional spatial structure of nonlinear subunits in the receptive fields of complex cell, *Vision Res. 30*, 249–254.

Tyler, C. W., and Julesz, B. (1978). Binocular cross-correlation in time and space. *Vision Res. 18*, 101–105.

von der Heydt, R., Adorjani, C. S., Haenny, P., and Baumgartner, G. (1978). Disparity sensitivity and receptive field incongruity of units in cat striate cortex. *Exp. Brain Res. 31*, 523–545.

Wheatstone, C. (1838). Contributions to the physiology of vision. Part the first. On some remarkable, and hitherto unobserved, phenomena of binocular vision. *Phil. Trans. Roy. Soc. 2*, 371–393.

Zeki, S. M. (1974). Cells responding to changing image size and disparity in the cortex of the rhesus monkey. *J. Physiol. 242*, 827–841.

Part II

Visual Texture

Andrei Gorea

The study of texture processing may be traced back to the statistical approaches of the 1940s meant to quantify the information limiting characteristics of "photographic granularity" (the computational perspective), or to the Gestalt school in the 1920s (the biological perspective; see Bergen, 1991; Sagi, 1991). Along these same lines, the modern era in the study of texture perception was most certainly set off in the 1960s by Julesz (1962) and Beck (1966).

Three decades later many aspects of texture processing have been elucidated. Nonetheless, some fundamental questions remain unanswered. For example, there is still some debate in the literature on what a texture actually is (the *definition* problem) and, as a corollary, whether the study of texture processing involves novel theoretical approaches relative to the classical "channel approach" of the 1970s. While there is a wide consensus on the parallel processing of textured stimuli at different spatial scales, we still need to understand how these parallel processes cooperate or interact (the *multiple scale* or *local/global* problem) and whether the choice of one specific scale may be determined by higher order processes such as attention (the *top-down* problem). We definitely do not know much about the *neural substrate* of the many different processes and computational algorithms proposed in the theoretical literature to account for the psychophysical results, nor do we have a clear idea of the actual scope of the now established *plasticity* of these neural mechanisms. The five contributors to this section address these and some other unsolved problems in texture processing. Since the meaningfulness of asking unanswered questions cannot be valued out of context, the contributors also provide relevant overviews of the literature which all build at some point or other upon the pioneering work of Bela Julesz.

What do we mean by visual "texture"? Building on Watt's, Caelli's, and Sagi's answers to this question (see also Bergen, 1991), one might come up with the following stratified definition: Visual texture is a 2D visual stimulus characterized by a visible *grain*. Visual grain consists in local modulations along dimensions such as luminance, color, and shape, which may or may not be discriminable. Two textures are visually different if they do not share the same grain and/or if they do not share, in the statistical sense, the same grain distributions across space.

Given this definition, any model of texture perception should account for the processing of both granularity and grain distribution. Extracting the granularity of a texture necessarily involves some form of local, nonlinear processing such as "texton" extraction. Estimating the statistical properties of the grain requires some global operation across the outputs of the local detectors. This reflects one aspect of the local–global issue in texture processing.

A related aspect is quite intuitive: segregation of two grain populations requires that the variance *within* these populations be smaller than the variance *across* populations. Computation of this form of "within/across" ratio may be implemented in different ways. One may argue that the most natural implementation, in the biological sense, is to equate "within" and "across" operators with small and large scale "double-opponent" units, respectively. Such units would compute a form of *generalized contrast* along an arbitrary (*n*th-order) dimension such as luminance, chroma (first order), orientation, spatial frequency, disparity, direction of motion (second order), etc. (Gorea and Papathomas, 1993).

The requirement of multiple scaling processing in texture segregation leads to a third aspect of the local–global issue, namely the fact that "what is [grain] at one [spatial] scale is texture at another" (Caelli, chapter 8).

To illustrate some of these and other issues raised by the study of texture perception, Watt (chapter 6) takes us on a walk "into the rugged hills near [his] home" and exemplifies how texture processing at different spatial (and temporal) scales serves different adaptive behaviors such as "choosing goals" for the walk (largest scale), deciding on whether "ordinary walking or scrambling" is the appropriate next move (intermediate scale) and picking up the right spot for placing our foot at each step (smallest scale). This approach to natural images enables segregation of relevant image surfaces and the assessment of some of their critical characteristics such as their overall slant (at the intermediate scale) and their roughness (at the smallest scale). However, beyond segregation and some sort of (partial) identification of surfaces, texture analysis also has more hidden *processing functions*. Such functions, the author argues, "do not serve a perceptual end in their own right." Rather, they make possible further processing of the visual image. In particular, they enable efficient representations of the critical spatial relationships in the image and, in coordination with attentional processes, determine the most relevant spatial scale in the image space at which further processing is needed.

Sagi's chapter (7) provides a more formal discussion of the different computational approaches used to account for texture segregation performances as they have been assayed psychophysically. Sagi introduces us to a generic texture segregation model (mostly based on his own work) and discusses each of its building blocks in relation to both the theoretical and experimental literature. He thus highlights some critical turning points and the advent of new concepts in the modeling of texture perception during the last three decades.

One of the major features shared by the different approaches discussed in this chapter is that they all assume a hard-wired system whose components immutably perform the very same computation. The second part of Sagi's contribution reminds us that this view is certainly not correct. Recent findings from the author's laboratory strongly support the claim that the neural mechanisms subserving human texture segregation may display a plastic behavior or, in other words, they may learn. The author discusses some specifics of such learning processes, their time-course and their possible physiological substrate.

Caelli (chapter 8) focuses his discussion on three types of problems encountered in texture processing, namely *discrimination*, *segmentation*, and *classification* (or identification). Under most circumstances, one may argue, spatial discrimination (i.e., "same" or "different") and segmentation are equivalent processes insofar as any discrimination will entail a segmentation and vice versa. The discrimination/segregation relationship is of a different nature altogether if the textures to be compared are displayed in temporal succession. Under such circumstances, one may argue that discrimination and classification are one and the same.

Caelli starts with a brief overview of the biological-vision literature and draws attention to the fact that the modeling efforts in this field have always used a passive filtering approach (see Sagi's chapter for a more detailed discussion). He then introduces some leading ideas having guided the machine-vision approach. Among those, the author discusses the theoretical derivation of optimal local texture feature operators (of which the *Markov Random Field* models are an example), the statistical methods involving covariance matrices (both local and global) and leading to rotation-invariant segmentation and classification, the region-based clustering, and the neural network approach to the classification problem.

The chapters by Gallant et al. (9) and by Victor et al. (10) provide insights into the neural substrate of texture processing. Using unitary recording techniques, Gallant et al. demonstrate that a significant subpopulation of V1 cells responds strongly to texture borders void of first order cues (i.e., luminance and/or color) that may be displayed outside of their classical receptive field. Thus, texture segmentation occurs at the earliest cortical processing stage. This view is supported by Victor et al.'s work involving scalp and epicortical visual evoked potentials as well as local field potentials. Basing their analysis on the statistical properties of the stimuli they constructed (a family of even, odd and random isodipole textures), these authors conclude that the nonlinearities required to account for the visual discrimination of such textures (as assayed both psychophysically and electrophysiologically) can already be found in the primary visual cortex. Moreover, the authors advance with some confidence that the spatial pooling required to account for visual sensitivity to long-range spatial correlations in the stimulus domain also takes place at this early processing level. Gallant et al. speculate on the potential involvement in texture processing of higher order nonlinearities as they are revealed in area V4. Cells in this area display marked preferences for one of three distinct families of stimuli, namely classical (Cartesian) 2D gratings, and polar and hyperbolic (non-Cartesian) gratings. Within the latter two categories, which are dominant, cells in V4 display well-behaved tuning profiles to complex dimensions combining frequency and orientation. The "non-Cartesian" cells, the authors believe, may be regarded as primitives in highly complex representations of the visual world.

References

Beck, J. (1966). Perceptual grouping produced by changes in orientation and shape. *Science 154*, 538–540.

Bergen, J. R. (1991). Theories of visual texture perception. In D. Regan, (Ed.), *Spatial Vision* (pp. 114–139). New York: CRC Press.

Gorea, A., and Papathomas, T. V. (1993). Double-opponency as a generalized concept in texture segregation illustrated with stimuli defined by color, luminance and orientation. *J. Opt. Soc. Am. A 10*, 1450–1462.

Julesz, B. (1962). Visual pattern discrimination. *IRE Trans. Inform. Theory 8*, 84–92.

Sagi, D. (1991). Spatial filters in texture segmentation tasks. In B. Blum, (Ed.), *Channels in the Visual Nervous System: Neurophysiology, Psychophysics and Models* (pp. 397–424). Tel-Ariv: Freund Publishing House.

6

Some Speculations on the Role of Texture Processing in Visual Perception

Roger J. Watt

The perceptual phenomena of texture perception have been explored in great detail over the last few years. This exploration has, to a large extent, centered on two questions. The first is related to *what* textures we can discriminate from each other, generally by investigating what textures can be segregated "effortlessly" in a single image (Beck, 1982; Caelli, 1985; Hallett and Hofman, 1991; Julesz, 1981; Landy and Bergen, 1991; Nothdurft, 1985a, 1990, 1991; Sagi, 1990; Sagi and Julesz, 1987). Subsequent research has focused on *how* such textures are discriminated (Julesz, 1981), and an understanding of the mechanisms responsible for texture processing is emerging. Another main area of research in texture perception concerns the use of surface markings of various sorts to provide information from which surface orientation and shape can be deduced (Gibson, 1979; Beck, 1982; Julesz, 1981, 1986; Nothdurft, 1985b; Sagi and Julesz, 1987). This is generally achieved by examining the deformations that patches of texture undergo when the angle with which they are viewed changes—so-called texture gradients. The purpose of this chapter is to examine a different question about texture perception: not how it is done, but *why* it is a part of human visual perception. This question could, in a very strict sense, be regarded as the starting point for a theory of the computation of visible texture (Marr, 1982).

The question of why texture is a part of visual perception may seem like a gratuitous question to ask: all of our visual perceptual faculties have adaptive, survival value. The survival value of texture perception is more difficult to identify, as can be revealed by attempting to define texture.

An analogy with color perception can identify the difficulties in considering what a texture might be. Neglecting the role of the illuminant for these considerations (it is irrelevant for the analogy), we can say that

• A color is the psychological response of a visual system to the spectral characteristics of a surface.

• Different surfaces generally have different spectral characteristics, and these normally lead to the surfaces being perceived as having different colors.

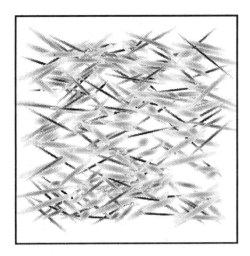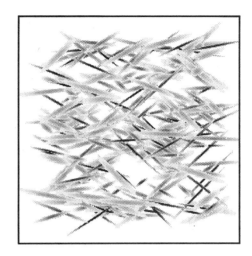

Figure 6.1
Two similar patches of texture. As textures, these are not distinguishable. They can, however, be distinguished by scrutiny. The sense in which the two stimuli are similar is the way in which they are seen as a texture.

• It is nevertheless, in principle, possible for two different surfaces with two different spectral characteristics to give rise to the same color response.

Likewise, we might say that

• A texture is the psychological response of a visual system to the spatial and structural characteristics of a surface.

• Different surfaces generally have different structural characteristics, and these normally lead to the surfaces being perceived as having different textures.

• It is nevertheless, in principle, possible for two different surfaces with two different structural characteristics to give rise to the same texture response.

The final point is where the analogy breaks down in its purest sense, because although it is probably true of texture, it is difficult to demonstrate. The basic fact of trichromacy is that two different surface characteristics can lead to the same color, the same perceptual effect. This can easily be demonstrated because the two surface characteristics can be silently substituted for each other without an observer noticing any change. This very strict criterion for equivalent perceptual effect cannot be applied to texture with the same force. When it is said that two patches of texture are indistinguishable, what is meant is that they are similar in a very particular way. They are not distinguishable without scrutiny, implying that they are similar only under one way of using the visual system.

An example of how two textures can be viewed in different ways with different consequences for their per-

ceived similarity is shown in figure 6.1. If the two images were placed together without any separating space, then the boundary between them would be invisible in both the sense that it could not be localized and also that its presence could not even be detected. In this sense they can be said to be similar textures. The two images are, however, different in the sense that one could not be substituted for the other without the process of substitution being visible. In this sense, they are different.

The starting point for a consideration of texture is the idea of similarity. This can be seen by noting that we only treat each image in figure 6.1 as a texture because each image is homogeneous—any one part of the image is similar to any other part. In very simplistic terms the textures are similar, and self-similar, because they are made up of a number of features, ellipsoids, drawn from a range of different sizes and orientations, and all positioned with few constraints. The features are individually similar, and their dispersion does not reliably create suprafeature patterns. For the present, this is a sufficient description of texture.

It is important to appreciate that this view of texture—namely, that it is a representation of a part of an image where the positioning of identifiable features does not matter and therefore has a homogeneous appearance—has a number of very awkward shortcomings. The most difficult one to deal with is the issue of spatial scale. The images in figure 6.1, for example, are clearly to our eyes homogeneous. This means that the distribution of blob parameters, such as length and orientation, is constant over the area of the texture. If we were to attempt to

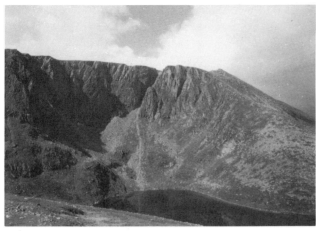

A

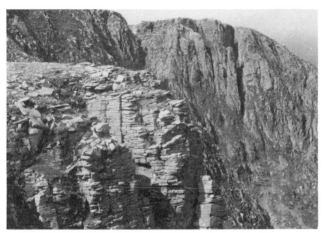

B

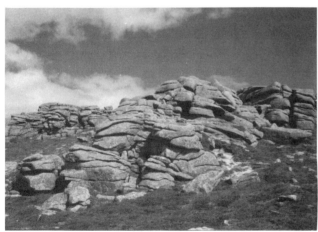

C

measure this, by computing the distribution of blob parameters locally at many different points in the image, we would discover that the extent to which the texture was homogeneous over the image depended on the size of the area around each point we chose to use in our calculations. The larger the area, the more homogeneous the texture would seem.

Examples of Texture Usage: A Walk

Imagine that you are coming along with me on a walk up into the rugged hills near my home. We will have to walk across very rough ground, choosing our own route around rocks, heather, and bog, while maintaining the general direction toward the goal. Such an expedition makes a number of very significant uses of visual perception, and in examining these we will be able to discover something of the role of texture in visual perception.

Three basic decision stages are involved in such a walk. We can illustrate these stages by representative images, as shown in figure 6.2.

- The first decision stage can be expressed as choosing a series of destinations, the main points on the walk. The first image (figure 6.2A) from the walk is a panoramic view of the hills that we wish to explore. Likely targets are the major landmarks such as promontories, ridges, corries, and rocky crags.

- The second decision stage is concerned with finding the routes that avoid "body-sized" obstacles, such as trees

Figure 6.2
The three images represent the three stages of visual decisions during a walk through rough country. Two points are illustrated: first, the decisions are made at a range of different scales, represented by the three images. At any one scale, two different types of information are required. Initially, (A) it is important to establish which parts of the landscape offer possibilities. This must be based on an appreciation of the local nature of the ground. Certain parts of the hillside are covered in wet bog, other parts are covered in loose stones, and only some parts are suitable for walking on. These parts are identified by examining the texture. Following from this, geometrically valid information about the direction of the route is needed. At the next stage (B) certain parts of the hillside will support a human body, and other parts will not. In this figure, much of what is seen is too vertical to be useful in this respect. The parts that are useful can be identified by examining the texture. The second type of information required concerns the spatial relationships between the parts of the hillside that are useful. At the third stage (C) of decision making on the walk, it is necessary to determine, from the accessible parts of the hillside, the track to be followed. The choices at this stage are determined by the nature of the ground and obstacles such as large boulders. Here the considerations are about the friction offered by the ground.

Table 6.1
Summary of the decision stages on the walk

Decision	Scale	Texture used for	Geometry used for
1	Journey (day)	Choosing goals for the day's walk	Planning the walk: how to link areas of easy ground
2	Body (2 hr)	Walking or scrambling?	How to get to the next area of easy ground
3	Foot (1 min)	Will my foot slip?	Step forward 0.75 m; turn right after 4 paces

and gullys. The second image (figure 6.2B) is a view of a specific hillside. This view shows some steep crags that must be avoided. It also shows a flat promontory that can be reached.

• The third decision stage is concerned with identifying ground that is suitable for stepping onto. The third image (figure 6.2C) is a view of a potential track to be followed. This image shows some large boulders that must be circumnavigated or climbed over.

Each of these images has some very characteristic and natural visible textures. With this example, the role of texture in visual processing will now be examined. A summary is given in table 6.1.

First Stage

As we set out, we are initially confronted with a view rather like that presented in figure 6.2A. The first task, on the basis of the visual information available in such an image, is to determine the general route. The decisions at this level are informed by the geometric layout of the features in the landscape, as represented in the image. Which parts of the image are cliffs, or loch, or scree slope can be identified by nature of the texture in different parts of the image. The differences in texture between the crags and the scree are clearly seen left of center in the image.

The visual processing of this image that is taking place offers several significant aspects for our purposes. We can imagine that a rough partition of the image into areas of homogeneous texture takes place. On the basis of the spatial characteristics of the texture within each area, the nature of the underlying land can be identified. This provides the raw material for the route selection decisions. Once this process has taken place, certain parts of the image can be given a more detailed scrutiny.

In making a judgment about the landscape, many of the details do not matter in a particular way. The response to the scree slope would not be changed, so far as route

decisions are concerned, by a rearrangement of the boulders. The scree slope is defined, for these purposes, by its general statistical properties, not its specific geometric details. This is a property of the decision, not a property of the physical object in the landscape. It also happens to correspond closely to the intuitive description of texture above.

Once a general decision about where the route should go has been made, the route has to be compiled into a sequence of moves. This sequence of moves requires spatial information. For example, a fine walk would be had by descending to the level of the base of the low crags on the left one-third of the way up from the loch to the ridge, by traversing over to the right side of the scree slope, and then making a way up through the deep gully and onto the ridge, leading to the summit at the far right end of the ridge. This description involves spatial relationships of two different types. There are qualitative relationships, such as "left of," "above," "descending." There are also quantitative relationships, such as "one-third of the way up."

The important point to note is that the visual description of the image that is implied by these considerations has a simple structure. The blocks of texture that are important have a characteristic size determined by the nature of the visual task. At the scale of this size and coarser, spatial information is required and must be represented; at finer scales than this, surface quality information, corresponding perhaps to visible texture, is required and must therefore be represented. In essence, there is a scale at which a discontinuity in the visual representation occurs, with spatial-relationships information being computed at coarser scales, and texture information being computed at finer scales. The scale itself is determined by the visual task, the decision to be made, and perhaps the nature of the image itself.

Second Stage

As progress is made along the route, a further sequence of decisions needs to be made. The (more detailed) route has to follow those parts of the hillside surface that are suitable for walking on. Generally this means that those parts of the hillside that have the right surface properties such as not being too wet, too crumbly, too steep are chosen. The conditions to be avoided are determined by the physical properties of the surface at physical spatial scales that are in correspondence with the size and structure of the human body.

The image shown in figure 6.2B contains a number of important features for decisions at this stage in the walk. Much of the image depicts hillside that is inaccessible.

This can be seen from the nature of the texture in the image. The prominent crag in the foreground has a texture that clearly indicates vertical hillside. The top of the crag has a different form of texture that clearly indicates horizontal hillside. The former is to be avoided, the latter to be walked on.

Once again, the visual processing that is occurring here has several significant features. First, the image is being split up into areas of homogeneous texture. These areas are then being analyzed to determine which offer safe ground for walking on. Then a route across the safe areas is planned. As before, the distinction occurs between the spatial-relationship information required for the route and the texture information required for the decisions about suitability for each part of the image.

As in the previous stage of decision making, there is a characteristic spatial scale at which a discontinuity exists between spatial representation and texture representation. The scale at which this split occurs is determined by the demands of the task, which at this level is itself determined by the size and structure of the human body.

Third Stage

Once a general route across safe ground has been selected, as described in the previous stage, then choices have to be made about leg- and foot-sized aspects of the route. The image shown in figure 6.2C illustrates this stage. Any route across the small section of hillside shown here would be feasible. However, only one route can be selected and so a decision has to be made. The decision will determine what type of walking will be required, as can be appreciated from the illustration where the choices are between scrambling and ordinary walking.

This is the stage where specific choices are made about where the foot is actually placed. While this does not generally require much visual processing (at least consciously) for walking over smooth and flat ground, for a walk of the type we have been considering it is a major preoccupation. The foot has to be placed on a piece of ground that will allow the foot to provide appropriate balance and thrust forces.

These forces will be produced effectively provided that the foot does not slip, which in turn requires that the area of contact between the foot and the ground match the friction offered by the ground. Vision therefore has to identify a place where a suitable area of the ground has the right friction. Visible texture will obviously provide a good (but not infallible) means of identifying the frictional nature of the ground.

Once again, there is a split in spatial scale between the two different types of processing, for spatial relationships

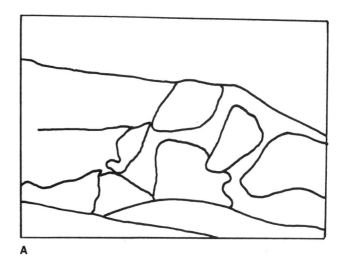

A

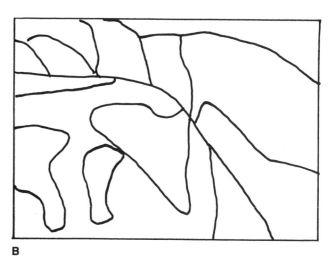

B

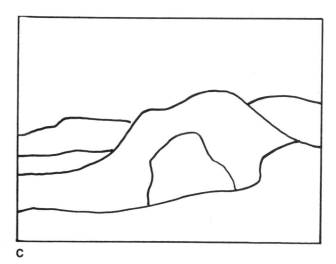

C

Figure 6.3
Sketches (A–C) of figure 6.2, which are intended to show the coarse-scale areas of texture. Within any one such area, geometric calculations are not needed, but between them, geometric calculations are required.

and for texture. Scales coarser than some critical value are processed to create representations of useful spatial relations, whereas finer scales contribute to a representation of surface texture characteristics (figure 6.3). In this case, the scale is determined by the size and structure of the leg and the foot.

Observations from the Walk

The purpose of describing the sequence of visually based decisions that are involved in a typical walk across rough ground was to illustrate the various functions that the visual representation of texture can serve. These will now be briefly listed. The most obvious uses are the following three:

• Image patches that correspond to different types of surface can be segregated.

• Surface orientation (especially horizontal versus vertical in the example) can be discriminated from the visible texture of the surface.

• Surface friction characteristics can be computed with some degree of certainty from visible texture.

There are some less obvious, and perhaps more important, functions that representations of visible texture are serving in the examples described above.

• Considering the number of discrete items that were involved in the reasoning about each image, the spatial relationships that need to be represented are kept relatively simple by assigning areas of the image to texture representation processes.

• The discussion above has implied that there exists, somehow and unexplained, a spatial scale at which an image can be split into useful pieces. It has been suggested that the actual scale at which this occurs will depend on both the visual task being undertaken and the actual image. The manner in which texture type representations can be used to discover this spatial scale will be described below.

These two latter uses of texture can be regarded as processing functions of texture. Processing functions make some other type of visual processing available, more efficient, or more suitable for the task in hand, but do not serve a perceptual end in their own right. These two processing functions will now be explored.

Spatial Relationships

The major proposition of this section of the chapter is that the computation of a full representation of spatial relationships within an image is potentially very time consuming, and is generally to be avoided. One function of texture is to provide a quick alternative form of representation that, while being less complete, is adequate for many purposes. A fuller version of the argument can be found in Watt (1988).

There are two temptations to be avoided in considering the computation of spatial relations within a biological visual system. It is tempting to assume that the location of each receptor within the visual field, and the location of each processing element thereafter, is given to the visual system. This is certainly the case in a machine vision system, where the computer-memory address of each pixel can be converted by a simple linear formula into the direction from which that pixel receives light information. Given this, the angular distance between any two image points can be calculated by using Euclidean geometry. To suppose that this might be the case for biological visual systems would be only an assumption and a rather unlikely one.

The second temptation to be avoided is the supposition that the actual function of spatial aspects of vision is to compute a representation of spatial locations (in the coordinate system of the two angular directions of the retinal image, or any other system). Certainly at the early stages of visual processing that are of interest in this chapter, such a representation is neither required nor desired. Much more useful at these stages of processing would be a representation that made explicit the distances and orientations between events in the image space.

A more reasonable assumption is that the visual system computes spatial relationships between a selected set of features in the image and that these features are then used as the basic information, the representational primitives, for further processes acting on the image. The set of features that is used needs to be a selected set, because the combinatorial demands posed by attempting to use a large set of features would be prohibitive. The number of distinct distances that would be needed to be represented is a rapidly accelerating function of the number of features ($n!$ for n features).

In fact it is possible to make some degree of simplification in the number of feature relations that must be calculated, if the relations are additive in some sense, so that given the distance and orientation of B from A, and of C from B, the relation of C to A can be calculated, if required. Provided that every feature entered into some relations, and that the relations encompassed the set, such a system of deferring a proportion of the calculations could be used to save time. This would save time only if the initial choices for calculating spatial relations were the most appropriate ones.

If the features are elements to which an orientation and a length can be applied, then even a representation of these feature attributes, while not making explicit the geometric structure of the image, will nonetheless be a representation that has certain spatial information. This form of representation, it is hypothesized, is the form of representation used for texture.

This argument applies to the complete set of some putative features. A full geometric representation can be calculated for such a set, but the time taken would be prohibitive. Instead, the calculation can be applied to a small subset of such features or to a small subset of the possible feature relations. Just which subset is the topic of the next section.

Texture and Attention

Implied in the considerations on the walk was a split between those (coarse) spatial scales at which the visual image is analyzed fully, and especially geometrically, and finer scales at which the visual image is analyzed in a different, texture-based manner. The utility of this split for the reduction in the resulting spatial relations is clearly very significant. However, such a utility would be very largely negated if the actual spatial scale used for the split were inappropriate.

Inspection of the illustrations from the walk could suggest that the same fixed spatial scale might be appropriate for finding the texture patches in all of them. This is, in part at least, an accident due to the preferences for composition that a photographer employs and the use of an optical zoom lens. However, a series of simple speculative calculations can be used to establish something like an universal range of patch sizes of interest.

The physical world, for the purposes of our walk, has a range of spatial scales that should be expressed in linear distance terms (meters). These scales will be called objective spatial scales. When projected into the plane of an image, these objective spatial scales become converted into image spatial scales. For a lens of fixed magnification, the appropriate measure of image spatial scales is linear visual angle. There then exists the familiar approximate linearity between objective spatial scale and image spatial scale, determined by the viewing distance.

The next footfall will be placed somewhere around 2 m away from the walker's eyes, and the relevant objective spatial scale might be 25 cm. The next obstacle to be avoided, in the sense of the third stage decision, will be somewhere around 8 m away, with a relevant objective spatial scale of around 1 m. The next landmark to be reached will be somewhere around 32 m away, with a relevant objective spatial scale of about 4 m. There may be a linear relation between the distance (and therefore optical projection size) and the objective scale of the relevant information. Within limits, this must be approximately the case, as can be deduced by taking the distances to extremes.

The implication of this linear relationship between distance and relevant objective spatial scale is interesting. If the relationship were a deterministic relationship, then the retinal scale at which spatial relationships should be calculated, and within which texture should be calculated, would have a fixed value. This precise state of affairs seems extremely unlikely, and at any one viewing distance, it is more likely that the range of retinal spatial scales of geometric interest might cover 1 order of magnitude or so. This line of reasoning is extremely reassuring, given that the range of objective scales for this walk (approx. 10 cm to 1 km) is about 4 orders of magnitude.

A range of an order of magnitude is a plausible account of the range of spatial scales actually processed by the human visual system (the bulk of the contrast sensitivity function, for example, lies within 1–10 c/deg and the spatial scales selected in the walk images corresponds roughly to about 3 c/deg). However, a range of a factor of 10 over potentially relevant spatial scale is far too wide to be usable. Details of the image and expectations about the image must be employed to select a narrower range. This, it is hypothesized, could be one very important role for visual attention.

Two general approaches can be distinguished of identifying which spatial scale should be used for the geometric information. The first is to start with a very coarse scale (at the extreme or near to it) and then to proceed through spatial scales, nesting each scale within its preceding one. This is explored in Watt (1988, 1990). A second, which will be considered here, is to use a particular version of the representation of texture to guide the selection of scale. In this case, the initial scale would need to be very coarse, but then, texture characteristics within that scale can be used to select which scales subsequently to use.

Suppose that any image, or part of an image, is given some form of analysis to discover the orientations and spatial scales of the structures that it contains. To be concrete, suppose that an image is filtered through a range of orientation and spatial scale selective filters, and that the resultant filtered images are parsed into a large set of zero-bounded blob regions. Each blob can be described as having an orientation, a length and a width (or an aspect ratio and a spatial scale), and a mass. This provides a set of descriptions from which we can determine how the mass is distributed across any of the parameters of the blob description. We can go one step further and for each value of aspect ratio, for example, determine a measure of its probability of occurrence in a normal diet of stimulation or its probability of occurrence on the null hypothesis that the image contains only noise. Either way it is then possible to identify which spatial scales contain the least likely distribution of structures. Clearly such scales are those that are likely to contain the most useful information and that might be the most suitable ones at which geometric representation would be desirable. This is explained in more detail in Watt (1991).

In this case, visual attention can be seen as being a process that regulates how a geometric representation of the image is created by determining, from information available in a texture representation, which spatial scales to use. The power of a texture representation to deliver sufficiently discriminative information to select between spatial scales will depend critically on the extent to which unusual structures occur and fail to occur in the texture representation. At this time, this is an open question, although the distribution of response values in a filtered image will certainly not adequately discriminate between spatial scales. The distributions of orientations and aspect ratios might be sufficiently sensitive to be suitable.

Conclusions: A Vision of Texture Vision

The concept of texture processing in the human visual system that emerges from these considerations has a number of significant features. The discussion of the walk highlighted direct functions of texture, where the visible texture of a surface is presumed to be a measure of the physical properties of the surface. It also revealed the need for the more generally understood indirect functions of texture, when, for example, the orientation of a surface is judged from the variations in the texture in the optical image of that surface. Neither of these functions is particularly surprising.

The speculation that texture may serve two interrelated processing functions is somewhat novel. The first of these functions is that texture may serve as a mechanism for representing certain types of (useful) spatial information, without the need to undertake time-consuming (and possibly unnecessary) geometric computations. The second function is that it may be used to provide the necessary information to indicate which spatial scale should be used for calculations of geometric relations between features. The key to how successful such a system would be lies in the nature of the features and feature attributes that are used to calculate the texture. For the first function, the more sophisticated the features and feature attributes, the more there will be of implicit geometric information. For the second function, a balance is required between having feature attributes that are too simple to reveal anything unexpected, and having feature attributes that are too complex and will always be revealed as unexpected. In the limit, if the feature were the entire image, then every image is equally unexpected in the sense that it will not have occurred before. Just where this limit might lie is an open question.

Acknowledgments

The work described in this paper was supported by a grant from the Science and Engineering Council (GR/H53181). I acknowledge my gratitude to Ben Craven and Ben Cruachan, on whom the arguments of this chapter were first tried out. I would also like to acknowledge the continued interest that Bela Julesz has shown in this work—this has been the main encouragement for writing this highly speculative chapter. The Scottish mountain used for the walk is known as Lochnagar.

References

Beck, J. (1982). Textural segmentation. In J. Beck (Ed.), *Organization and Representation in Perception.* Hillsdale, NJ: Lawrence Erlbaum.

Caelli, T. (1985). Three processing characteristics of visual texture segmentation. *Spatial Vision 1,* 19–30.

Gibson, J. J. (1979). *The Ecological Approach to Visual Perception.* Boston: Houghton-Mifflin.

Hallett, P. E., and Hofman, M. I. (1991). Segregation of some mesh-derived textures evaluated by free-viewing. *Vision Res. 31,* 1701–1719.

Julesz, B. (1981). Textons, the elements of texture perception and their interactions. *Nature (London) 290,* 91–97.

Julesz, B. (1986). Texton gradients. The texton theory revisited. *Biolog. Cybern. 54,* 245–251.

Landy, M. S., and Bergen, J. R. 1991. Texture segregation and orientation gradient. *Vision Res. 31,* 679–691.

Marr, D. C. (1982) *Vision.* San Francisco: Freeman.

Nothdurft, H.-C. (1985a). Orientation sensitivity and texture segmentation in patterns with different line orientations. *Vision Res. 25,* 551–560.

Nothdurft, H.-C. (1985b). Sensitivity for structure gradient in texture discrimination tasks. *Vision Res. 25,* 1957–1968.

Nothdurft, H.-C. (1990). Texture segregation by associated differences in global and local luminance distribution. *Proc. R. Soc. London B 239,* 295–320.

Nothdurft, H.-C. (1991). Texture segmentation and pop-out from orientation contrast. *Vision Res. 31,* 1073–1078.

Sagi, D. (1990). Detection of an orientation singularity in Gabor textures: Effect of signal density and spatial frequency. *Vision Res. 30,* 1377–1388.

Sagi, D., and Julesz, B. (1987). Short range limitations on detection of feature differences. *Spatial Vision 2, 39–49.*

Watt, R. J. (1988). *Visual Processing: Computational, Psychophysical and Cognitive Research.* Hillsdale, NJ: Lawrence Erlbaum.

Watt, R. J. (1990). Visual analysis and the representation of spatial relations. *Mind Lang. 5,* 267–288.

Watt, R. J. (1991). *Understanding Vision.* London: Academic Press.

7

The Psychophysics of Texture Segmentation

Dov Sagi

Texture segmentation involves breaking an image into different regions having some internal regularities. The first attempt to understand perceptual processes involved in texture segmentation was made by Julesz (1962), who also constrained the problem to early vision. Technically, this was made possible by using meaningless high-contrast random-dot patterns, exposed briefly (for less then 160 msec and followed by visual noise) so as to avoid eye movements. It is assumed that shortening stimulus duration does not affect acuity so much as it avoids high-level (top-down) processes having a high degree of complexity. Experimental results show that human observers can locate some texture boundaries within this brief presentation time even when visual attention is not available for the task (Braun and Sagi, 1990). Most experiments involving textures were designed to find the differences that make textures discriminable, or their boundary (when put next to each other) detectable. Theories of texture perception differ in the similarity measure they adopt to predict discrimination. Since textures can be only statistically defined (within a given area), the task of texture border localization imposes contradicting demands on the mechanisms involved, and probably involves processes operating on different scales. Different scientific approaches to human texture segmentation differ in the scale they adopt for the problem. Early texture models attempted to define global texture properties that would enable discrimination between two given textures. Julesz (1962) defined the problem in statistical terms, thus using global concepts to account for human performance. Only later, after discovering the limitations of global accounts (Julesz, 1980), along with the introduction of local geometric features into the texture process (Beck, 1982; Caelli and Julesz, 1978; Julesz, 1981), was the emphasis shifted to local processes. However, these local "feature" or "texton" detectors were assumed to be followed by a global process, which computes their global statistics (Julesz, 1981; Treisman, 1985). Global statistics can be useful for texture discrimination; however, segmentation requires border localization and thus some recovery of the lost location information by a top-down, probably attentive, process. As texture segmentation and boundary localization seem to be carried out without visual attention (Braun and Sagi, 1990) and without any detailed "feature" processing (Sagi and Julesz, 1985; Nothdurft, 1993), models assuming global statistics of local features should be rejected. Later theories assumed a local "textural gradient" detection stage, thus avoiding global processes (Beck, 1982; Nothdurft, 1985a,b; Sagi and Julesz, 1985, 1987), or transferring it to the final decision stage (Rubenstein and Sagi, 1990) and keeping a simple feedforward design. These recent theories of texture segmentation assume a few processing stages that are not strictly local. The different processing stages involve integration over different spatial extents, with the range of interaction increasing hierarchically.

A Theory of Texture Segmentation

Here we assume two filtering stages with a nonlinearity in between (Bergen and Adelson, 1988; Fogel and Sagi, 1989; Landy and Bergen, 1991; Malik and Perona, 1990; Rubenstein and Sagi, 1990; Sutter et al., 1989). At the first filtering stage the classic spatial filters (Daugman, 1980; Wilson and Bergen, 1979) are being used. Second-stage filters are defined as linear spatial filters and in most implementations are assumed to perform isotropic local bandpass filtering on a scale somewhat larger than that of first stage filters. Using well-defined linear filters as major ingredients makes the analysis of these models simpler and allows for quantitative predictions. These models can be designed to account for human performance on psychophysical tasks. I emphasize the psychophysical task since it plays a major role in the success of any model and it is being ignored in most models. Modeling the psychophysical task was made possible by the availability of a large amount of psychophysical data from four-alternative-forced-choice (4AFC) experiments carried out by Gurnsey and Browse (1987). Rubenstein and Sagi (1990) added a simple decision stage to the two filtering stages in an attempt to model the 4AFC task and to derive percentage of correct response as model prediction. Their model assumes four processing stages (figure 7.1):

1. *Filtering*: The input image is being filtered by localized spatial-frequency and orientation-selective filters like Gabor filters. A pointwise nonlinear operation is being applied at the filters' outputs. Possible nonlinearities may include squaring of filter output to provide an energy measure (Turner, 1986; Fogel and Sagi, 1989), a compressive nonlinearity (Caelli, 1985), or both (Rubenstein and Sagi, 1990). The output of this stage consists of a large number of filtered images (maps).

2. *Gradient detection*: Each filter map is being filtered again using a low resolution isotropic bandpass filter. A classical center-surround (DOG) filter can be used here. This second stage of filtering can be viewed as a two-stage process: energy integration across space (averaging), resulting in a "texture energy" measure, followed by a gradient detection (local inhibition). This filtering operation results in enhanced activity in locations where local filter energy changes.

3. *Combination stage*: All filter maps are combined into one master map where gradients from all maps are represented. The combination process may not necessarily imply summing up responses across maps, however, it does imply the loss of identity or label of individual maps.

4. *Decision stage*: Given the responses generated by the previous combination stage, a decision has to be reached in order to fulfill the psychophysical task.

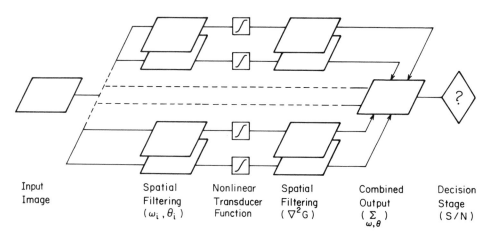

Figure 7.1
A model for texture segmentation. See text for description.

All model processing stages are based on current knowledge of the visual system; however, the application of this knowledge to problems involving texture discrimination and search is controversial.

The First Filtering Stage

The first stage consisting of spatial filters is being objected by popular feature-based theories (Julesz, 1990; Treisman and Gelade, 1980). In addition, data from search experiments support the notion that orientation and spatial frequency are processed separately and can be conjoined only by attentive processes (Walters et al., 1983), while our model predicts a conjoined processing of both dimensions. However, these experiments were using the Treisman and Gelade (1980) search paradigm where nontarget elements are of two types, thus producing irrelevant feature gradients in the background. This would confuse the decision-making stage since it relies on gradient information only and not on filter label. Sagi (1988), using a modified stimulus without background gradients, showed that the conjunction of orientation and spatial frequency can be effortlessly detected.

The Second Stage of Filtering

Evidence for a second stage of filtering comes from experiments concerning the perceived contrast of suprathreshold patterns (Cannon and Fullenkamp, 1991; Chubb et al., 1989; Sagi and Hochstein, 1985) and the detection of low-contrast targets in the presence of spatially displaced masks (Polat and Sagi, 1993). This stage can be viewed as consisting of local inhibitory connections between adjacent spatial filters having similar properties. These connections are assumed to operate above filter threshold only and their spatial range scales with filter size so that they connect filters separated by a distance of at most six times their typical wavelength (Polat and Sagi, 1993; Sagi, 1990). Polat and Sagi (1994a) also showed that second stage interactions are not isotropic but rather concentrated along the first stage filter orientation and a direction orthogonal to it. Note that at this stage only filters having similar properties are connected to each other, thus gradients are measured for each filter type separately. It is still possible that filters with different properties interact. Rubenstein and Sagi (1993), using periodic Gabor textures, found some evidence for nonisotropic excitatory interactions between filters having orthogonal orientations. These interactions seem to extend over a range somewhat larger than the in-between-same-type excitatory interactions. Interactions between spatially adjacent filters of different orientations can contribute to the detection of orientation gradients and are consistent with the experimental results of Nothdurft (1985a,b, 1991, 1993). In the model described here in-between-different-type filter interactions are not assumed.

The Combination Stage

The end product of the second filtering stage (stage 2 above) consists of many filter gradient maps, each indicating local energy changes within a specific spatial frequency and orientation band. This representation contains labeling of both the locations and the identity (the specific band) of gradients. To account for the insensitivity of the texture segmentation process for feature identity (Sagi and Julesz, 1985) we have to collapse all maps into a single master map where each location signals a combined local gradient value. Experimental evidence supporting the existence of a master map comes also from studies showing interference in tasks involving two or more maps (Nothdurft, 1993; Pashler, 1988; Sagi, 1991; Wertheim, 1981). This end product has properties similar to that of a feature gradient map, although without performing local comparisons between detectors having different feature values (there is no direct measurement of local orientation differences). The saliency map suggested by Koch and Ullman (1985) represents a similar concept.

The Decision Stage

Finally, we need a decision stage in order to generate a response, a stage that is a necessity in all psychophysical models. This stage is task dependent and has access to the combined map only. Detection of a texture target can be carried out by looking for above threshold activity in the combined map; localization of a texture target can be performed by looking for the location having highest activity (strongest gradient). This stage is the only stage having access to all locations in the visual field and thus has the ability to perform global computations. These computations may involve assigning different weights to different locations according to the statistical reliability of the activity at the different locations. However, since filter labels (orientation and spatial frequency) are lost in the previous stage, there is no way to differentially weight different filter maps (Sagi, 1991).

Theory Prediction and Experimental Data

The success of the model can be judged according to its ability to predict human performance on texture discrimination tasks. We claim that linear filters with the nonlinearities introduced in stages 1 and 4 can replace the geometric feature detectors suggested before (Caelli and Julesz, 1978) to account for the discriminability of iso-second-order statistics textures. Turner (1986) showed that some texture pairs having the same second-order statistics, and hence power spectra, may produce filter responses (Gabor energy) with different first-order statistics. Fogel and Sagi (1989) used the Gabor energy measure to compute filter response differences between target and background elements in search tasks. Calculations based on this energy measure were applied to stimuli used by Kröse (1987) and were compared with Kröse's experimental data yielding an excellent correlation. However, among the 12 target-background pairs tested one was found to be an exception; the model predicted no discrimination while psychophysically the pair was discriminable. This pair, consisting of triangular and arrow-shaped elements (figure 7.2), was shown to generate texture pairs having iso-dipole statistics (Caelli and Julesz, 1978) and, as can be appreciated from the energy curves in figure 7.2, have the same energy only when energy *is averaged across all orientations*. The failure of the Fogel and Sagi (1989) computations to account for this specific iso-dipole case resulted from the use of global energy averages; since orientation was randomized across space in the Kröse (1987) experiments, energy was averaged across all orientations without taking into account local energy variations. Once local energy variations are considered, one can base detection on the observation that the target energy differs from its neighboring elements' energy in most occasions. Thus local energy differences can contribute to the detection process. However, once gradients are considered one may expect false gradients to occur between adjacent background elements, forcing us to use a decision rule that separates signal from noise.

Rubenstein and Sagi (1990) analyzed the statistical distribution of local energy gradients in connection with the signal detection problem posed by the psychophysical task. In particular, they modeled the four-alternative-forced-choice task used by Gurnsey and Browse (1987). In this task the observer had to indicate the display quadrant in which the foreground texture was most likely to appear. Gurnsey and Browse (1987) tested 18 texture pairs in psychophysical experiments, taking every pair twice by using each pair member as foreground element and background element in turn (totaling 36 cases). Most importantly, they found that exchanging pair members between foreground and background can have a dramatic effect on psychophysical performance. Since this exchange does not affect the energy difference at the foreground-background border, this finding may be taken as evidence against any spatial gradient-based model, in-

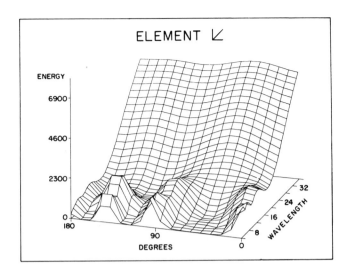

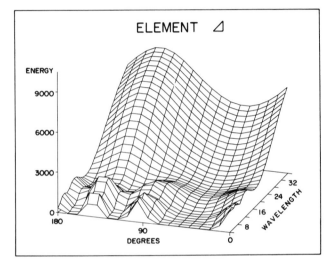

Figure 7.2
Gabor energy distribution of two texture elements used by Caelli and Julesz (1978) to demonstrate effortless discrimination of textures having identical power spectra. Gabor energies were computed using pairs (sine and cosine) of Gabor signals of different orientations and wavelength, and texture elements of size 17 × 17 (as in Rubenstein and Sagi 1990). Note that the two elements differ in the way energy is distributed across the different orientations (at longer wavelength). Only when energies are averaged across all orientations (or space when in textures) are elements' energies equal at all wavelengths.

cluding ours. However, as noted above, energy differences at the foreground-background border have to be considered in respect to energy differences existing in the background (the signal detection problem), thus performance should depend on background properties allowing for the foreground-background symmetry to be broken. Rubenstein and Sagi (1990) found that the most important source for background variability is the orientation randomization employed in most texture experiments. Using Gabor energy distributions across orientation at

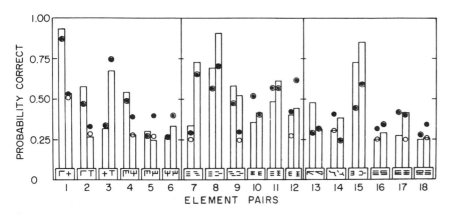

Figure 7.3
The predictions of the Rubenstein and Sagi (1990) model (circles) compared with the experimental data (histogram bars) of Gurnsey and Browse (1987). The figure (from Rubenstein and Sagi, 1990) is presented in groups of two elements, representing a particular stimulus. Each histogram rectangle represents the psychophysical performance level with the element depicted below it in the foreground and the adjacent element in the background. Filled circles represent the predic-tion obtained by selecting the spatial frequency yielding the highest performance for each pair ($r = 0.8$). The open circles represent predictions for Gabor filters having only larger wavelength ($r = 0.83$). The model accounts for performance asymmetries whenever they are significant. Note that pair 13 is an elongated version of the pair depicted here in figure 7.2, thus producing lower performance levels; however, experimental asymmetry seems to exist.

different spatial frequencies, they were able to model the Gurnsey and Browse (1987) findings (figure 7.3). The computations of this model rely heavily on the conjoined dependence of filter response on spatial frequency and orientation. What is relevant for discrimination is the low-frequency part of the energy spectra where filter wavelength is approximately equal to texture element size. At this wavelength different elements have different energy distribution across the orientation spectra, and in most cases these distributions have different averages. Figure 7.2 shows a case where the average energies across orientations are equal but the energy variance is different; thus the element having a flat energy curve will create a uniform background while the other one will create a noisy background (when randomly oriented). Since most textures used by Gurnsey and Browse (1987) are best discriminated by the same range of spatial frequencies the model predictions are not very sensitive to the assumptions made on the combination map (processing stage 3). While the Rubenstein and Sagi (1990) analysis considers the signal-in-noise problem within a single map (both signal and noise are in the same filter map), the combination stage predicts that detection is affected by noise in other maps. Recent experimental results indicate also the existence of intermap interactions (Rubenstein and Sagi, 1993).

Something is Still Missing

While the histograms depicted in figure 7.3 show a nice qualitative fit between theory and data, some critical problems are still left open. Asymmetry in performance exists also in cases where texture elements orientation is not randomized. For example, consider the detection of tilted line segments (foreground) in a background of vertical line segments; here, an exchange of the foreground and background elements produces a decreased performance level (Treisman and Gormican, 1988; Foster and Ward, 1991). Size-based texture segmentation shows also an asymmetric performance, with the larger texture elements being more salient (Gurnsey and Browse, 1989). Texture targets generated from open forms (broken circles, arrows as in figure 7.2) are easier to detect when coupled with closed forms (circles and triangles, respectively) (Treisman and Gormican, 1988; Williams and Julesz, 1992). The existing two-stage-filtering models can account for discrimination in these cases but not for asymmetries. The signal-in-noise framework allows for asymmetries even when no external noise is introduced into the system (e.g., orientation variability) by assuming internal noise that depends on the specific input. Thus, vertical lines may generate less internal noise than tilted lines as would be expected from their finer internal representation, and large texture elements may produce more noise than small ones (it is also possible that low-frequency filters are noisier than high-frequency filters). In the same way, broken shapes may be expected to generate more internal noise than closed ones. As for now, this assumption is not supported by independent experimental evidence. More than that, consider the triangle-arrow pair depicted in figure 7.3 that produces asymmetric performance with an advantage for the arrows in the foreground. This asymmetry holds with or without orientation randomization (Rubenstein, 1994), while orientation variability would predict an advantage for triangles when in the foreground (see in figure 7.2 where the triangle energy spectrum is more variable along the orientation dimension). Thus, if internal noise is the source of asymmetry in these cases, it should be powerful enough to override the noise resulting from the orientation variability. Williams and Julesz (1992) suggested, when using closed circles and open circles as texture elements, that broken forms tend to be closed by "subjective contours." This "subjective closure" would be more distractive when operating on open circles in the background due to their higher frequency of occurrence (background area is assumed to be larger than foreground area). While this account for closed/opened form asymmetry is very attractive, it is difficult to see how it can be applied to the general case, in particular to shapes like arrows (figure 7.2).

One interesting aspect of the Williams and Julesz (1992) data is that the same asymmetry exists for stimuli consisting of only two elements, pointing toward a nontexture type of asymmetry, or for some attentive sources. Attention may also be involved in orientation- (and size-) based asymmetries, as these asymmetries occur only for small orientation differences (Sagi and Julesz, 1987) and thus can be viewed as a threshold phenomenon. As most texture experiments described in the literature do not monitor observers' attention, it is possible that visual attention plays an important role when texture pairs differ by a small change on one parameter (orientation, size, or gap length). Braun (1993) showed, using a dual task paradigm, that detection of a small target within an array of somewhat larger distractors depends on the availability of attentive resources, while the reversed task can be performed without attention. Using a similar paradigm, Rubenstein (1994) could demonstrate the involvement of attention in gap/closure-based segmentation tasks, but not in triangle/arrow-based texture segmentation tasks. Sireteanu and Rettenbach (1993) showed, using reaction time experiments, that orientation-based asymmetries and closure-based asymmetries disappear with practice, when keeping the orientation difference (or gap size) constant. It would be interesting to see how practice improves performance on orientation, size, and gap (closure)-based segmentation and to examine the correlation between discrimination thresholds and asymmetry.

While second-stage filters proved to be very useful in modeling the segmentation process, there is no clear evidence supporting a specific or a unique filter type. The default structure assumes an isotropic DOG (summation and inhibition) type spatial filter operating on first stage filter maps (Malik and Perona, 1990; Rubenstein and Sagi, 1990); however, there is no direct psychophysical evidence to support this filter type. Contrast detection experiments support nonisotropic second-stage filters where integration of first stage-filter activity is performed along the first-stage filter principal orientation and, to a somewhat lesser extent, in a direction orthogonal to it (Polat and Sagi, 1994a). Data from these contrast detection experiments can be modeled by assuming either excitatory or inhibitory interactions (or both), though later experiments (Polat and Sagi, 1994b) favor excitatory interactions. Texture segmentation experiments suggest summation along the first-stage filter principal orientation, in addition to sideway excitatory interactions with orthogonal filters (Rubenstein and Sagi, 1993). Some models (Landy and Bergen, 1991; Malik and Perona, 1990) assume both within-map inhibition and between-maps inhibition, though in these models the intermap inhibition can be replaced by some nonlinear transducer function. It is certainly possible that the visual system employs different types of second-stage filters and that first-stage filters may interact in different, not necessarily simple, ways. It is also possible that these interactions have some adaptive properties and change according to the task and stimulus type.

Perceptual Learning in Preattentive Vision

Surprisingly enough, although practice effects are generally known, little research has been published on learning effects in simple visual tasks (Ball and Sekuler, 1982; Fiorentini and Berardi, 1980; Ramachandran and Braddick, 1973). Fiorentini and Berardi (1980) describe practice effects in tasks involving phase discrimination. They found learning to be specific for orientation, spatial frequency, and location (hemifields), implying a low-level site for the neuronal changes; however, this learning effect showed interocular transfer, implying neural modifications at a processing level where the information originating from the two eyes is already combined. Karni and Sagi (1991) examined performance improvement for a task involving detection of texture gradients. The task involves either detection of three disparate lines (differing in orientation from the background) or identification of the global orientation created by these three lines (being vertical or horizontal). These tasks were shown to be preattentive or inattentive in the sense that they do not rely on any attentive resources (Braun and Sagi, 1990). In such an experiment the target appears in a random location so that observers are forced to collect information from a relatively large visual field. On the other hand, the relevant information is local in the sense that observers have to detect orientation gradients. Also note that although an identification task is being used, the task does not involve pattern identification (of local elements) but rather an identification of a structure defined by feature gradients that, in turn, is the limiting factor in the task. This situation is quite different from the one in the learning studies described above, in which observers were presented with spatially uniform stimuli where any part of the visual field can be used for the task. This procedure allows for attention to be focused, directed, and to be used. Our situation can be better described as a task where observers have to detect a small signal of an unknown location within a larger field of noise.

The main finding of Karni and Sagi (1991) is that learning is specific for

1. Location in the visual field. Learning does not transfer from one quadrant to another.

2. Background orientation but not target orientation. Once observers have learned one target orientation, they can perform as well for the orthogonal orientation. This is not true for background orientation.

3. Eye. Learning does not transfer between eyes.

The above properties of the learning phenomena imply that learning takes place at an early stage of visual processing, at a level similar to that of spatial filters or of their lateral interactions. The structure that is being modified is local, has orientation specificity, and is monocular. These constraints do not leave us much choice in identifying the physiological correlate to the modified structure. Monocular and orientation-selective cells have been found so far only in some layers of visual area V1 (Zeki, 1978). More so, cells at this level of processing were also found to be sensitive to orientation gradients as implied by our task (Van Essen et al., 1989; Gallant et al., this volume). Though the actual changes occur at the preattentive level of processing, they are probably gated (Karni and Sagi, 1991) or controlled (Ahissar and Hochstein, 1993; also this volume) by some task-dependent process, or by cognitive set (Shiu and Pashler, 1992).

Another interesting feature of the texture learning data is the time course of learning (Karni and Sagi, 1993). The results show improvement over a time period of 4 to 5 days, although our observers performed a few hundred trials on each daily session. This is quite a slow time course compared with the earlier studies mentioned above. However, once observers learned the task they could maintain their improved level of performance for at least 3 years without further practice. Even more interesting is the observation (Karni and Sagi, 1993) that observers do not improve much during each daily session and up to 8 hours after a training session (except for a fast phase of learning at the beginning of their training, which is local but shows interocular transfer). This implies some incubation period in which changes induced by the repetitive performance of the task take place. During this period of 8 hours, the observers were not doing any activity related to the psychophysical task; however, in most cases the time interval between two sessions included night sleep. In later experiments, observers were tested in the evening, before sleep, and then again in the morning after sleep. Experimental results show that observers do not significantly improve performance of the task if deprived of REM (dream) sleep, whereas deprivation of other sleep stages (slow wave sleep) only minimally affects consolidation (Karni et al., 1994). It should be noted that REM deprivation affects performance only for tasks that are being learned (or being consolidated), while tasks that are already learned are not affected by sleep deprivation. This recent result may contribute to our understanding of the biological mechanisms involved in memory consolidation.

We suspect that the learning phenomena we observed involve modification at the filter level or at a level where adjacent filters interact (second-stage filters). Modifications at the lateral interaction level can increase inhibition between adjacent filters and thus reduce the response level for the background, and noise in general. This increased inhibition is also consistent with the general principle of "redundancy reduction" where the sensory system tries to ignore redundant information (Barlow, 1990). Evidence for plasticity at the level of filter interactions (connections) is provided by lateral masking experiments.

Plasticity of Lateral Interactions

While texture experiments can be considered as the "royal road" to understanding preattentive pattern discrimination, a finer method is required for exploring detailed neuronal interactions. Polat and Sagi (1993) used a lateral masking paradigm to explore spatial interactions. In these experiments observers had to detect the presence of a Gabor target when flanked by two high-contrast Gabor patches (masks) at variable separations. Results showed a decrease of target sensitivity at small target to mask separations, and an increase of target sensitivity at larger separations, up to six times the target wavelength. In later experiments, we allowed observers to practice on the lateral masking experiments for a few weeks. The effect of practice is strikingly uniform across observers; all of them increased their enhancement range, up to 20 times the target wavelength, practically showing interactions on all distances tested (Polat and Sagi, 1994b). This learning phenomenon was also found to be monocular; that is, practicing with one eye did not generate any range increase for the other eye. In addition, the range increase was found to be specific for spatial frequency and orientation. Thus, it is reasonable to assume that the increase in interaction range, as observed in our lateral masking experiments, occurs at the same level of processing as texture learning, probably at a level corresponding to visual area V1.

The long-range interactions obtained after a few weeks of practice may imply the existence of long-range connections in the cortex. However, this is probably not the case. The data can be better explained by assuming a chain of connections, where activity from distal regions can spread through intermediate cells to the target cell. This chain can be developed only continuously, that is, longer range interactions cannot be developed before intermediate range interactions take place (Polat and Sagi, 1994b). Moreover, the chain can be broken by repetitive stimulation of an intermediate region. This implies that neighboring elements in the chain must be activated during the same period of practice in order to develop their connections, while activation of only one of them, without the other, may reduce the connection efficacy. Thus we can induce new associations by introducing correlations between the Gabor masks and dissociations by breaking these correlations. In light of these findings we should view preattentive vision as an associative feedback network, rather than as a feedforward system capable of increasing sensitivity due to repetitive stimulation.

Conclusion

Thirty years after the pioneering study of Julesz (1962) we seem to have reached a good understanding of processes underlying human texture perception. As we enter the fourth decade of texture research, we will probably see more quantitative models of texture segmentation, producing a better understanding of texture perception and of the architecture underlying preattentive visual processes. But probably the most unexpected outcome of this research is the recent finding that preattentive vision is not a rigid sensory module. The picture emerging from the studies described here is of a dynamic visual system in which early representations keep changing as the environment changes. The high degree of plasticity we

observed raises the possibility that almost any pattern of spatial interactions can be obtained in early vision by direct or indirect connections. Global shape properties, as closure and figure/ground assignment, may be captured by this system via chains of connections, as indicated by the recent findings of Kovács and Julesz (1993). Reaching an understanding of the visual system and of texture perception will therefore involve understanding the learning rules of the system and the constraints put on it by the system architecture. As these learning rules are expected to apply to brain processes in general, we can view the study of texture discrimination as the royal road to understanding, not only preattentive pattern discrimination, but cognitive processes in general.

References

Ahissar, M., and Hochstein, S. (1993). Attentional control of early perceptual learning. *Proc. Natl. Acad. Sci. U.S.A. 90,* 5718–5722.

Ball, K., and Sekuler, R. (1982). A specific and enduring improvement in visual motion discrimination. *Science 218,* 697–698.

Barlow, H. B. (1990). Conditions for versatile learning, Helmholtz's unconscious inference, and the task of perception. *Vision Res. 30,* 1561–1571.

Beck, J. (1982). Textural segmentation. In J. Beck (Ed.), *Organization and Representation in Perception* (pp. 285–317). Hillsdale, NJ: Erlbaum.

Bergen, J. R., and Adelson, E. H. (1988). Early vision and texture perception. *Nature (London) 333,* 363–364.

Braun, J. (1994). Visual search among items of different salience: Removal of visual attention mimics a lesion in extrastriate area V4. *J. Neurosci. 14,* 554–567.

Braun, J., and Sagi, D. (1990). Vision outside the focus of attention. *Percept. Psychophys. 48,* 45–48.

Caelli, T. M. (1985). Three processing characteristics of visual texture segmentation. *Spatial Vision 1,* 19–30.

Caelli, T., and Julesz, B. (1978). On perceptual analyzers underlying visual texture discrimination: Part I. *Biol. Cybern. 28,* 167–175.

Cannon, M. W., and Fullenkamp, S. C. (1991). Spatial interactions in apparent contrast: Inhibitory effects among grating patterns of different spatial frequencies, spatial positions and orientation. *Vision Res. 31,* 1985–1998.

Chubb, C., Sperling, G., and Solomon, J. A. (1989). Texture interactions determine perceived contrast. *Proc. Natl. Acad. Sci. U.S.A. 86,* 9631–9635.

Daugman, J. D. (1980). Two dimensional spectral analysis of cortical receptive field profiles. *Vision Res. 20,* 847–856.

Fiorentini, A., and Berardi, N. (1980). Perceptual learning specific for orientation and spatial frequency. *Nature (London) 287,* 43–44.

Fogel, I., and Sagi, D. (1989). Gabor filters as texture discriminator. *Biol. Cybern. 61,* 103–113.

Foster, D. H., and Ward, P. A. (1991). Asymmetries in oriented-line detection indicate two orthogonal filters in early vision. *Proc. R. Soc. London B 243*, 75–81.

Gurnsey, R., and Browse, R. A. (1987). Micropattern properties and presentation condition influencing visual texture discrimination. *Percept. Psychophys. 41*, 239–252.

Gurnsey, R., and Browse, R. A. (1989). Asymmetries in visual texture discrimination. *Spatial Vision 4*, 31–44.

Julesz, B. (1962). Visual pattern discrimination. *IRE Transact. Inform. Theory IT-8*, 84–92.

Julesz, B. (1980). Spatial nonlinearities in the instantaneous perception of textures with identical power spectra. *Phil. Transact. R. Soc. London B 290*, 83–94.

Julesz, B. (1981). Textons, the elements of texture perception and their interactions. *Nature (London) 290*, 91–97.

Julesz, B. (1990). AI and early vision. In R. Blake and T. Troscianko (Eds.) *AI and the Eye* (pp. 9–20). New York: Wiley.

Karni, A., and Sagi, D. (1991). Where practice makes perfect in texture discrimination—evidence for primary visual cortex plasticity. *Proc. Natl. Acad. Sci. U.S.A. 88*, 4966–4970.

Karni, A., and Sagi, D. (1993). The time course of learning a visual skill. *Nature (London) 365*, 250–252.

Karni, A., Tanne, D., Rubenstein, B. S., Askenasi, J. J. M., and Sagi, D. (1994). Overnight improvement of a perceptual skill is critically dependent on REM sleep. *Science*, in press.

Koch, C., and Ullman, S. (1985). Shifts in visual attention: Towards the underlying neural circuitry. *Hum. Neurobiol. 4*, 219–227.

Kovács, I., and Julesz, B. (1993). A closed curve is much more than an incomplete one: Effect of closure in figure-ground segmentation. *Proc. Natl. Acad. Sci. U.S.A. 90*, 7495–7497.

Kröse, B. J. A. (1987). Local structure analyzers as determinants of preattentive pattern discrimination. *Biol. Cybern. 55*, 289–298.

Landy, S. L., and Bergen, J. R. (1991). Texture segregation and orientation gradient. *Vision Res. 31*, 679–691.

Malik, J., and Perona, P. (1990). Preattentive texture discrimination with early vision mechanisms. *J. Opt. Soc. Am. A7*, 923–932.

Nothdurft, H. C. (1985a). Orientation sensitivity and texture segmentation in patterns with different line orientation. *Vision Res. 25*, 551–560.

Nothdurft, H. C. (1985b). Sensitivity for structure gradients in texture discrimination tasks. *Vision Res. 25*, 1957–1968.

Nothdurft, H. C. (1991). Texture segmentation and pop-out from orientation contrast. *Vision Res. 31*, 1073–1078.

Nothdurft, H. C. (1993). Saliency effects across dimensions in visual search. *Vision Res. 33*, 839–844.

Pashler, H. (1988). Cross-dimensional interaction and texture segregation. *Percept. Psychophys. 43*, 307–318.

Polat, U., and Sagi, D. (1993). Lateral interactions between spatial channels: Suppression and facilitation revealed by lateral masking experiments. *Vision Res. 33*, 993–999.

Polat, U., and Sagi, D. (1994a). The architecture of spatial interactions. *Vision Res. 34*, 73–78.

Polat, U., and Sagi, D. (1994b). Spatial interactions in human vision: From near to far via experience dependent cascades of connections. *Proc. Natl. Acad. Sci. U.S.A. 91*, 1206–1209.

Ramachandran, V. S., and Braddick, O. (1973). Orientation specific learning in stereopsis. *Perception 2*, 371–376.

Rubenstein, B. S. (1994). *Image Gradients and Performance Asymmetries in Early Vision*. Ph.D. dissertation, The Weizmann Institute of Science, Rehovot, Israel.

Rubenstein, B. S., and Sagi, D. (1990). Spatial variability as a limiting factor in texture discrimination tasks: Implications for performance asymmetries. *J. Opt. Soc. Am. A 7*, 1632–1643.

Rubenstein, B. S., and Sagi, D. (1993). Effects of scale in texture discrimination tasks: Performance is size, shape, and content specific. *Spatial Vision 7*, 293–310.

Sagi, D. (1988). The combination of spatial frequency and orientation is effortlessly perceived. *Percept. Psychophys. 43*, 601–603.

Sagi, D. (1990). Detection of an orientation singularity in Gabor textures: Effect of signal density and spatial-frequency. *Vision Res. 30*, 1377–1388.

Sagi, D. (1991). Spatial filters in texture segmentation tasks. In B. Blum (Ed.), *Channels in the Visual Nervous System: Neurophysiology, Psychophysics and Models* (pp. 397–424). London: Freund Publishing House.

Sagi, D., and Hochstein, S. (1985). Lateral inhibition between spatially adjacent spatial frequency channels? *Percept. Psychophys. 37*, 315–322.

Sagi, D., and Julesz, B. (1985). "Where" and "What" in vision. *Science 228*, 1217–1219.

Sagi, D., and Julesz, B. (1987). Short range limitations on detection of feature differences. *Spatial Vision 2*, 39–49.

Sireteanu, R., and Rettenbach, R. (1993). Serial search can become parallel with practice. *Perception 22* (Suppl.), 36.

Shiu, L., and Pashler, H. (1992). Improvement in line orientation discrimination is retinally local but dependent on cognitive set. *Percept. Psychophys. 52*, 582–588.

Sutter, A., Beck, J., and Graham, N. (1989). Contrast and spatial variables in texture segregation: Testing a simple spatial-frequency channels model. *Percept. Psychophys. 46*, 312–332.

Treisman, A. (1985). Preattentive processing in vision. *Comput. Vis. Graphics Image Proc. 31*, 156–177.

Treisman, A., and Gelade, G. (1980). A feature integration theory of attention. *Cog. Psychol. 12*, 97–136.

Treisman, A., and Gormican, S. (1988). Feature analysis in early vision: Evidence from search asymmetries. *Psychol. Rev. 95*, 15–48.

Turner, M. R. (1986). Texture discrimination by Gabor functions. *Biol. Cybern. 55*, 71–82.

Van Essen, D. C., DeYoe, E. A., Olavarria, J. F., Knierim, J. J., Fox, J. M., Sagi, D., and Julesz, B. (1989). Neural responses to static and moving texture patterns in visual cortex of the Macaque monkey. In D. M. K. Lam and C. Gilbert (Eds.), *Neural Mechanisms of Visual Perception* (pp. 137–154). The Woodlands, TX: Portfolio Publishing.

Walters, D., Biederman, I., and Weisstein, N. (1983). The combination of spatial-frequency and orientation is not effortlessly perceived. Supplement to *Invest. Opthalmol. Visual Sci. 24*, 238.

Wertheim, A. H. (1981). Distraction in visual search. Report IZF 1981–7, Institute for perception TNO, Soesterberg (The Netherlands).

Williams, D., and Julesz, B. (1992). Perceptual asymmetry in texture perception. *Proc. Natl. Acad. Sci. U.S.A. 89*, 6531–6534.

Wilson, H. R., and Bergen, J. R. (1979). A four mechanism model for threshold spatial vision. *Vision Res. 19*, 19–32.

Zeki, S. (1978). Functional specialization in the visual cortex of the rhesus monkey. *Nature (London) 274*, 423–428.

8

A Brief Overview of Texture Processing in Machine Vision

Terry Caelli

In the areas of biological and machine vision the study of texture processing is typically restricted to three types of problems. In the first, *texture discrimination*, interest lies in predicting how two textures are perceived/registered as the "same" or "different" given that the sensor or observer knows where the possibly different texture could be. The second, *texture segmentation*, involves the automatic partitioning of an image into regions defined as having different (at least two, usually many) textural structures, without any prior knowledge of where the different regions may be. In the third, *texture classification*, a given texture is classified as belonging to one of a number of known (from training) texture types. Texture discrimination and segmentation are defined as "early vision" problems insofar as the underlying processes are presumed not to involve previous training or adaptation processes. For this reason these two paradigms have played important roles in understanding human vision and the types of computational procedures necessary for machines to encode images in ways which permit higher-level image understanding.

Of course, these different texture-processing problems presume that we have an agreed definition of texture and, fortunately, there is a commonly accepted necessary condition for the existence of texture, that is, the regular occurrence of a pattern (structure) over a spatial region. However, what makes our understanding of textures complex are two additional observations. One, the predicate "texture" usually applies to the complete region containing the texture, including all spatial regions between the basic texture pattern and their elements. That is, our percept of a textural region is contiguous. Two, texture and pattern are relative to the spatial scale of analysis: what is pattern at one scale is texture at another.

The ability of human observers to segment images into such contiguous regions has been of great interest in the biological vision literature. This, in turn, has motivated the development of many machine vision systems that actually segment textures to various degrees of success consistent with human perception. This convergence of interest has led to a large number of models that share a set of common processing components (see, in this volume, the chapters of Gallant, Van Essen, and Nothdurft, and Sagi). These components correspond to

1. Initial texture feature extraction

2. The extraction of evidence for different textured regions

3. The actual segmentation or classification of textured regions

What differentiates these models is just how the various components are implemented. The aim of this chapter is to examine some of these different models, particularly as they occur in the machine vision literature, while retaining reference to some of the biologically based models. We will consider each component of the systems in order.

Initial Texture Feature Spaces

Rather than concentrate on "global" texture measures, as used before the late 1970s, recent texture encoders are typically defined "locally." That is, the texture features are determined from the covariation of pixels and such correlations are stored as local features. That is, such features can be evaluated at each pixel (position) in the image. Using the above-mentioned definition of texture as that which involves the regular occurrence of a spatial structure over an image region (see Dunn et al., 1994), then all local measures are typically focused on describing the (regular) micropattern structures that define the texture.

These initial textural features are usually found by using moving windows over at least one spatial scale (see, for example, Bergen and Adelson, 1988, in biological vision; Haralick, 1973, in machine vision), and include responses to both first- (individual pixel intensity values) and second-order (relational) textural properties. In biological vision, the underlying texture feature detectors are usually formulated as fixed sets of filters (isotropic or orientation-specific Gabor filters) followed by nonlinear transducers/rectification (recent examples, Malik and Perona, 1990; Sagi, 1991, see also Sagi's chapter, this volume). In machine vision (and sometimes in biological vision; see Caelli, 1988) such detectors are often derived from the textures, per se, and by the use of additional constraints. Further, the detectors may not even take the form of filters insofar as the local texture statistics could include, for example, covariance (see below) or co-occurrence (Haralick, 1973). Such constraints include the ability to derive a set of orthogonal filters (Ade, 1983), minimizing within- and maximizing between-textural differences (Geman and Geman, 1984). That is, what differentiates such detectors (textons) are

1. Whether the detectors are derived adaptively from the images and other types of self-organizing principles, or whether they are fixed and invariant to the image properties

2. The types of measures that are used to register the outputs of such detectors and so the evidence for specific textural information, to result in the registration of local textural features

As will be shown below, this latter problem is nontrivial insofar as the local texture features have to be derived in such a way that textural subregions that have no local textural information, and yet form a part of the perceived textural region, must be encoded as belonging to the same texture. This problem is typically ignored in many biological texture processing models as they do not actually compute what is perceived, but, rather, a prediction of discriminability, per se (see, for example, Sagi, 1991).

In our very first studies on texton enumeration (Caelli et al., 1978) we were concerned with generating texton differences under identical texture power spectra. From these studies we were still able to generate detectors signaling lines, corners, and closure differences. However, once this isopower spectra condition was relinquished, the constraints on texton generation were not so clear, at that stage. Indeed, soon after these studies, Laws (1980) successfully implemented a texture classification scheme based on the outputs of an arbitrary set of edge and bar detectors.

As it emerged, the two most common encoders were (and still are) those determined by *convolution* (*filter-based*) *methods* and those determined by the extraction of *local second-order statistics* from textures. In the former case, then, the initial texton "output" is defined by

$$O(x, y) = \sum_{u, v \in R} d(u, v) I(x + u, y + v)$$

where the "texton" detector, $d(u, v)$, is either determined from the textures themselves (as from the eigenfilter method of Ade, 1983) or on the use of filters, selected for other reasons, including their response to different orientations and sizes of texture micropatterns. Here, $I(x, y)$ corresponds to the full textured image. Summation is defined within the neighbourhood, R, of each position or pixel, (x, y), and indexing of the neighborhood elements is defined by $u, v \in R$.

Filter-Based Methods

The two more common representations used in the literature today are those based on sets of bandpass filters such as orientation-specific Gabor (see Caelli, 1988; Dunn et al., 1994) or adaptive filters derived to minimize a cost function such as those that can minimize within, and maximize between, the region variances (Caelli, 1988; Dunn et al., 1994). However, it should be noted that such outputs, as a result of bandpass filtering, are typically rectified into energy values, as used, for example, by Laws (1980). This type of rectification has also been used in the biological vision models for almost a decade (see, for example, Caelli, 1985; Sagi, 1991).

Perhaps the most important trend in the recent machine vision literature has been to develop a theoretical basis that underpins the process of deriving such optimal local texture feature operators. Such approaches, as, for example, the Markov random field (MRF) models of Geman and Geman (1984) and Nababar and Jain (1992) are aimed at deriving local features that minimize some global error or energy function under the assumption that the texture is stochastic and the similarities of textural regions accord to Gibbs distribution: pixels close to each other are much more likely to have the same covariance structures, at a given scale, than those that are farther away. What differentiates the MRF models from adaptive filtering, per se, is that the MRF, if assumed to hold, justifies the use of simulated annealing to determine these local support functions or filters (see Geman and Geman, 1984, for more details). To this stage, however, there has been no evidence for such types of constraints to operate in human texture processing, though this does not imply that biological texture processing is unconstrained!

Local Statistical Methods

In contrast, texture features derived from local statistical methods result in texture characterizations from statistics of fixed or moving windows that compute various types of relationships between image pixel intensities, as with symmetrical co-occurrence or covariance matrices. Global (expected) covariance matrices are computed by moving a window over the full texture region and computing the covariation of all pixels within a moving window. The (expected) neighborhood pixel variances constitute the diagonals, and the types off-diagonal covariance values define the correlations present in the region. The eigenvalues and eigenvectors of such matrices capture the predominant texture structures similar to the outputs of different filters. In fact, in Ade's (1983) eigenfilter method texture filters are derived from the eigenvectors of this (windowed) covariance statistic:

$$\text{cov}(u, v) = \text{cov}[(n - 1)i + j, (n - 1)k + l]$$
$$= \sum_{x, y} [I(x + i, y + j) - \bar{I}][I(x + k, y + l) - \bar{I}]$$

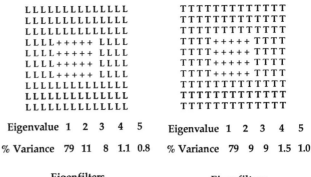

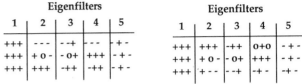

Eigenvalue	1	2	3	4	5
% Variance	79	11	8	1.1	0.8

Eigenvalue	1	2	3	4	5
% Variance	79	9	9	1.5	1.0

Figure 8.1

(*Top*) "+" embedded in "L" and "T" textures. (*Bottom*) The 3 × 3 eigenfilters for each texture pair, depicted in terms of the signs of the filter kernels; also shown is the variance explained by each filter (from the square of each eigenvalue). Note the differences between the derived texture features (filters) for each texture pair.

where n corresponds to the (square) window size (the two sets of indices, i, j, k, l, are necessary to enable the covariance to be defined with respect to each pixel compared to every other) and resulting in a symmetric $n^2 \times n^2$ matrix. The eigenvectors of this matrix are $n^2 \times 1$ in size, or, when properly reformatted into raster form, $n \times n$. In this form they can be used as filters to encode each texture; an example is shown in figure 8.1.

Notice here that the "line," "edge," and "corners" features, and their relative strengths as defined by their eigenvalues, all result from this method of analysis. The observed lack of symmetry in texture discrimination (see Gurnsey and Browse, 1989) may well be due to such differences in texture feature statistics, which, as can be seen from this example, come from the actual densities of each texture type. This explanation for such asymmetries is different from Sagi (1991) and Rubenstein and Sagi (1990) who propose that the difference is due to internal noise in the encoding of different features.

A local covariance structure can also be defined in another way. The local covariance matrix can be determined with respect to the covariance of the $[x, y, \text{and } z = I(x, y)]$ values around a position. This results in a 3×3 covariance matrix whose eigenstructures define the predominant intensity gradients and curvatures (see the section "A Current Example"; Madiraju et al., 1993).

By definition, these types of texture "signatures" are derived from the textures and a large number of such features have been proposed over the past 20 years from the co-occurrence matrices of Haralick (1973), to recent ensemble covariance techniques used by Ade (1983) and, more recently, the local covariance technique recently briefly defined above (Madiraju et al., 1993; see the section "A Current Example"). In all cases such statistics can be used to optimize classes of associated filters in contrast to the simple use of fixed sets of filters for texture feature extraction. One benefit of not using the filter versions is that if the filters are bandpass, as they typically are, their outputs need to be rectified or transformed to constitute textural feature evidence measures. In this way energy rectification (Caelli, 1985), variance around zero-crossings (Watt, 1987), and the use of Hilbert transforms, or "energy" transforms, consisting of the energy outputs of even and odd filters, have all been used to overcome this problem. This is one reason why most texture filter-based texture processing models have a nonlinear transducer after filtering (see, for example, Sagi, 1991).

Determining Texture Region Measures

Perhaps one of the more difficult problems for texture feature extraction is the fact that textures, by definition, though regular at a given scale, are nonstationary. This means that independently of whether the texture features are generated from detectors derived from the image or not, the outputs of such detectors, even for a single texture, will vary across space. This point has been mostly neglected in the biological vision literature as most models are not concerned with identifying the texture regions as much as they are with segmenting the image. However, it is a problem in machine vision.

The two solutions to this problem are to derive filters or statistics directly from larger windows, and to derive their size to attain this goal (as, for example, with Dunn et al., 1994). The second approach is to use two windows: one for the initial texture feature extraction and a larger one to compute the statistics of these features over larger regions. This latter approach is more common in the biological vision literature where the second window is used as a basis for relaxation-type operations (Caelli, 1985, 1988) or for broader filtering processes (see, for example, Bergen and Adelson, 1988; Sagi, 1991). All approaches have specific benefits and have one common theme: that to capture texture differences it is necessary to have second-order texture feature difference encoding that is tuned to maximize between- and minimize within-textural differences. This has sometimes been referred to as texture "gradient" detection (Nothdurft, 1990) and, in general, there seems to be a need for such processing due to the

heterogeneity of the texture feature maps over the image regions. In the section "A Current Example" we will deal with an example of this aspect of texture segmentation in the context of rotation-invariant texture processing.

Segmentation and Classification

Once a texton map (a texture feature vector-valued function evaluated at each image pixel) has been attained, classification or segmentation follow naturally, though the actual decision processes need to be explicated. For classification, traditional statistical methods can be used where each pixel is classified as belonging to one of a set of training textures by a suitable classifier. Again, for this case, the texture features must be derived after the second level of processing in order to obtain a representation that has the least variability within a given textured region. As already discussed, global texture statistics—yielding those features derived by integrating over the complete image—have been replaced by local texture features and so the texture classification problem, again, is typically translated into pixel labelling.

For segmentation, in machine vision, there are essentially two approaches: texture gradient or boundary detection, or region-based clustering. In the former case the essential task is to determine the boundaries ("texton gradients") that sufficiently divide textures into different types. Such operators have been proposed by Nothdurft (1990) and others. Indeed, some recent neurophysiological results support this type of encoding occurring within the vertebrate visual cortex (see Gallant's et al., this volume). The other approach, that of clustering, has had some deal of recent success with segmenting both range and intensity information (see Besl and Jain, 1988; Hoffman and Jain, 1987). In such an approach pixels are typically grouped according to their feature similarities and the clustering algorithms differ in terms of the types of functions to be minimized. Such functions are usually measures of within-to-between class feature distance statistics.

Before dealing with an example, a final theoretical comment needs to be made on the neural network approaches to texture processing. It is also possible, within the context of texture classification, to train a neural network to classify textures having trained them on examples of the target texture types. Typically the input layer consists of an $n \times n$ moving window with at least one hidden layer. The network would learn to tune the window function to best discriminate the textures. This is accomplished by determining the weights in the network. However, as already pointed out in the literature by Lippmann (1987) and, more recently by Caelli et al. (1993), this is formally equivalent to developing least-squares filters and linear discriminant function-type classifiers. The reason for this is that the weights produce both orthogonalization of the signals and clustering of the weights. This is not to say that neural nets should not be used to solve such problems. Rather, it simply states that the representation is the same as past models and the only issue is whether gradient descent (as used in backpropagation) helps in the estimation of the texture feature weights.

A Current Example: Invariant Texture Segmentation and Classification

Our new covariance texture features are based upon the local covariance of intensity in the neighborhood of a pixel. That is, in contrast to Ade's (1983) method, our new covariance method determines the covariance of the image position and intensity values $\{x, y, I(x, y)\}$ as a 3×3 covariance matrix *at each pixel* and determined with respect to a neighborhood square window. The eigenvectors and eigenvalues of such covariance matrices determine the orientation and magnitudes of best-fitting planes (in the 3D position $[x, y]$) and intensity $[I(x, y) = z]$ space) and the eigenvalues are invariant to rotations and shift. Consequently, they can be used as initial features for invariant texture registration. It is also possible to determine "second-order" covariance, defined by the rate of change of the first eigenvectors, and such statistics determine the equivalent to the magnitudes of (unscaled) surface normal and curvatures at a position (see Berkmann and Caelli, 1994, for more details). In this application we use the rotation-invariant property of such eigenvalues to enable rotation invariant texture segmentation and classification.

Rotation invariant texture classification has already been addressed in the literature, as, for example by Haralick (1973) and Kashyap and Khotanzad (1986). The former uses a number of differently oriented co-occurrence matrices while the latter approach uses circular symmetric autoregressive models for texture encoding. Our approach is somewhat related to the latter in so far as invariant descriptors are determined by a linear model based on the relationships between neighboring pixels. The difference, however, lies in how these relations are measured. Here the covariance matrix is defined by

$$C(x, y) \equiv C = \frac{1}{N} \sum_{m=1}^{N} [w_m - \overline{w}(x, y)][w_m - \overline{w}(x, y)]^T$$

where w_i corresponds to the $(x, y, z = I(x, y))$ coordinate vector for position i in the texture, T corresponds to the transpose, and

$$\overline{w}(x, y) = \frac{1}{N} \sum_{i=1}^{N} w_i,$$

computed over the local $n \times n$ window, where $N = n^2$.

The matrix, C, is symmetric and its three eigenvectors correspond to the best-fitting plane and "normal" to the intensity surface, while its eigenvalues determine the magnitudes of the major directions of these vectors. These eigenvalues capture roughness and structural properties of the local texture information. The third eigenvalue simply corresponds to the sampling density, and so is constant over the image, and was omitted in further analysis.

Since they are defined at every pixel, they vary over the texture regions. For this reason, as occurs in most other texture processing algorithms, a second window is required. That is, if we were to simply compute these invariant descriptors over larger regions then the averaging effects would destroy the encoding of the specific textural information. Rather, we compute means, variances, and kurtosis moments over the larger window to then produce more representative texture features. The resultant texture feature space was therefore six dimensional with three moments determined over a larger square window, for each of the two texture-specific eigenvalues.

Texture Classification

We have found that a simple discriminant function (two-layered neural network) was adequate for classification. The classifier was developed by randomly selecting 31×31 texture samples, determining the eigenvalues (over 7×7 windows) and texture features (over the 15×15 larger window), and the discriminant function for the two-class problem shown in figure 8.2 (left and center columns). At runtime, a moving 15×15 window was taken, and eigenvalues and features were computed. Each pixel, centered in the window, was then classified by the discriminant function, as shown in figures 8.2 and 8.3.

Texture Segmentation

Segmentation differs from classification in so far as there is no prior knowledge of texture region types. As already discussed, solutions to this more difficult problem are either based on region boundary detection, per se, or the use of region clustering procedures. In this example we have chosen the latter approach.

The algorithm first involves sampling the image and selecting the maximum number (k) of clusters. From these samples we then compute eigenvalues (3×3 matrix) and texture features over a larger window, in this case of variable size for comparison purposes. We then run the cluster procedure CLUSTER (Jain and Dubes, 1988) to cluster feature samples into the specified clusters.

This technique (CLUSTER) uses a minimum within-squared error criterion, as is the case with K-means clustering (Jain and Dubes, 1988). However, it differs from this latter method in so far as it also determines the number of clusters that best fits the data. The algorithm starts with two clusters and then forms an additional cluster by selecting the sample further away from the centroids of all clusters, as with divisive clustering methods. K-means clustering is then performed on these ($n + 1$) clusters.

The process iterates with an additional, interleaved reverse agglomerative phase. The process alternates till cluster increases or decreases do not change the within-to-between distance cost function as is used in normal K-means clustering.

Some Experimental Results

Figures 8.2 and 8.3 show classification and segmentation results for a number of different textures—using the techniques described above—including the 15×15 larger window size for texture feature extraction. The effect of this latter window size on classification performance is shown in figure 8.4.

It should be noted that although we have used the eigenvalues of the covariance matrix for the purposes of

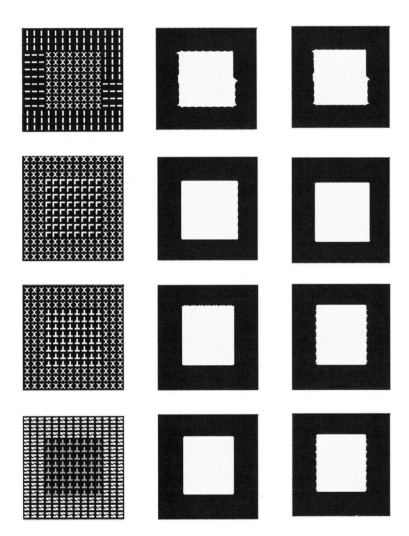

Figure 8.2
Rotation-invariant texture pixel classification (center column) and segmentation (right column) for four different synthetic texture pairs. Here different intensity values correspond to different textured regions as a result of either classification or segmentation methods (see text for details).

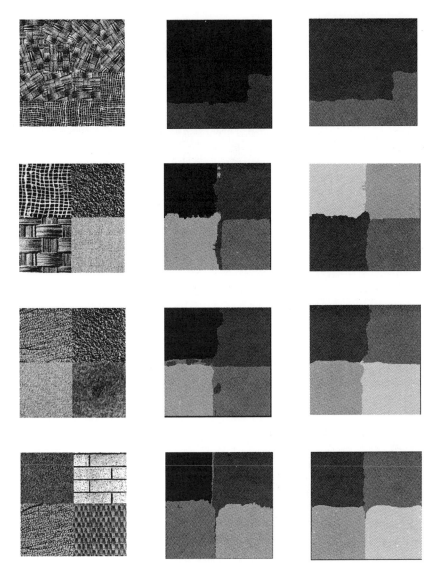

Figure 8.3
Rotation-invariant texture pixel classification (center column) and segmentation (right column) for four different collections of natural textures [the textures were taken from the Brodatz (1956) collection]. Here different intensity values correspond to different textured regions as a result of either classification or segmentation methods (see text for details).

rotation and shift-invariant classification and segmentation, the full eigenvectors supply a texture signature that is orientation-specific in so far as the eigenvectors correspond to oriented planes in the joint position-intensity space so defining oriented intensity ramps that capture the main intensity gradients in the neighborhood of a pixel. This constitutes a more powerful texture code and, as is well known, is analogous to the local Fourier phase space, while the eigenvalues correspond to the local Fourier power spectrum—together constituting the spectral decomposition of a matrix. However, for these studies it was not necessary to use the full spectral decomposition to obtain reasonable performance.

Conclusions

As can be seen from the results, the difference between classification and segmentation is not that great, particularly if the feature extraction, and related processes, enable clear differentiation of the different texture types in texture feature space (see figures 8.2 and 8.3). This finding is not necessarily specific to these examples. Indeed, given adequate texture features that can index the inherent feature structures and a method that can minimize within and maximize between the texture feature projections, robust texture segmentation can be more-or-less guaranteed

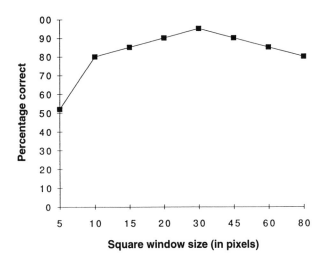

Figure 8.4
The effect of the larger texture feature window size (abscissa, square window sizes, in pixels) on classification performance (ordinate, PC, percentage correct pixel classification).

without using supervised learning (classification) methods. Here we have endeavored to present a brief overview of the types of processes required to build texture segmenters (and classifiers) as typically occur in current machine vision systems, and which are reasonably reliable, with the more well-known texture types (see figures 8.2 and 8.3).

What has not been accomplished is to bind these ideas with the more "natural" segmentation problems that present to the human perceiver in everyday life. Such questions are also discussed in the chapter by Watt (this volume). It may even be the case that, in the area of passive sensing, as in human vision, textures may be somewhat peripheral to our understanding of 3D objects and other world structures in the following sense. Textural information, simply as one form of nonzero intensity covariance within the neighborhood of a pixel, is essential for the direct inference of depth, whether using shape-from-stereo, focus, motion, or texture perspective, per se. However, such information, qua textures, may serve no other particular purpose in "ecological" vision and further interpretations of the perceived world may occur with respect to the perceived 3D surface shape and surface materials of objects. From this perspective, image-based textures would play a part in scene understanding only if they reflect surface material properties of importance to given recognition problems.

Much like the work completed in biological vision, machine vision research into texture processing has been largely theoretical and based on more or less synthetic textures. However, machine vision algorithms for texture segmentation typically have a different goal compared to most biological models. The latter are more concerned with predicting psychophysical data while the former is concerned with producing an image of what may be perceived. Such a "production system" approach to understanding visual processing often raises subtle issues that, otherwise, would not be seen from the other perspective.

However, in both cases, research must move to more realistic textures and we must endeavor to more rigorously understand how texture processing fits within the broader problem of image understanding.

Acknowledgment

This project was funded by a grant from the Centre for Intelligent Decision Systems.

References

Ade, F. (1983). Characterization of textures by "Eigenfilters." *Signal Process. 5*, 451–457.

Bergen, J., and Adelson, E. (1988). Visual texture segmentation based on energy measures. *J. Opt. Soc. Am. A 3*(13), 98–101.

Berkmann, J., and Caelli, T. (1994). On the relationship between surface covariance and differential geometry. In A. Toet (Ed.) *Shape in Picture* Springer-Verlag, Series F: Computer and Systems Sciences, Vol. *126*, 343–352.

Besl, P., and Jain, R. (1988). Segmentation through variable-order surface fitting. *IEEE: Transact. Pattern Anal. Machine Intelligence 10*, 167–192.

Brodatz, P. (1956). *Texture: A Photographic Album for Artists and Designers.* New York: Dover.

Caelli, T. (1985). Three processing characteristics of visual texture segmentation. *Spatial Vision 1*, 19–30.

Caelli, T. (1988). An adaptive computational model for texture segmentation. *IEEE Transact. Syst. Man Cybern. 18*(1), 9–17.

Caelli, T., Julesz, B., and Gilbert, E. (1978). On perceptual analyzers underlying visual texture discrimination. *Biol. Cybern. 29*, 201–214.

Caelli, T., Squire, D., and Wild, T. (1993). Model-based neural networks. *Neural Networks 6*(5), 613–627.

Dunn, D., Higgins, W., and Wakeley, J. (1994). Texture segmentation using 2-D Gabor elementary functions. *IEEE: Transact. Pattern Anal. Machine Intelligence 16*, 130–149.

Geman, S., and Geman, D. (1984) Stochastic relaxation, Gibbs distribution, and the Baysian restoration of images. *IEEE Transact. Pattern Anal. Machine Intelligence 6*, 721–741.

Gurnsey, R., and Browse, R. (1989). Asymmetries in visual texture discrimination. *Spatial Vision 4*(1), 31–44.

Haralick, R. M. (1973). Statistical and structural approaches to texture. *IEEE Transact. Syst. Man Cybern. 3*, 610–621.

Hoffman, R., and Jain, A. K. (1987). Segmentation and classification of range images. *IEEE Transact. Pattern Anal. Machine Intelligence 9*(5), 608–620.

Jain, A. K., and Dubes, R. C. (1988). *Algorithms for Clustering Data.* Englewood Cliffs, NJ: Prentice Hall.

Kashyap, R., and Khotanzad, A. (1986). A model-based method for rotation invariant texture classification. *IEEE Transact. Pattern Anal. Machine Intelligence 8*(4), 472–481.

Laws, K. (1980). Rapid texture identification image processing for missile guidance. *SPIE 238*, 376–380.

Lippmann, R. (1987). An introduction to computing with neural nets. *IEEE: ASSP Mag.* April, 4–22.

Madiraju, S., Caelli, T., and Liu, C. C. (1993). On the covariance technique for robust and rotation invariant texture processing. *Proc. First Asian Comput. Vision Conf.* Osaka, 171–174.

Malik, J., and Perona, P. (1990). Preattentive texture discrimination with early vision mechanisms. *J. Opt. Soc. Am. A 7*, 923–932.

Nababar, S., and Jain, A. (1992). Edge detection and labelling by fusion of intensity and range images. *SPIE Proc. Appl. Artificial Intelligence,* Orlando, April, 33–40.

Nothdurft, H. C. (1990). Texton segregation by associated differences in global and local luminance distribution. *Proc. R. Soc. London B239,* 295–320.

Rubenstein, B. S., and Sagi, D. (1990). Spatial variability as a limiting factor in texture discrimination tasks: Implications for performance asymmetries. *J. Opt. Soc. Am A 7*, 1632–1643.

Sagi, D. (1991). Spatial filters in texture segmentation tasks. In E. Blum (Ed.), *Channels in the Visual Nervous System: Neurophysiology, Psychophysics and Models* (pp. 397–424). London: Freund.

Watt, R. (1987). An outline of the primal sketch in human vision. *Pattern Recog. Lett. 5*, 139–150.

9

Two-Dimensional and Three-Dimensional Texture Processing in Visual Cortex of the Macaque Monkey

Jack L. Gallant,
David C. Van Essen, and
H. Christoph Nothdurft

Computer-generated textures have many of the properties we associate with natural images, yet they can be easily controlled. Texture stimuli are therefore well suited to experiments on basic issues in vision (Julesz, 1991). Two issues that have benefited from the psychophysical or computational use of texture are image segmentation (Bovik et al., 1990; Julesz, 1981, 1984, 1986; Malik and Perona, 1990; Nothdurft, 1990a; Sagi, this volume; Stevens, 1981; Sutter et al., 1989; Victor et. al., this volume) and the representation of three-dimensional shape (Bajcsy and Lieberman, 1976; Blake et al., 1993; Cumming et al., 1993; Gibson, 1966; Todd and Akerstrom, 1987; Todd and Mingolla, 1983; Witkin, 1981). However, there have been relatively few neurophysiological studies of texture (Hammond and MacKay, 1975, 1977; Nothdurft, 1990b; Nothdurft and Li, 1984, 1985), especially when compared to the large number of studies using conventional bar and grating stimuli to assess basic mechanisms of neural coding.

Our laboratories have explored several aspects of the neural basis of texture perception. First, we have examined the neural mechanisms underlying classic texture-based perceptual phenomena such as texture pop-out and texture segmentation (DeYoe et al., 1986; Knierim and Van Essen, 1992; Nothdurft and Li, 1984, 1985; Olavarria et al., 1992; Van Essen et al., 1989). Second, we have investigated the neural mechanisms underlying the perception of natural scenes and three-dimensional (3D) shape, and have used texture as a tool in our studies. In this report we discuss recent results concerning the responses of area V1 neurons to texture borders. Area V1 is the first major cortical processing station for visual information. V1 neurons have fairly small receptive fields, and one class of cells in this area gives remarkably linear responses to stimuli falling within the classical receptive field. (Other V1 cells display relatively simple nonlinearities.) We also discuss the responses of area V4 neurons to textured surfaces oriented in 3D and to a novel class of grating-based stimuli. Area V4 lies on the prelunate gyrus, and is a major visual processing station between area V1 and the inferotemporal complex. V4 receptive fields are many times larger than those found in area V1. Cells in both V1 and V4 are selective for simple visual dimensions such as retinal disparity, color, orientation, and frequency, but cells in V4 are generally selective for more complex stimulus characteristics than those in V1. There have been few studies of the responses of V4 cells to rich stimuli, however, and much remains to be discovered.

Methods

The techniques used in our single-unit neurophysiological recordings are described in detail elsewhere (Gallant et al., 1993a; Olavarria et al., 1992). In brief, recordings were carried out on adult macaque monkeys that were anesthetized with Sufentanil and immobilized to prevent eye movements. Appropriate anesthesia doses were determined for each animal before paralysis, and throughout the experiment anesthesia was monitored and adjusted according to standard electrocardiographic and electroencephalographic criteria. Single units were isolated using Levick-style or tungsten microelectrodes inserted through a sealed recording chamber and into striate cortex, or into area V4 on the prelunate gyrus. In most experiments, stimuli were presented on a Silicon Graphics workstation controlled by a Macintosh computer using customized software for stimulus generation, experimental control, and data analysis.

Results

Neural Responses to Texture Borders in Area V1

Effortless or preattentive texture segmentation can occur when a texture region differs from its surround along a salient dimension such as orientation. The limiting case of texture segmentation, called texture pop-out, occurs when a single texture element differs from its surround (Bergen and Julesz, 1983; Luschow and Nothdurft, 1993; Nothdurft, 1991; Treisman and Gelade, 1980). Previous experiments have examined the neural basis of texture pop-out in area V1 (Knierim and Van Essen, 1992; Van Essen et al., 1989). About a third of the cells tested produced a significantly larger response when the texture element within the receptive field was part of a pop-out display than when it was part of homogeneous texture field, suggesting that the signal necessary for pop-out is present as early as area V1 (see also Victor et al., this volume). Because texture pop-out shares many properties with perceptual segmentation involving larger regions of texture (Nothdurft, 1991), we decided to evaluate

the neural representation of extended texture borders in area V1.

The behavioral importance of texture borders (and pop-out) lies in the fact that these structures draw attention to themselves, so that such a border is more salient than the surrounding texture. If cells in area V1 are involved in this process, their responses might be enhanced near texture borders, relative to their responses in homogeneous texture regions. We therefore designed an experiment in which the responses of isolated cells were assessed at many different positions in a large texture display.

The stimuli for these experiments consisted of a texture bar composed of many elements with identical orientations, surrounded by a texture field whose elements had the orthogonal orientation (see figure 9.1A and B). The orientation of the elements within the bar was optimized for each cell, and the size was chosen so that only one element fit within the classical receptive field of the cell. The spacing between elements was randomized slightly, to minimize spacing artifacts. The texture bar was between five and nine elements wide, and was oriented diagonally relative to the cell's preferred orientation. Thus the texture border was oriented at 45° relative to the texture elements. Across trials each of the elements composing one row of the texture bar, and several elements in the same row but lying outside the bar, were centered on the receptive field of the cell. The positions were tested in random order, and each display was flashed for 0.5 sec. Thus the texture field was, in effect, scanned across the receptive field of the cell along a line crossing the texture bar.

We recorded from 156 cells in area V1 using these stimuli (Nothdurft et al., 1992). We found that the responses of some cells increased significantly when a texture border was near the receptive field, versus when the nearby texture field was homogeneous. Figure 9.1C illustrates the responses of one such cell tested with a bar nine elements wide; the response at the texture border was more than double the response within the central portion of the texture bar. Altogether, 93 of the 156 cells (about three-fifths) showed a significant increase in responses near a texture border, for at least one border orientation. When the four border conditions used for each cell (two sides of the texture bar at each of two bar orientations) were averaged together, 23 of the cells (about one-seventh) showed a significant increase in responses.

To quantify the changes in responses near a texture border, we calculated a border enhancement index for each cell. This index was computed by taking the difference between a cell's mean response to an optimally ori-

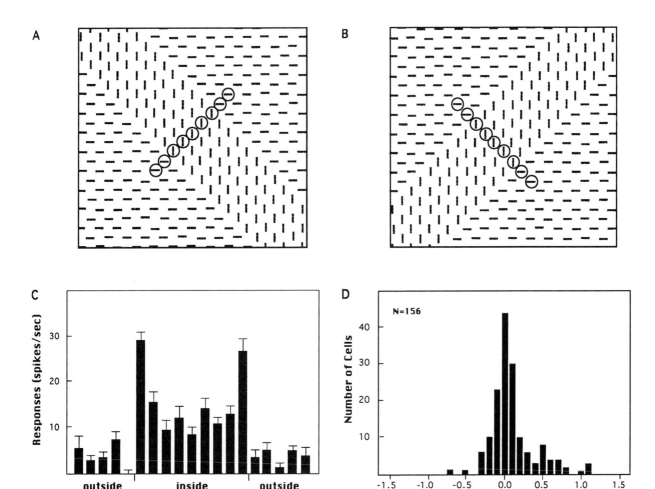

Figure 9.1

(*A*) Example of a texture bar used in texture border experiments. The texture bar was between five (as shown here) and nine elements wide. The bar was surrounded by a field of texture elements at the orthogonal orientation. The orientation of the elements was optimized individually for each cell, and the borders of the texture bar were always oriented at 45° relative to the orientation of the elements. Textures were shown using the optimal color for each cell, and were displayed for 0.5 sec on a dark background. During the test each element falling along a single row in the texture bar, and a few elements in the surround, were centered on the cell's receptive field (shown here by circles centered on nine elements within the texture). (*B*) Example of a texture bar orthogonal to that shown in A. The orientation of the elements in the bar and the surround is the same as in A. (*C*) Responses of a single V1 cell when the receptive field was

centered on various locations within and outside of a texture bar. This cell gave the largest response when a texture element of the optimal orientation was within the receptive field, and a texture border was next to the receptive field. The responses in the middle of the texture bar were suppressed, and were very low outside of the texture bar, where the elements were orthogonal to the cell's preferred orientation. (*D*) Border enhancement index for 156 cells tested in the texture border experiment. The index was computed by taking the difference between a cell's mean response to an optimally oriented texture element at the edge of the texture bar and in the middle of the texture bar, and normalizing this value with respect to the cell's response to a homogeneous texture field. Positive values indicate enhanced responses near the texture border.

ented texture element adjacent to the border and at a distance from the border, and normalizing this value with respect to the cell's responses within a homogeneous texture field (far from the border). The distribution of border enhancement indices for the 156 cells in our sample is presented in figure 9.1D. Positive values indicate enhanced responses near the texture border, while negative values indicate reduced responses near the border. The modal index value is zero, but the distribution is skewed toward positive index values, indicating a large general border enhancement effect for a subpopulation of cells.

Many cells in area V1 produce a larger response near a texture border than in a homogeneous region of texture. Most of these cells appear to have a preferred border orientation, but in a significant subpopulation border orientation is not important. Thus area V1 does contain information about texture borders that could aid in image segmentation. Though the responses obtained near a texture border are larger than those obtained in the center of a uniform texture field, they are usually smaller than the responses to a single bar placed within the classical receptive field and no surrounding texture elements. This confirms previous findings that stimuli outside the classical receptive field generally have a suppressive effect (cf. Gulyas et al., 1987; Knierim and Van Essen, 1992).

Neural Responses in Area V4 to 3D Textured Surfaces

The representation of perceptually significant borders in the retinal image is an important visual function, but this process is just one part of a system whose ultimate aim is the construction of a rich internal representation of the visible external world. There is as yet no consensus on the form of this representation. On one extreme are proposals that the visual system constructs an internal 3D model of the shapes and positions of objects in the world (Marr, 1982; Pentland, 1985, 1989). On the other extreme are proposals that recognition is inherently 2D, based on complex template-matching between the incoming image and a library of stored 2D images (Lowe, 1990; Poggio and Edelman, 1990; Ullman, 1990). The models that have been proposed for the neural representation of objects are so diverse, and often so abstract, that testing them is difficult (see Plaut and Farah, 1990). One testable proposal is that the visual system explicitly represents the viewer-centered orientation of visible surfaces in the environment, in what Marr (1982) called the $2\frac{1}{2}$ D sketch.

We sought to test this hypothesis by searching for cells that were tuned for local values of surface orientation. The visual system generally represents physical dimensions according to a local value coding principle, in which relevant dimensions such as color or frequency are represented by a population of cells, each of which responds to a limited range of values along the relevant dimension. Planar surfaces, for example, can be parameterized by two dimensions, slant and tilt. Slant refers to the angle between the surface normal and the line of sight, while tilt refers to the rotation of the surface normal around the line of sight. If the visual system contains an explicit representation of 3D surface orientation, cells should be tuned for specific values of slant and tilt, and the population of cells should span the permissible range of these two dimensions. We decided to record in area V4, where cells' receptive fields are several degrees across and selectivities are complex enough so that an explicit representation of surface slant and tilt might be viable.

Responses to 3D Textured Surfaces

One of the most common means of rendering simple surface shapes is to use textured surfaces in which the texture elements are mapped onto the surface and then rendered in 3D through projective geometry. Such 3D textured surfaces have been studied intensively, using both psychophysical (Blake et al., 1993; Cutting and Millard, 1984; Todd and Akerstrom, 1987) and theoretical (Bajcsy and Lieberman, 1976; Stevens, 1981; Witkin, 1981) techniques. Because a great deal of work has already been done using 3D textured surfaces, and because they are fairly easy to render and control, we chose to use them in our study.

The stimuli used for these experiments were textures composed of many circular elements. Cells in area V4 are generally selective for both color and spatial frequency (Desimone and Schein, 1987; Gallant et al., 1993a; Schein and Desimone, 1990), so the color of the texture gradient and the size of the texture elements were optimized for each cell. To make the textures appear more irregular, the positions and sizes of the individual texture elements were randomized slightly within each display. The textures were mapped onto a plane, and the plane was oriented in 3D space by perspective projection (figure 9.2A and B). Surfaces were constructed for many combinations of slant and tilt, and in most cases for three different texture element sizes bracketing the optimal spatial frequency for a cell. For some cells the texture gradients were confined to the classical receptive field, while for others the gradients extended into the nonclassical surround. The results obtained with both types of stimuli were qualitatively similar, however, so they are treated together here.

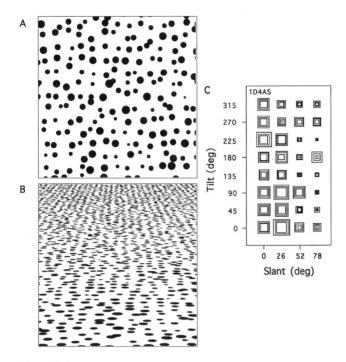

Figure 9.2

(*A*) Example of a texture used in 3D textured surface experiments. Each texture was composed of circular elements whose mean size was optimized individually for each cell. Textures were shown using the optimal color for each cell, and were displayed for 0.5 sec on a dark background. The texture shown here is parallel to the image plane, and so has a slant of 0° and a tilt of 0°. (*B*) Example of a 3D texture surface with slant of 80° and tilt of 90°. The surface appears to be receding away from the viewer. (*C*) Responses of a single V4 cell to 3D textured surfaces varying in slant and tilt. Surface slant is given on the abscissa, while surface tilt is given on the ordinate. Data were averaged across the three texture sizes used, 0.5, 1.0, and 2.0 times the texture size corresponding to the best grating frequency for the cell. Squares give the normalized firing rates, and standard errors, to each combination of slant and tilt. This cell responded best to low slant values, and gave a fairly uniform response to different tilts.

We recorded from 90 cells in area V4 using these stimuli (Gallant et al., 1991) and found that the responses of some cells were significantly modulated by varying slant and tilt. Figure 9.2C illustrates the responses of one cell that responded best at small slants (0° and 26°) and across a range of tilts. (The 2-D histograms in figure 9.2C are meant to indicate the effects of slant and tilt, and the sizes of the squares indicate the responses of the cell to each combination of slant and tilt.) To quantify the effects of slant, tilt, and texture size on cells' responses, we evaluated the normalized stimulus response rates of 73 of these cells with a three-factor analysis of variance (ANOVA). Varying surface slant produced significant changes in the response rates of 18 of the 73 cells examined (about one-fourth), whereas varying tilt produced significant changes in the response rates of only 11 cells (about one-eighth).

By far the largest effect was obtained by varying texture size, which produced significant changes in the response rates of 38 of 73 cells (about one-half). Of the 18 cells whose firing rate was significantly modulated by varying slant, 16 were also significantly modulated by varying texture size. In general, the largest responses were obtained when the slant angle was zero (i.e., when the surface was parallel to the image plane), but often the slant producing the largest response varied with texture size. These observations suggest that responses were determined primarily by texture size, and only secondarily by surface slant and tilt.

The unexpectedly large effects of texture size prompted us to investigate these effects more carefully. We had originally varied texture size by altering the sizes of the elements within a texture before any projective transformations. The effective *retinal size* of the elements after projection, however, is a function of both the specified texture size and the slant of the surface. We computed the median retinal texture size of our stimuli (taking both specified texture size and slant into account) for 14 cells. Variation in retinal size produced significant changes in the response rates of 9 of these cells (about two-thirds). Thus it appears that the projected retinal texture size may account for a larger proportion of the variance of cells' firing rates than either surface slant or specified texture size considered alone.

Responses to Frequency Modulated (FM) Gratings

As part of our preliminary testing, we assessed cells' responses to sinusoidal gratings having a range of spatial frequencies and orientations. (Such gratings are known to be particularly effective in driving cells in area V1; De Valois and De Valois, 1990.) We found that gratings were generally more effective than textures in driving cells in area V4. We therefore designed a new stimulus set in which a 2D sinusoidal grating was projected into 3D, using the same methods employed for generating textured 3D surfaces (see figure 9.3A and B). Thus these 3D frequency-modulated (FM) gratings had, in addition to their 2D frequency and orientation, a defined slant and tilt. The 2D orientation was always selected so as to be either orthogonal or parallel to the direction of tilt. When the 2D orientation and 3D tilt were orthogonal, grating frequency was modulated along the direction of tilt (figure 9.3A). When they were parallel, the modulation was more complex (owing to perspective projection), but was mainly orthogonal to the direction of tilt (figure 9.3B). In most cases several different 2D frequencies were tested that bracketed the optimal frequency for a cell.

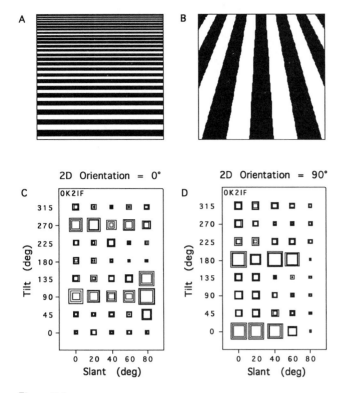

Figure 9.3

(*A*) Example of a 3D frequency modulated (FM) grating with a slant of 80° and a tilt of 90°. The 2D orientation of this grating was selected so that the direction of frequency modulation was parallel to the direction of slant. Gratings used in the experiments were quantized to 250 luminance levels and were displayed for 0.5 sec on a dark background. (*B*) Example of a 3D frequency modulated (FM) grating with a slant of 80° and a tilt of 90°, but whose 2D orientation is rotated 90° from the grating shown in A. The 2D orientation of this grating was selected so that the direction of frequency modulation was orthogonal to the direction of slant. The perspective projection of such a grating into 3D produces a complex frequency modulation. (*C*) Responses of a single V4 cell to 3D FM gratings whose 2D modulation (4 c/deg) was parallel to the direction of slant (as A). Slant is given on the abscissa, and tilt is given on the ordinate. Squares in the two-way plot give normalized relative firing rates and standard errors. This cell responded best to a wide range of slants when the tilt was either 90° or 270°. (*D*) Responses of the same V4 cell shown in C to 3D FM gratings whose 2D orientation was orthogonal to the direction of slant (as in B). The cell responded best to a wide range of slants when the tilt was either 0° or 180°. The pattern of responses for this cell indicates that it was tuned for a specific retinal orientation, but did not distinguish between various slants or tilts.

We tested 22 cells in area V4 using FM gratings. The 2D orientation of the gratings had by far the largest effect on firing rate. Figure 9.3C and D illustrates the responses of a cell whose firing rate was significantly modulated both by varying 2D orientation and by varying tilt. Note that the pattern of responses obtained with the two 2D grating orientations is shifted in phase by 90° with respect to tilt, indicating that the cell's responses were determined primarily by the effective retinal orientation of the grating, not the 3D tilt of the grating. In addition, the cell was fairly insensitive to changes in tilt of 180°, indicating that it was not selective for the absolute sign of 3D orientation. These features were present, to some degree, in the responses of most of the cells that were significantly modulated in this test. Of the 22 cells tested, 2D orientation had a significant effect on the firing rate of 13 (slightly more than one-half). Varying tilt apart from 2D orientation had a significant effect on the firing rates of 9 cells (about two-fifths), and varying slant produced significant changes in the firing rates of 4 cells (about one-fifth).

If cells in area V4 represent 3D surface orientation explicitly, different cells should be tuned for a wide range of slants and tilts spanning the range of possible orientations. In addition, any such tuning should not be due to variation along some simpler dimension, such as spatial frequency, which covaries with 3D orientation under some circumstances. We found no cells in our sample that had these characteristics. Therefore neither these experiments nor our preliminary studies employing more complex textured shapes (such as textured spheres) have provided significant support for the hypothesis that the visual system explicitly encodes the 3D orientation of visible surfaces. Instead, our results suggest that the responses of V4 cells to texture patterns may result largely from these cells' complex, nonlinear responses to spatial frequency and orientation.

Neural Responses to Non-Cartesian Gratings in Area V4

The large effects of texture size obtained in our studies of 3D textured surfaces prompted us to reassess our approach to surface representation in area V4. We reasoned that if V4 responses are in large part a complex function of the spatial frequency and orientation spectrum, it might be profitable to investigate a different stimulus domain in which frequency and orientation information were both rich and easily controlled. We developed a new stimulus set consisting of sinusoidal gratings whose orientation and frequency are modulated according to several different basis functions. These gratings fall into three classes: conventional 2D sinusoidal gratings, polar gratings,

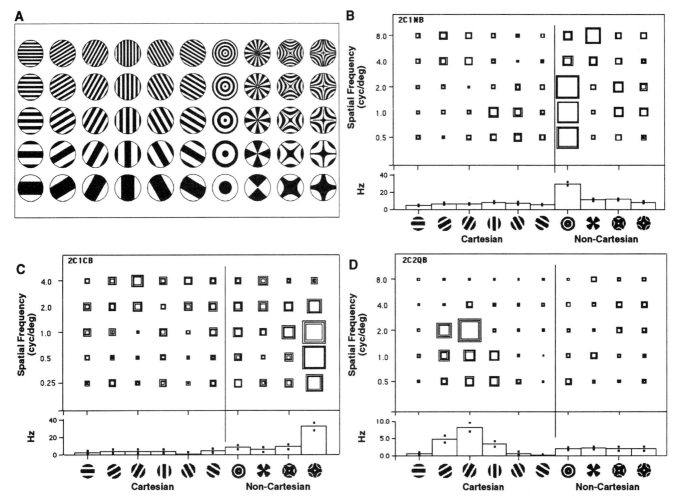

Figure 9.4

(*A*) Stimulus set consisting of Cartesian and non-Cartesian (polar and hyperbolic) gratings. For clarity square wave gratings are shown (though stimuli were sinusoidally modulated), and the frequency of high-frequency gratings has been reduced. Gratings used in the experiments were quantized to 250 luminance levels and were displayed for 0.5 sec on a neutral gray background. (*B*) Responses of a single V4 concentric cell to Cartesian and non-Cartesian gratings. The abscissa specifies grating type (six Cartesian grating orientations, concentric and radial gratings, and two hyperbolic grating orientations). The ordi-

nate specifies spatial frequency. The marginal histogram gives the mean firing rates and standard errors of the means collapsed across spatial frequency. Squares in the two-way plot give normalized relative firing rates and standard errors. (*C*) Responses of a single V4 hyperbolic cell to Cartesian and non-Cartesian gratings. (*D*) Responses of a single V4 Cartesian cell to the same stimulus set. When cells are tested with larger non-Cartesian stimulus set, Cartesian tuning such as this is quite rare. (Reprinted, with permission, from Gallant et al., 1993a.)

and hyperbolic gratings (see figure 9.4A). We refer to the conventional gratings as Cartesian stimuli, and the polar and hyperbolic gratings together as non-Cartesian stimuli. The various Cartesian and non-Cartesian stimuli are each correlated with different 3D texture shapes. Cartesian stimuli correspond most closely to planar textured surfaces, polar stimuli to textured spheres, and hyperbolic stimuli to textured saddles.

We recorded from 225 neurons in area V4 using these stimuli (Gallant et al., 1993a,b). The most striking finding was that some cells gave a highly selective response to certain non-Cartesian stimuli. Figure 9.4B illustrates the responses of one cell that was selective for concentric

gratings at several different frequencies, while figure 9.4C shows the responses of a cell that was selective for hyperbolic gratings having a particular orientation and a narrow range of frequencies. For comparison, figure 9.4D illustrates the responses of a cell that, according to our original tests, was selective for Cartesian gratings having a narrow range of orientations and frequencies. Overall, about one-fifth of the cells in our sample were significantly more responsive to the best non-Cartesian grating than to the best Cartesian grating. This one-fifth figure may be deceptively low, due to the conservative statistical test we used; the majority of cells gave a larger response to non-Cartesian than to Cartesian gratings.

More recent experiments using a much larger repertoire of non-Cartesian gratings (including spirals and a larger range of hyperbolic gratings) suggest that cells in area V4 that give a significantly greater response to Cartesian than non-Cartesian stimuli are surprisingly rare. We have used cluster analysis and multidimensional scaling techniques to categorize the responses of our 85 most thoroughly tested cells (Gallant et al., 1993b). The cluster analysis produces two primary cell classes, one whose exemplar (the average response vector of all the cells in the cluster) is highly selective for hyperbolic stimuli, and one whose exemplar is selective for polar stimuli. The polar class is further divided into several subclasses, and the exemplar of each subclass emphasizes a different region of the polar stimulus space. There appears to be a small subcluster that is highly selective for high-frequency radial gratings, and these responses may reflect the length- and width-tuned cells previously reported in area V4.

The non-Cartesian selectivity of cells in area V4 was unexpected given previous results obtained in area V1, where virtually all cells are reported to be highly selective for Cartesian gratings (De Valois and De Valois, 1990; but see Lehky and Sejnowski, 1992). The V4 responses also possess important spatial nonlinearities. For example, many of the cells are insensitive to either the local spatial position of patterns or their local phase. Though some cells are highly selective for spiral gratings, they are often not particularly selective for the sign of the spiral (left or right). Very few cells are selective for radial patterns. We are currently investigating the possibility that cells preferring radial stimuli correspond to a previously reported subpopulation that responds best to narrow bars (Desimone and Schein, 1987).

Cells in area V4 appear to be much more selective for members of our Cartesian and non-Cartesian stimulus set than to any of the 3D textured surfaces used in our earlier experiments. In addition, the overall responses elicited by the grating patterns are generally much larger than those elicited by the surface textures. We suspect that the effects of texture frequency and orientation obtained in our earlier experiments were due to the Cartesian and non-Cartesian tuning characteristics of cells in area V4. Furthermore, it is possible that these properties play a role in the perception of complex natural texture patterns, and of artificial textures such as Glass patterns (Glass, 1969).

Conclusion

Visual image segmentation and border identification appear to be carried out by a distributed and somewhat redundant system that can detect and represent borders based upon a wide variety of stimulus dimensions. Such mechanisms have previously been reported in areas V2 (DeYoe et al., 1986; von der Heydt, 1989), MT (Albright, 1992; Olavarria, 1992), and IT (Sary et al., 1993). Our experiments on texture borders demonstrate that mechanisms responsible for representing non-luminance-based borders exist in area V1 as well, and are probably related to those responsible for texture pop-out (Knierim and Van Essen, 1992). The system responsible for representing borders is organized around a few basic principles, one of which is linear filtering followed by nonlinear processes optimized so as to convert small narrow-band border signals into a larger broad-band border representation (Chubb and Sperling, 1988; von der Heydt and Peterhans, 1989; Malik and Perona, 1990; Sutter et al., 1989; Van Essen and Anderson, 1990; Victor et al., this volume). This process is analogous to the way amplitude-modulated signals are decomposed into carrier and modulator signals (Pelli, 1987). Our results suggest that areas V1 and V2 contain mechanisms sufficient for this type of processing.

Our experiments on 3D textured surfaces were meant to test proposals that one stage of visual processing involves the creation of a viewer-centered representation of visible surfaces. Unfortunately our experiments did not provide significant evidence in support of this hypothesis. Instead, the responses of V4 cells to 3D textured surfaces appeared to be related to their orientation and spatial frequency spectra. The results of the 3D FM grating experiments were somewhat clearer; responses were determined primarily by the 2D retinal orientation of the gratings.

It is possible that an explicit representation of surface orientation does exist in area V4, but our stimuli were insufficient to reveal it. Though this possibility could be examined with more sophisticated stimulation techniques (such as rendered stereo surfaces), we are not optimistic that such an experiment would produce substantially different results. A general representation of surface orientation should operate across a variety of different cues, and so its presence should be revealed with the 3D textured surfaces used here. On the other hand, certain cues such as stereo and motion parallax may be less cognitive than the texture cues used here, and so might reveal mechanisms of 3D representation that are not sensitive to texture stimuli.

The 2D frequency and orientation selectivity of area V4 cells were studied more systematically in our experiments using Cartesian and non-Cartesian gratings. These experiments suggest that the selectivity of V4 cells for frequency, and particularly for orientation, can be very complex, and yet can lead to well-behaved tuning profiles once the appropriate stimulus dimensions have been identified. We do not yet understand the visual function of these complex responses (but see Hoffman, 1966). Though there are several different functions that could conceivably be mediated by non-Cartesian cells (Gallant et al., 1993a), the focus of this chapter on texture brings one possibility to the fore: if natural images and texture have many attributes in common, perhaps we should regard non-Cartesian responses as a form of higher order texture processing. These responses might, for example, reflect complex local energy measurements underlying the processes of image segmentation and similarity grouping. These measurements could form the input to an essentially 2D image recognition system, or could be the basis for more sophisticated structural scene analysis.

Acknowledgments

We gratefully acknowledge many valuable discussions with Drs. B. Julesz and C. H. Anderson during the course of this research. These experiments were supported in part by grants from the Office of Naval Research, NATO, and the National Institutes of Health.

References

Albright, T. D. (1992). Form-cue invariant motion processing in primate visual cortex. *Science 225*, 1141–1143.

Bajcsy, R., and Lieberman, L. (1976). Texture gradient as a depth cue. *Comput. Graphics Image Process. 5*, 52–67.

Bergen, J. R., and Julesz, B. (1983). Parallel versus serial processing in rapid pattern discrimination. *Nature (London) 393*, 696–698.

Blake, A., Bulthoff, H. H., and Sheinberg, D. (1993). Shape from texture: Ideal observers and human psychophysics. *Vision Res. 33*, 1723–1737.

Bovik, A. C., Clark, M., and Geisler, W. S. (1990). Multichannel texture analysis using localized spatial filters. *IEEE Transact. Pattern Anal. Machine Intelligence 12*, 55–73.

Chubb, C., and Sperling, G. (1988). Drift-balanced random stimuli: A general basis for studying non-Fourier motion perception. *J. Opt. Soc. Am. A 5*, 1986–2007.

Cumming, B. G., Johnston, E. B., and Parker, A. J. (1993). Effects of different texture cues on curved surfaces viewed stereoscopically. *Vision Res. 33*, 827–838.

Cutting, J. E., and Millard, R. T. (1984). Three gradients and the perception of flat and curved surfaces. *J. Exp. Psychol. General 113*, 198–216.

Desimone, R., and Schein, S. J. (1987). Visual properties of neurons in area V4 of the macaque: Sensitivity to stimulus form. *J. Neurophysiol. 57*, 835–868.

Desimone, R., Albright, T. D., Gross, C. G., and Bruce, C. (1984). *J. Neurosci. 4*, 2051–2062.

De Valois, R. L., and De Valois, K. K. (1990). *Spatial Vision.* New York: Oxford.

DeYoe, E. A., Knierim, J. J., Sagi, D., Julesz, B., and Van Essen, D. C. (1986). Single unit responses to static and dynamic texture patterns in macaque V2 and V1 cortex. *Invest. Ophthalmol. Visual Sci. Suppl. 27*, 18.

Gallant, J. L., Braun, J., and Van Essen, D. C. (1991). Responses of cells in area V4 of macaque visual cortex to simulated 3D surfaces. *Soc. Neurosci. Abstr. 17*, 525.

Gallant, J. L., Braun, J., and Van Essen, D. C. (1993a). Selectivity for polar, hyperbolic, and Cartesian gratings in macaque visual cortex. *Science 259*, 100–103.

Gallant, J. L., Connor, E. C., Rakshit, S., and Van Essen, D. C. (1993b). Selectivity for polar and hyperbolic gratings in macaque visual area V4: Multivariate classification and anatomical distribution. *Soc. Neurosci. Abstr. 19*, 771.

Gibson, J. J. (1966). *The Senses Considered as Perceptual Systems.* Boston: Houghton-Mifflin.

Glass, L. (1969). Moire effects from random dots. *Nature (London) 223*, 578–580.

Gulyas, B., Orban, G. A., Duysens, J., and Maes, H. (1987). The suppressive influence of moving textured backgrounds on responses of cat striate neurons to moving bars. *J. Neurophysiol. 57*, 1767–1791.

Hammond, P., and MacKay, D. M. (1975). Differential responses of cat visual cortical cells to textured stimuli. *Exp. Brain Res. 22*, 427–430.

Hammond, P., and MacKay, D. M. (1977). Differential responsiveness of simple and complex cells in cat striate cortex to visual texture. *Exp. Brain Res. 30*, 275–296.

Hoffman, W. C. (1966). The Lie algebra and visual perception. *J. Math. Psychol. 3*, 65–98.

Julesz, B. (1981). Textons, the elements of texture perception, and their interactions. *Nature (London) 290*, 91–97.

Julesz, B. (1984). Toward an axiomatic theory of preattentive vision. In G. Edelman, M. Cowen, and E. Gall (Eds.), *Dynamic Aspects of Neocortical Function* (pp. 585–612). New York: Wiley.

Julesz, B. (1986). Texton gradients: the texton theory revisited. *Biol. Cybern. 54*, 245–251.

Julesz, B. (1991). Early vision and focal attention. *Rev. Modern Phys. 63*, 735–772.

Knierim, J. J., and Van Essen, D. C. (1992). Neuronal responses to static texture patterns in area V1 of the alert macaque monkeys. *J. Neurophysiol. 67*, 961–980.

Lehky, S. R., Sejnowski, T. J., and Desimone, R. (1992). Predicting responses of nonlinear neurons in monkey striate cortex to complex patterns. *J. Neurosci. 9*, 3566–3581.

Lowe, D. G. (1990). Visual recognition as probabilistic inference from spatial relations. In A. Blake and T. Troscianko (Eds.), *AI and the Eye* (pp. 261–279). New York: Wiley.

Luschow, A., and Nothdurft, H. C. (1993). Pop-out of orientation but no pop-out of motion at isoluminance. *Vision Res. 33*, 91–104.

Malik, J., and Perona, P. (1990). Preattentive texture discrimination with early visual mechanisms. *J. Opt. Soc. Am. A 7*, 923–932.

Marr, D. (1982). *Vision*. San Francisco: Plenum.

Milewski, A., and Yonas, A. (1977). Texture size specificity in the slant aftereffect. *Percept. Psychophys. 21*, 47–49.

Nothdurft, H. C. (1991). Texture segmentation and pop-out from orientation contrast. *Vision Res. 31*, 1073–1078.

Nothdurft, H. C. (1990a). Texton segregation by associated differences in global and local luminance distribution. *Proc. R. Soc. London B 239*, 295–320.

Nothdurft, H. C. (1990b). Texture discrimination by cells in the cat lateral geniculate nucleus. *Exp. Brain Res. 82*, 48–66.

Nothdurft, H. C., and Li, C. Y. (1984). Representation of spatial details in textured patterns by cells of the cat striate cortex. *Exp. Brain Res. 57*, 9–21.

Nothdurft, H. C., and Li, C. Y. (1985). Texture discrimination: Representation of orientation and luminance differences in cells of the cat striate cortex. *Vision Res. 25*, 99–113.

Nothdurft, H. C., Gallant, J. L., and Van Essen, D. C. (1992). Neural responses to texture borders in macaque area V1. *Soc Neurosci. Abstr. 18*, 1275.

Olavarria, J. F., DeYoe, E. A., Knierim, J. J., Fox, J. M., and Van Essen, D. C. (1992). Neural responses to visual texture patterns in middle temporal area of the macaque monkey. *J. Neurophysiol. 68*, 164–181.

Pelli, E. (1987). Perception of high-pass filtered images. *Proc. SPIE 845*, 140–146.

Pentland, A. (1985). *Perceptual Organization and the Representation of Natural Form* (Note 357). Menlo Park, CA: SRI International.

Pentland, A. (1989). Shape information from shading: A theory about human perception. *Spatial Vision 4*, 165–182.

Plaut, D. C., and Farah, M. J. (1990). Visual object representation: Interpreting neurophysiological data within a computational framework. *J. Cog. Neurosci. 2*, 320–343.

Poggio, T., and Edelman, S. (1990). A network that learns to recognize three-dimensional objects. *Nature (London) 343*, 263–266.

Sary, G., Vogels, R., and Orban, G. A. (1993). Cue-invariant shape selectivity of macaque inferior temporal neurons. *Science 260*, 995–998.

Schein, S. J., and Desimone, R. (1990). Spectral properties of V4 neurons in the macaque. *J. Neurosci. 10*, 3369–3389.

Stevens, K. A. (1981). The information content of texture gradients. *Biol. Cybern. 42*, 92–105.

Sutter, A., Beck, J., and Graham, N. (1989). Contrast and spatial variables in texture segregation: Testing a simple spatial-frequency channels model. *Percept. Psychophys. 46*, 312–332.

Tanaka, K., Saito, H.-A., Fukada, Y., and Moriya, M. (1991). Coding of visual images of objects in the inferotemporal cortex of the macaque monkey. *J. Neurophysiol. 66*, 170–189.

Todd, J. T., and Akerstrom, R. A. (1987). Perception of three-dimensional form from patterns of optical texture. *J. Exp. Psychol. Human Percept. Perform. 13*, 242–255.

Todd, J. T., and Mingolla, E. (1983). Perception of surface curvature and direction of ilumination from patterns of shading. *J. Exp. Psychol. Human Percept. Perform. 9*, 583–595.

Treisman, A. M., and Gelade, G. (1980). A feature-integration theory of attention. *Cog. Psychol. 2*, 97–136.

Ullman, S. (1990). Three-dimensional object recognition. *Cold Spring Harbor Symp. Quant. Biol. 4*, 889–898.

Van Essen, D. C., and Anderson, C. H. (1990). Information processing strategies and pathways in the primate retina and visual cortex. In S. F. Zornetzer, J. L. Davis, and C. Lau (Eds.), *Introduction to Neural and Electronic Networks* (pp. 43–72). Orlando, FL: Academic Press.

Van Essen, D. C., DeYoe, E. A., Olavarria, J. F., Knierim, J. J., Fox, J. M., Sagi, D., Julesz, B. (1989). Neural responses to static and moving texture patterns in visual cortex of the macaque monkey. In D. M.-K. Lam and C. Gilbert (Eds.), *Neural Mechanisms of Visual Perception* (pp. 137–154). Woodlands, TX: Portfolio.

von der Heydt, R., and Peterhans, E. (1989). Mechanisms of contour perception in monkey visual cortex. I. Lines of pattern discontinuity. *J. Neurosci. 9*, 1731–1748.

Witkin, A. (1981). Recovering surface shape and orientation from texture. *Artificial Intelligence 17*, 17–45.

10

Isodipole Textures: A Window on Cortical Mechanisms of Form Processing

Jonathan D. Victor,
Mary M. Conte, Keith Purpura,
and Ephraim Katz

Isodipole textures were introduced by Julesz as counter-examples to his conjecture concerning preattentive visual processing. Subsequently, a number of variations on the original isodipole textures have been developed. This chapter summarizes the theoretical basis of the isodipole texture technique and describes some of the insights that have resulted from its use in the analysis of cortical processing of form.

A Perspective on Isodipole Textures

Identification of borders between objects is a necessary step in the visual analysis of any scene. The visual system performs this task rapidly, seemingly effortlessly, and without the need for focused attention. One theme of Julesz' work is that such segmentations are based on statistical properties of neural population responses, rather than on the precise level of activity in individual neurons. More than 20 years ago, Julesz and co-workers (1973) hypothesized that a restricted set of statistics—"dipole statistics"—sufficed to account for preattentive segmentation and discrimination.

Dipole statistics are the second level in a hierarchy of statistical characterizations of visual textures. At the bottom of the hierarchy are first-order statistics, which describe the frequency with which points of an image have specific luminance values. First-order statistics thus constitute the distribution (histogram) of luminance values. Dipole statistics describe the frequency with which pairs of points of an image at a given relative separation have specific luminance values. Third-order statistics describe the frequency with which triplets of points of an image at given relative separations have specific luminance values. Fourth- and higher-order statistics are defined in an analogous fashion.

It is important to recognize that the Julesz conjecture applies to visual textures, not to specific images (see Yellott, 1993 and Victor, 1993 for additional discussion on this issue). The conceptual distinction is that a texture is a *family* of images that shares certain statistical properties. The concept of a texture is meant to capture the ability of the visual system to classify and process certain images in a manner that does not depend on the specific location of their individual features (see Caelli, this volume, and Watt, this volume).

The significance of the Julesz conjecture is most readily appreciated for visual textures composed of two luminance levels. For such textures, first-order statistics specify only the average luminance. Clearly, textures with the same average luminance may be readily distinguishable on the basis of the spatial distribution (i.e., granularity) of the luminance. Thus, sensitivity of first-order statistics alone cannot account for texture discrimination. Second-order (dipole) statistics begin to describe the spatial distribution of luminance values. For visual textures composed of two luminance levels, dipole statistics are equivalent to the global power spectrum. Thus, for such textures, the hypothesis that isodipole textures cannot be discriminated is equivalent to the claim that luminance and global power spectrum determine preattentive texture discrimination. In neurophysiologic terms, this would mean that texture discrimination is based on the overall level of activity in populations of neurons with common spatial-filtering properties. The neurophysiologic interpretation holds provided that one can consider visual neurons to be well approximated by *linear* spatial filters.

In 1978, Julesz and co-workers (Caelli and Julesz, 1978; Julesz et al., 1978; Victor and Brodie, 1978) identified several counterexamples to the claim that isodipole textures could not be discriminated. These examples showed that local processing must be more complex than linear spatial filtering, since all of these texture pairs would generate equal population-averaged responses in arrays of linear filters. While the idea that cortical neurons are nonlinear is certainly not a novel one, the psychophysical observations are important in two ways: they identify a functional significance for spatial nonlinearities, and they provide a rich stimulus set for further analysis of these nonlinearities (see Sagi, this volume).

We focus on the isodipole textures (Julesz et al., 1978) shown in figure 10.1a, b, and c. These textures consist of assignments of two luminance values (e.g., dark or light) to each check on a lattice. The assignment of a luminance value to a check is determined by the value of its state $a_{i,j}$, which is $+1$ or -1. The states of the checks in the initial row and column ($a_{0,j}$ and $a_{i,0}$) are assigned at random to $+1$ or -1. The states of the checks in the interior of the texture are defined recursively. For the even texture, the recursion rule is $a_{i+1,j+1} = a_{i,j}a_{i+1,j}a_{i,j+1}$, so that all 2×2 subregions contain an even number of checks in the state $+1$. For the odd texture, the recursion rule is $a_{i+1,j+1} = -a_{i,j}a_{i+1,j}a_{i,j+1}$, so that all 2×2 subregions contain an odd number of checks in the state $+1$.

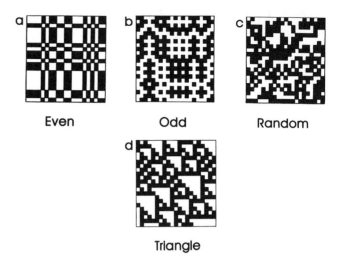

Figure 10.1
Examples of the even (*a*), odd (*b*), random (*c*) and triangle-glider (*d*) textures. These four textures have identical dipole statistics, and the first three textures have identical third-order statistics.

These textures, along with the texture in which all states are assigned at random ("the random texture"), have identical second-order statistics, and are therefore isodipole textures. Moreover, the third-order spatial correlation statistics of these textures are equal. These statistical properties, along with several extensions of the above construction, are key to our strategy for analyzing the spatial nonlinearities that underlie the neural processing of visual form.

Visual Evoked Potential Analysis

We chose to augment the psychophysical studies of texture discrimination with visual evoked potential (VEP) measurements (Victor, 1985; Victor and Zemon, 1985; Victor and Conte, 1989b). VEPs are the net result of neural activity in visual cortex as registered by scalp surface electrodes (Regan, 1989). There were two main reasons for choosing this approach: VEP analysis would allow direct examination of response dynamics, and would also allow an immediate bridge to animal studies. The stimuli for the VEP studies consisted of a sequence of sample textures drawn alternately from two texture classes. That is, a typical visual stimulus consists of (even texture example 1, random texture example 1, even texture example 2, random texture example 2, . . .), with each texture example presented for approximately 250 msec. VEP signals were averaged over a period, which included one sample of each texture.

This averaged VEP response was decomposed into two components: a symmetric component, which is the average of the response to each interchange, and an antisymmetric component, which is the difference between the response to the onset of the even texture and the onset of the random texture. The antisymmetric response component necessarily isolates neural mechanisms that respond differentially to the two texture classes. Because of the statistical properties of the isodipole textures, mechanisms that are sensitive merely to local luminance and contrast changes cannot contribute to the antisymmetric component, but only to the symmetric response component. The dynamics and contrast dependence of the symmetric response component resembled the traditional P-100 component of the VEP. The antisymmetric response component had a higher contrast threshold and more sluggish dynamics (Victor and Conte, 1987b), and was present only in response to *discriminable* isodipole pairs. We focus on the antisymmetric response component, and use its dependence on texture statistics to develop models for the neural computations underlying texture discrimination.

Models for the Generation of the Antisymmetric Response Component

The statistical properties of the even, odd, and random textures permit immediate elimination of certain classes of models—linear models and models whose formal order of nonlinearity is three or less, for example. However, one goal of this work is the development of plausible (and testable) models for the computations that underlie local form extraction, and not just the exclusion of various candidates. To constrain such models, we developed several variations on the even, odd, and random textures. Each of these variations led to guidelines for viable models.

Partially Decorrelated Textures

The even, random, and odd textures can be viewed as members of a continuum. Consider the probability $P_{1,1}$ that a 2×2 subregion of checks within one of these textures contains an even number of bright checks. In the even texture, this probability is 1. In the random texture, this probability is 0.5. In the odd texture, this probability is 0. This probability is directly related to the fourth-order correlation among these checks, $c_{1,1} = \langle a_{i,j} a_{i+1,j} a_{i,j+1} a_{i+1,j+1} \rangle$. With the convention that a bright check corresponds to state $+1$ and a dark check corresponds to state -1, the relationship is $c_{1,1} = 2P_{1,1} - 1$. Thus, $c_{1,1} = 1$ for the even texture, 0 for the random texture, and -1 for the odd texture.

There are several ways to create textures with intermediate values of the correlation $c_{1,1}$ that retain the isodipole property (Victor and Conte, 1989b). These textures not only share all statistics up to (and including) third-order, but also have identical *local* correlations at fourth order. They differ in the strength of long-range fourth-order correlations, and this difference allows an experimental analysis of the role of these long-range correlations.

One way of creating such textures is by "sporadic decorrelation." A texture with sporadic decorrelation is created from a standard even texture by inversion of the state of some randomly chosen fraction ε_{spor} of the checks. This leads to a new texture for which $c_{1,1} = (1 - 2\varepsilon_{spor})^4$. A second way of creating such textures is by "propagated decorrelation." To create a texture with propagated decorrelation, the usual recursion rule $a_{i+1,j+1} = a_{i,j} a_{i+1,j} a_{i,j+1}$ for the even texture is replaced by a stochastic rule: $a_{i+1,j+1} = a_{i,j} a_{i+1,j} a_{i,j+1}$ with probability $1 - \varepsilon_{prop}$, and $a_{i+1,j+1} = -a_{i,j} a_{i+1,j} a_{i,j+1}$ with probability ε_{prop}. That is, inversions are generated with probability ε_{prop}, and are propagated through the rest of the texture. This leads to a new texture for which $c_{1,1} = 1 - 2\varepsilon_{prop}$. By setting $(1 - 2\varepsilon_{spor})^4 = 1 - 2\varepsilon_{prop}$, one may generate sporadic- and propagated-decorrelation textures with identical short-range correlation $c_{1,1}$. The crucial point is that these textures differ in their long-range correlations. In textures with propagated decorrelation, long-range correlations decline exponentially with distance. In textures with sporadic decorrelation, long-range and short-range correlations are equal.

Sporadic and propagated decorrelation processes can be combined to create textures for which $c_{1,1} = (1 - 2\varepsilon_{spor})^4 (1 - 2\varepsilon_{prop})$. Furthermore, these processes are only two examples of a more general decorrelation strategy, which consists of random placement of multiple examples of a template of a specific size and shape on a standard even texture, followed by inversion of checks that lie in an odd number of these templates. The sporadic decorrelation process corresponds to templates that consist of single checks. The propagated decorrelation process is the limiting case of templates, which are large rectangles. All of these decorrelation processes do not change statistics up to order 3, and all result in ergodic textures. (Ergodicity is a statistical property that is required to guarantee that most individual texture examples typify the texture ensemble.)

Differences in responses to even textures with sporadic and propagated decorrelation can be used to identify the role of long-range correlations. If long-range correlations were required for generation of the antisymmetric response component, then the antisymmetric response component would disappear in textures with propagated decorrelation. Alternatively, if the antisymmetric response component depended only on short-range correlations, then textures that shared the same value of $c_{1,1}$ should elicit identical responses, independent of the nature of the decorrelation.

Experimental results (Victor and Conte, 1987a, 1989b) fell between these two extremes. Textures with propagated decorrelation were distinguishable from random textures by psychophysical and VEP measures, but the distinguishability of these textures was smaller than for textures with sporadic decorrelation and the same value of $c_{1,1}$. Qualitatively, this implies that long-range correlations are not required for texture discrimination, but that correlations are relevant over a distance that exceeds the smallest block (2×2) of checks.

For textures subjected to sporadic decorrelation, the amplitude of the antisymmetric response component was very nearly proportional to $c_{1,1}$, and the dynamics were independent of $c_{1,1}$. For textures with propagated decorrelation, dynamics were also independent of $c_{1,1}$, but VEP response size depended on $c_{1,1}$ in a more complex fashion. We used the details of this dependence to determine the relative importance of correlations at various distances. Response size was modeled as a convolution of an assumed weight $w(i,j)$ with the correlation strength $c_{i,j}$ among the corners of an $(i + 1) \times (j + 1)$ rectangle. For textures with sporadic decorrelation, $c_{i,j} = (1 - 2\varepsilon_{\text{spor}})^4$. For textures with propagated decorrelation, $c_{i,j} = (1 - 2\varepsilon_{\text{prop}})^4$. We found (Victor and Conte, 1989b) that a weight $w(i,j)$ that declines exponentially with distance provides a very good fit to the observed responses to both kinds of textures. Weights that were concentrated along a thin (nearly one-dimensional) region provided somewhat better fits, but the difference between one-dimensional and two-dimensional weights was not present in all subjects.

Thus, we concluded that an adequate model would require sensitivity to spatial interactions over a distance of several checks along a one-dimensional strip. Furthermore, over a modest range of check sizes (4 to 16 min), the inferred length of this strip was proportional to check size—consistent with the idea that texture processing is approximately scale-invariant.

Role of Spatial Phase

The isodipole condition guarantees equality of spatial frequency content (and autocorrelations) at the level of texture ensemble, and we have used this statistical property to constrain features for a local computational model. However, individual examples of even and random textures are not exactly matched for spatial frequency content. In principle, these small differences might support texture discrimination via global spatial frequency statistics. We (Victor and Conte, 1993) evaluated this possibility by another extension of the isodipole texture construction.

In this construction, even and random textures were manipulated in a way that preserved their power spectrum exactly, at the level of the individual texture *example*. The first step of the construction is a two-dimensional Fourier transform of example of even and random textures that have been smoothed to soften the edges. Then, each Fourier component is shifted in phase by an independently chosen random amount in the range $[-\Phi, \Phi]$. The Fourier transform is then inverted. (The preliminary step of low-pass filtering is to avoid "ringing" of these phase-jittered textures.) The resulting textures have the same power spectrum as the smoothed texture that were subjected to the initial Fourier transform, since the Fourier amplitudes are unchanged. Models based on a global analysis thus predict that discriminability of even and random textures would be unaffected by the phase jitter Φ.

We found (Victor and Conte, 1993) that the antisymmetric response component depended strongly on Φ. For the 4 min check size, responses were attenuated by a factor of 2 as Φ approached π radians (full randomization). For check sizes 8 min or greater, the antisymmetric response component was essentially zero for $\Phi \geqslant 0.5\pi$ radians. Since phase-jittering preserves the differences in the global power spectra of the texture examples, the absence of an antisymmetric component under phase-jittered conditions implies the global power spectral differences can play at most a minor role in the generation of the antisymmetric VEP component.

Conveniently, there is a common asymptotic limit for spatial-phase dependence of models based on local non-linear subunits. Provided that the subunit is smaller than the check, the dependence of the antisymmetric response component on the amount Φ of phase jitter is approximately $[(\sin \Phi)/\Phi]^4$. For checks of size 8 min or greater, the observed dependence on Φ was well-approximated by this formula. This is consistent with the results of the propagated-decorrelation experiments described above—which suggested a range of scales of computational units extending down to check sizes of 4 min, but not smaller.

Other Gliders, and a Model for the Local Computation

The analysis of spatial phase confirms the notion that the antisymmetric response component is generated by a local computation, rather than one that is sensitive to global statistics of individual texture examples. To constrain internal structures for candidate models, we used a third variation on the construction of the isodipole textures (Victor and Conte, 1989a, 1991). As Gilbert (1980) has shown, it is possible to use a wide variety of recursion relationships to generate additional textures, all of which have the isodipole property and all of which are ergodic. In all of these textures, the recursion relationship is specified by a template of checks (a "glider") whose parity is constrained. (Additionally, it is possible to apply the decorrelation and spatial-phase constructions described above to textures based on alternate gliders.)

We studied nine such isodipole textures—two third-order textures and seven fourth-order textures. Isodipole textures based on some gliders were readily distinguishable from the random texture, while isodipole textures based on other gliders required sustained visual attention to distinguish from the random texture. Visual salience assayed psychophysically correlated closely with the size of the antisymmetric response component elicited in response to alternation with the random texture.

Based on the studies with decorrelated textures, we proposed a provisional model for local form analysis (figure 10.2). The model consisted of two nonlinear stages: local band-pass filtering and partial rectification of these local signals, followed by cooperative pooling of these rectified signals over a narrow strip. This model accounted for which gliders led to textures with visually salient structure, and which did not. Essentially, the stage of cooperative pooling endowed the model with sensitivity to higher order interactions over a moderate spatial extent, as was shown to be necessary by the studies based on decorrelated textures. Alternative models—based on glider size, glider symmetry, and the information content of the texture (in the sense of Shannon, 1948)—failed to

account for which textures had visually salient structure, and which did not.

The salient features of the provisional model are (1) an initial array of N subunits in which a linearly filtered transformation of the visual input is locally rectified, and (2) a second stage in which these rectified outputs are summed and subjected to a second threshold set at Nh. We found (Victor and Conte, 1991) that at least $N = 6$ such subunits are required to provide reasonably texture-specific responses; further increases in the number of subunits increase specificity but only at the expense of response size. The second threshold h is also required to provide specificity, but too high a value for h produces an unreasonable loss in response size. Modeling could not determine whether the subunits must have an oriented internal structure, but, if the subunits are oriented, their axes must be perpendicular to the subunit array. Long-range cooperative interactions of units with similar orientation tuning is consistent with current concepts of long-range connections in primary visual cortex (Ts'o et al., 1986).

Previous investigators (Jones and Palmer, 1987; Movshon et al., 1978a,b; Spitzer and Hochstein, 1985) have proposed models of simple or complex-cell receptive field structure that consist of linear filters combined with a single nonlinearity. These models were constructed to account for responses to bars, gratings, and noise. For these stimuli, our two-nonlinearity model collapses to a one-nonlinearity model. This is because such stimuli would drive the subunits in synchrony (for a stimulus parallel to the long axis of the model), one at a time (for a stimulus perpendicular to the long axis of the model), or independently (for an uncorrelated noise stimulus). That is, the need for the second nonlinearity and the inadequacy of previous models are apparent only because we have used complex stimuli with spatial structure along two dimensions.

There are at least two ways in which this model framework must be incomplete. A detailed analysis of the VEP responses showed that textures based on triangular three-element gliders (figure 10.1d) generated an antisymmetric response component whose dynamics differed subtly from the dynamics of the responses generated by the other textures. This small but consistent difference suggests that it is an oversimplification to assume that all antisymmetric response components are generated by a single computational mechanism with stereotyped dynamics.

The second way in which the model is necessarily incomplete is related to its dependence on overall contrast. The model's specificity relies on the threshold of the second nonlinearity. As overall stimulus contrast increases,

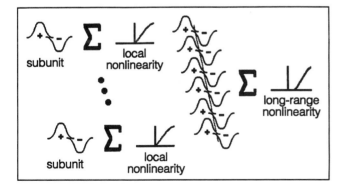

Figure 10.2
A provisional model for local form analysis, featuring two nonlinear stages.

the size of the signals generated by the first (local) nonlinearity will increase, and will eventually surpass the threshold of the second nonlinearity. Thus, the model would predict that specificity will be lost at higher contrasts. To avoid the loss of specificity with increasing contrast, it is necessary for the level of the second threshold (or, equivalently, the gain of the subunits) to be adjusted by overall stimulus contrast.

This kind of adjustment would be provided by a cortical contrast gain control, for which experimental evidence has already been obtained (Ohzawa et al., 1985). The maintenance of specificity over a range of contrasts is likely to be the main role of a cortical contrast gain control. The need for a contrast gain control to preserve tuning properties across a range of contrasts has also emerged from the more traditional view of cortical cells as spatial filters (Heeger, 1992). However, the stimulus specificity of this postulated gain control, and how it interacts with form analysis (i.e., feedforward vs. feedback, divisive vs. threshold elevating, etc.) remains an area for future work.

Animal Studies

The minimal requirements for a computational mechanism that could generate an antisymmetric response component include interactions of formal order 4 (or greater) among four locations in space. Because this degree of complexity was not part of existing views of simple or complex receptive fields (Hubel and Wiesel, 1968; Jones and Palmer, 1987; Movshon et al., 1978a,b; Spitzer and Hochstein, 1985), we initially hypothesized (Victor, 1985; Victor and Zemon, 1985) that these computations took place in extrastriate regions.

Initial studies in primates consisted of epicortical field potential recordings in the anaesthetized, paralyzed macaque monkey (Purpura and Victor, 1990a). In contrast to our expectations, epicortical potentials revealed strong antisymmetric response components over V1. The temporal configuration of these components, and their dependence on texture type were very similar to that of the antisymmetric response component observed in man.

One possibility is that the antisymmetric response component was generated by a specialized subpopulation of cortical neurons. Indeed, this would be one literal interpretation of the provisional model—the first nonlinearity (the local nonlinear subunits) represented one class of cortical cells, and the second nonlinearity (the long-range pooling) might represent another class in a processing hierarchy. We therefore examined the laminar organiza-

tion of the antisymmetric response to isodipole textures (Purpura et al., 1992). These studies were performed with a multichannel microelectrode (Schroeder et al., 1991) consisting of 15 electrodes spaced at 150 μm intervals and one distal contact at a spacing of 1000 μm.

To examine laminar profiles, local field potentials recorded along the electrode array were combined to generate current source density records (Freeman and Nicholson, 1975). Calculated current source densities elicited by texture interchange were decomposed into symmetric and antisymmetric response components in a manner analogous to the decomposition of VEP data. The symmetric response component elicited by texture interchange was essentially independent of which class of textures was used. The antisymmetric response component was large only for interchanges between different classes of textures, and the even/random and even/odd responses were larger than the odd/random responses. The symmetric response component had a more transient time course than did the antisymmetric response component. These were the same features we had previously seen in the scalp and epicortical records.

However, despite the differential dependence of the symmetric and antisymmetric response components on the stimulus, they had essentially identical laminar profiles. Based on evidence of ocular dominance and orientation tuning in other recordings with this electrode (Katz et al., 1992), we estimate an effective summing area for the current source density to be approximately 150 μm at each recording site. Thus, at this level of resolution, it does not appear that the antisymmetric response component is generated by a specific class of cortical neurons. Rather, the colocalization of the symmetric and the antisymmetric response components suggests that the computational complexity required to extract local form elements (and not just spatial filtering) is a frequent feature of the neurons of primary visual cortex. Along with other recent observations (Gallant et al., this volume), our findings make it difficult to continue to view primary visual cortex simply as a bank of spatial filters.

Applications of Isodipole Textures to Other Visual Modalities

The statistical properties of isodipole textures facilitate experiments that separate linear spatial filtering and extraction of local features. This distinction is important not just in the processing of static monochromatic textures. This section discusses applications of isodipole textures in the analysis of color and motion processing.

Color and Texture

Detection and processing of visual form are markedly reduced when luminance cues are removed from an image, leaving only chromatic differences—a finding that has been interpreted as a separation of central processing of color and form signals (Livingstone and Hubel, 1987). An alternative explanation is that the apparently minor nature of chromatic input to form analysis is merely a consequence of a difference in the overall sensitivities of luminance and chromatic pathways (Mullen, 1985).

Isodipole textures provide a way to address this issue. As described above, the antisymmetric component of the VEP, by definition, is generated only by neural mechanisms that are differentially sensitive to the even and random texture classes, and thus measures sensitivity to some aspects of visual form. Simultaneously, the symmetric component of the VEP provides a measure of sensitivity to luminance or contrast.

These considerations hold equally well for textures in which the black and white regions are replaced by regions which differ in color. We (Purpura and Victor, 1990b; Victor and Purpura, 1992) examined the VEPs elicited by such stimuli to determine whether the antisymmetric component was selectively eliminated when only chromatic signals were present. VEP responses to checkerboard pattern appearance were used as a control for changes in the spatial filtering properties of the visual system under near-isoluminant conditions. Though the experimental design is simple in principle, there are a variety of technical issues, such as the chromatic aberration of the eye and spatial inhomogeneities in both the retina and a CRT display, which need to be considered. To circumvent these problems, we (1) blurred the stimuli to eliminate high spatial frequencies, and (2) used a sequence of texture stimuli that swept a range of color and luminance values, in order to ensure that we closely bracketed the point at which luminance signals were most nearly eliminated. The results of this study were striking: near isoluminance, the antisymmetric response component was essentially absent, while the pattern appearance response persisted, or even enlarged.

On the basis of these results, it is tempting to postulate that form processing simply has no access to chromatic signals, consistent with a strict interpretation of the concept of separate processing of color and form. However, another series of experiments clearly demonstrated that processing of form is strongly influenced by the chromatic composition of the input, even though the response to isodipole interchange cannot be driven by chromatic signals alone. These studies compared the adapting effects of a monochromatic adapting field on the response to isodipole interchange (K. Purpura, J. D. Victor, and J. Gordon, unpublished results). Under the hypothesis that the isodipole response is driven only by luminance inputs, the adapting effects of the monochromatic field should be proportional to its luminance, independent of its wavelength. However, suppression of the antisymmetric component by adapting fields of short wavelengths (490 nm or less) was threefold greater than would be expected from luminance alone. Adapting fields in the range 560 to 590 nm also produced a greater attenuation of the antisymmetric response than would be expected from their luminance. The wavelength-dependent effect of the adapting field is clear evidence of chromatic input to form processing. The short-wavelength effect is consistent with a blue-cone input to form processing, but the 560–590 nm effect suggests a role for opponent mechanisms as well.

In sum, when luminance signals are absent, chromatic signals alone fail to support form processing. However, when luminance signals are present, chromatic and luminance signals interact strongly in form processing.

Motion and Texture

Standard models for the extraction of visual motion are based on cross-correlation (Reichardt, 1961; Nakayama, 1985). In the context of the Fourier representation of an image as a superposition of drifting gratings, cross-correlation translates into an analysis of the energy contained in the various Fourier components (Adelson and Bergen, 1985).

Cross-correlation and Fourier energy models account for the perception of motion in most stimuli that appear to be moving. However, Chubb and Sperling (1988) devised several families of stimuli that elicit the strong sense of motion but produce no net motion signal from standard motion models. Since the percept of motion in these stimuli cannot be extracted from the energy in its individual Fourier components, these stimuli have been called "non-Fourier motion stimuli." A simple example of a non-Fourier motion stimulus is a gray occluder drifting in front of a random black and white noise field. For this stimulus, cross-correlations between the occluder and the background become zero when the luminance of the stimulus matches the mean luminance of the background, yet motion remains prominent under this condition.

Chubb and Sperling (1989) modified the standard cross-correlation model by adding a preliminary stage of local filtering and rectification prior to standard motion analysis. This preliminary stage can be thought of as a preprocessor that extracts (unsigned) contrast and temporal contrast changes, and presents these signals to the cross-correlation stage. The modified model properly extracts motion signals from a wide variety of non-Fourier stimuli that elicit a strong percept of motion.

Consider next a visual stimulus consisting of alternating bands of textures, with the borders between the bands drifting uniformly from frame to frame. The preprocessing stage postulated by Chubb and Sperling (1989) would be insensitive to borders defined by isodipole textures, and thus their model would predict that motion perception would be significantly reduced for a stimulus whose bands were alternately examples of the even and the random textures (even though the texture boundaries would be readily apparent). Indeed, this somewhat counterintuitive result is exactly what we (Victor and Conte, 1990) found! Although direction of motion in such stimuli could be determined, this determination required approximately 300 msec of observation. The subjective impression was that the task was performed by judging positional changes with time, and not by judging motion as such. These observations support the notion that the preprocessor involved in non-Fourier motion processing is not sensitive to form as such, but just to spatial-frequency and temporal-frequency content.

Summary

We have described many of the salient findings that have resulted from the use of isodipole texture stimuli. Discrimination of isodipole textures implies analysis based on local (nonlinear) extraction of features, and not simply spatial-filtering operations. The spatial scale of these operations was identified by introduction of sporadic and propagated errors into the texture construction. Manipulation of spatial phase and modification of the recursion "glider" provided additional constraints for the spatial structure of form analysis. From these constraints and notions of biological plausibility, we developed a two-stage model for cortical form analysis, in which locally rectified signals are combined by a second nonlinear stage of larger spatial extent. Field potential and single-unit studies in the macaque indicate that these processes take place in V1, and colocalize with signals reflecting linear spatial filtering.

Investigation of the chromatic inputs to local feature processing through the use of chromatic isodipole textures and field adaptation studies leads to a complex picture of interaction of luminance and chromatic mechanisms. Incorporation of isodipole textures into motion stimuli provides an upper limit for the complexity of texture information that is available for motion processing.

The provisional model for local form analysis requires a dynamic adjustment of gains (or thresholds) based on local contrast. Exploration of the mechanism of this adjustment is likely to provide insight into interactions of visual submodalities and the operation of the cortical contrast gain control.

Acknowledgments

Supported in part by NIH grants EY1428, EY7977, and EY9314, The McDonnell-Pew Foundation, The Revson Foundation, and The Hirschl Trust.

References

Adelson, E. H., and Bergen, J. (1985). Spatiotemporal energy models for the perception of motion. *J. Opt. Soc. Am. A 2*, 284–299.

Caelli, T., and Julesz, B. (1978). On perceptual analyzers underlying visual texture discrimination. Part I. *Biol. Cybern. 28*, 167–175.

Chubb, C., and Sperling, G. (1988). Drift-balanced random stimuli: a general basis for studying non-Fourier motion perception. *J. Opt. Soc. Am. A 5*, 1986–2006.

Chubb, C., and Sperling, G. (1989). Two motion perception mechanisms revealed through distance-driven reversal of apparent motion. *Proc. Natl. Acad. Sci. U.S.A. 86*, 2985–2989.

Freeman, J. A., and Nicholson, C. (1975). Experimental optimization of current source density technique for anuran cerebellum. *J. Neurophysiol. 38*, 369–382.

Gilbert, E. N. (1980). Random colorings of a lattice on squares in the plane. *SIAM J. Alg. Disc. Meth. 1*, 152–159.

Heeger, D. J. (1992). Normalization of cell responses in cat striate cortex. *Visual Neurosci. 9*, 181–197.

Hubel, D. H., and Wiesel, T. N. (1968). Receptive fields and functional architecture of monkey striate cortex. *J. Physiol. 195*, 215–243.

Jones, J. P., and Palmer, L. A. (1987). The two-dimensional spatial structure of simple receptive fields in cat striate cortex. *J. Neurophysiol. 58*, 1187–1211.

Julesz, B., Gilbert, E. N., Shepp, L. A., and Frisch, H. L. (1973). Inability of humans to discriminate between visual textures that agree in second-order statistics—revisited. *Perception 2*, 391–405.

Julesz, B., Gilbert, E. N., and Victor, J. D. (1978). Visual discrimination of textures with identical third-order statistics. *Biol. Cybern. 31*, 137–149.

Katz, E., Purpura, K., Mao, B., Schroeder, C., and Victor, J. D. (1992). Responses to broad-band and band-limited noise in V1: dependence on spatial frequency, color and orientation. *Soc. Neurosci. Abstr. 18*, 295.

Livingstone, M. S., and Hubel, D. H. (1987). Psychophysical evidence for separate channels for the perception of form, color, movement, and depth. *J. Neurosci. 7*, 3416–3468.

Movshon, J. A., Thompson, I. D., and Tolhurst, D. J. (1978a). Spatial summation in the receptive fields of simple cells in the cat's striate cortex. *J. Physiol. 283*, 53–77.

Movshon, J. A., Thompson, I. D., and Tolhurst, D. J. (1978b). Receptive field organization of complex cells in the cat's striate cortex. *J. Physiol. 283*, 79–99.

Mullen, K. T. (1985). The contrast sensitivity of human color vision to red-green and blue-yellow chromatic gratings. *J. Physiol. 359*, 381–400.

Nakayama, K. (1985). Biological image motion processing: a review. *Vision Res. 25*, 625–660.

Ohzawa, I., Sclar, G., and Freeman, R. D. (1985). Contrast gain control in the cat's visual system. *J. Neurophysiol. 54*, 651–667.

Purpura, K., and Victor, J. D. (1990a). Processing of form in monkey visual area V1. *Soc. Neurosci. Abstr. 16*, 293.

Purpura, K., and Victor, J. D. (1990b). Dissociation of cortical form mechanisms and spatial filtering at isoluminance. *Invest. Ophthalmol. Vis. Sci. 31* (suppl.), 265.

Purpura, K., Katz, E., Mao, B., Canel, A., and Victor, J. D. (1992). Responses to broad-band and texture stimuli in V1: evidence for spatial and temporal interactions. *Soc. Neurosci. Abstr. 18*, 295.

Regan, D. (1989). *Human Brain Electrophysiology*. New York: Elsevier.

Reichardt, W. (1961). Autocorrelation, a principle for the evaluation of sensory information by the central nervous system. In W. A. Rosenblith (Ed.), *Sensory Communication* (pp. 303–317). New York: Wiley.

Schroeder, C. E., Tenke, C. E., Givre, S. J., Arezzo, J. C., and Vaughan, H. G., Jr. (1991). Striate cortical contribution to the surface-recorded pattern-reversal VEP in the alert monkey. *Vision Res. 31*, 1143–1157.

Shannon, C. E. (1948). A mathematical theory of communication. *Bell Sys. Tech. J. 27*, 379–423.

Spitzer, H., and Hochstein, S. (1985). A complex-cell receptive-field model. *J. Neurophysiol. 53*, 1266–1286.

Ts'o, D. Y., Gilbert, C. D., and Wiesel, T. N. (1986). Relationships between horizontal interactions and functional architecture in cat striate cortex as revealed by cross-correlation analysis. *J. Neurosci. 6*, 1160–1170.

Victor, J. D. (1985). Complex visual textures as a tool for studying the VEP. *Vision Res. 25*, 1811–1827.

Victor, J. D. (1994). Images, statistics, and textures: a comment on "Implications of triple correlation uniqueness for texture statistics and the Julesz conjecture." *J. Opt. Soc. Am. A*, in press.

Victor, J. D., and Brodie, S. (1978). Discriminable textures with identical Buffon needle statistics. *Biol. Cybern. 31*, 231–234.

Victor, J. D., and Conte, M. M. (1987a). Local and long-range interactions in pattern processing. *Invest. Ophthalmol. Vis. Sci. 28 (Suppl.)*, 362.

Victor, J. D., and Conte, M. M. (1987b). Visual evoked potentials elicited by simple and complex textures: Distinct components with similar scalp topographies. In C. Barber and T. Blum (Eds.), *Evoked Potentials III: The Third International Evoked Potentials Symposium* (pp. 183–189). Boston: Butterworths.

Victor, J. D., and Conte, M. M. (1989a). What kinds of high-order correlation structure are readily visible? *Invest. Ophthalmol. Vis. Sci. 30 (Suppl.)*, 254.

Victor, J. D., and Conte, M. M. (1989b). Cortical interactions in texture processing: Scale and dynamics. *Visual Neurosci. 2*, 297–313.

Victor, J. D., and Conte, M. M. (1990). Motion mechanisms have only limited access to form information. *Vision Res. 30*, 289–301.

Victor, J. D., and Conte, M. M. (1991). Spatial organization of nonlinear interactions in form perception. *Vision Res. 31*, 1457–1488.

Victor, J. D., and Conte, M. M. (1993). Lack of global power spectral contributions to isodipole texture discrimination, as assessed by manipulations of spatial phase. *Invest. Ophthalmol. Vis. Sci. 34 (Suppl.)*, 1238.

Victor, J. D., and Purpura, K. (1992). Alterations of form vision at isoluminance identified through the use of visual textures. In R. Pinter and B. Nabet (Eds.), *Nonlinear Vision: Determination of Neural Receptive Fields, Function, and Networks* (pp. 243–264). Cleveland: CRC Press.

Victor, J. D., and Zemon, V. (1985). The human visual evoked potential: Analysis of components due to elementary and complex aspects of form. *Vision Res. 25*, 1829–1844.

Yellott, J. (1993). Implications of triple correlation uniqueness for texture statistics and the Julesz conjecture. *J. Opt. Soc. Am. A 10*, 777–793.

Part III

Motion Perception

Charles Chubb

When we think of the domains in which Bela Julesz has changed the course of research in visual perception we think first of stereopsis and second of preattentive texture segregation. However, it is no less true that the advent of the random-dot cinematogram (Julesz and Payne, 1968) revolutionized the way in which we now think about motion perception. A random-dot cinematogram is a movie, each of whose frames comprises a field of random dots. Of course, if all the dots in such a movie are independently painted either white or black, the result is a field of randomly flickering visual noise. However, if a rectangular subfield of the dots retains its initial (random) pattern across frames of the movie, that subfield will emerge quite clearly as a randomly patterned, nonflickering rectangle against a background of flickering noise. If, in addition, this rectangle is shifted, say one texture element to the right with each frame in the movie, the result is a random-dot cinematogram; the percept elicited is of a randomly patterned rectangle moving smoothly to the right against a background of flickering noise. This rectangle emerges quite vividly even though it is defined solely by its motion.

Prior to the research prompted by the introduction of the random-dot cinematogram, most work in the perception of "apparent movement" was rooted in paradigms inherited from the Gestalt school. In these studies, subjects were asked to judge the strength of apparent motion elicited by displays in which something appears at one place in the visual field at one time, and then something else appears somewhere else at a slightly later time. For a range of offsets in space and time, subjects can make fairly reliable assessments of the strength of motion elicited from the first presentation to the second.

It was a seminal sequence of experiments with random-dot cinematograms (Braddick, 1973, 1974) that led Oliver Braddick to draw the distinction between the "long-range" and "short-range" motion mechanisms. These two mechanisms were required to account for the percepts elicited, on the one hand, by classic apparent movement displays ("long-range motion"), and on the other hand, by random-dot cinematograms ("short-range motion"). This distinction has dominated thinking about motion perception ever since. In particular, Braddick's experiments dramatically underscored the fundamental message of the random-dot cinematogram: Human visual processing incorporates a motion sensing system (the "short-range" system) that operates directly on the raw intensities in the dynamic visual image. Paradoxical as it might seem, this system does not need to know *what* it is computing the motion *of*. It works automatically (one might even say *blindly*) to register local shifts in pattern over space and time, without regard to the precise structure of the patterns whose motion it is detecting. Indeed, the fact that one vividly perceives the shape of the motion-defined figure in a random-dot cinematogram indicates that the output of this "short-range" mechanism is itself used in segmenting the visual field.

In the two decades that have passed since Braddick's experiments, a vast body of empirical results (e.g., Anstis, 1970; Lappin and Bell, 1976; Bell and Lappin, 1979; Baker and Braddick, 1982a,b; Chang and Julesz, 1983a,b, 1985; Ramachandran and Anstis, 1983; Nakayama and Silverman, 1984; van Doorn and Koenderink, 1984) has led to a remarkable consensus in the computational modeling of short-range motion perception. A host of prima facie different models was proposed (Horn and Schunck, 1981; Marr and Ullman, 1981; Watson and Ahumada, 1983a,b, 1985; Adelson and Bergen, 1985; van Santen and Sperling, 1984, 1985; Fleet and Jepson, 1985; Heeger, 1987). However, researchers soon realized that these models were very closely related in the computational ends they achieved (Adelson and Bergen, 1986; Simoncelli and Adelson, 1991). All of these models conformed to the *motion-from-Fourier-components (MFFC) principle* (Watson et al., 1986), which dictates that the apparent motion elicited by a stimulus should be consonant with the distribution of energy in the spatiotemporal Fourier transform of the stimulus. Thus, for instance, if most of the energy in a stimulus resides in rightward-drifting Fourier components (drifting sinusoidal gratings), then the MFFC principle dictates that the motion elicited by that stimulus should be predominantly rightward.

The existence of a generally accepted computational model to account for the motion of random-dot cinematograms opened the door to the systematic study of other sorts of visual motion—sorts of motion that were essentially *inconsistent* with the MFFC principle (Ramachandran, Rao, and Vidyasagar, 1973; Sperling, 1976; Lelkens and Koenderink, 1984; Derrington and Badcock, 1985; Green, 1986; Pantle and Turano, 1986; Derrington and Henning, 1987; Chubb and Sperling, 1988; Cavanagh and Mather; 1989; Cavanagh, Arguin, and Von Grunau, 1989; Turano and Pantle, 1989; Victor and Conte, 1990; Zanker, 1993;

Gorea, Papathomas, and Kovacs, 1993). At least two of the chapters in this section deal directly with questions concerning varieties of such *second-order motion* (as opposed to the *first-order motion* elicited by random-dot cinematograms). Chapter 15 by Zanker focuses primarily on second-order motion defined by first-order motion. Such *theta motion* (Zanker, 1993) is elicited, for instance, by a moving patch, defined by random texture that is itself translating, but in a direction different from the direction of the patch. Zanker models the detection of such motion computationally, and shows that the the computations required to detect *theta* motion will also detect other sorts of *second-order motion*.

Cavanagh's chapter (chapter 11) is concerned with the role of attention in detection of second-order motion. Much of the modeling of second-order motion (e.g., Chubb and Sperling, 1988, 1991) proposes that second-order motion is detected by (1) applying to the input stimulus some grossly nonlinear transformation (such as linear filtering followed by rectification), and then (2) submitting the transformed stimulus to spatiotemporal Fourier energy analysis similar to that applied directly to the (untransformed) stimulus by the short-range motion mechanism in detecting the motion of random-dot cinematograms. However, an alternative possibility is that such motion is detected by *attentional tracking*. Cavanagh uses a variety of empirical methods to investigate this possibility for a range of different sorts of second-order motion.

Farell's chapter (chapter 12) focuses on the role of color in motion perception, and more generally on the interaction between color and luminance in pattern perception. Despite early indications that the spatiotemporally varying chromaticity of the stimulus was not analyzed for motion by the visual system (e.g., Ramachandran and Gregory, 1978; Livingstone and Hubel, 1987), evidence to the contrary is now accumulating (e.g., Krauskopf and Farell, 1990; Stromeyer, Eskew, and Kronauer, 1990; Gorea and Papathomas, 1989; Papathomas, Gorea, and Julesz, 1991). The results reported by Farell provide striking new proof that motion and pattern perception are mediated by complex interactions between chromatic and luminance mechanisms.

In considering the question of how the visual system detects first-order or second-order motion, we are concerned with the rudimentary processes by which two-dimensional motion is detected in the visual field over time. However, it has long been realized (Wallach and O'Connell, 1953) that the visual system can use such low-level, two-dimensional motion information to rapidly assign depths in three-dimensional space to moving components of the visual display. The chapters of Lappin, Craft, and Tschantz (chapter 14) and also of Sperling and Dosher (chapter 13) are both concerned with this *kinetic depth effect*.

Lappin, Craft, and Tschantz focus their attention on stimuli composed of moving dots. In all cases the dots are randomly embedded in some invisible, curved surface, and their motion is generated by moving that implicit surface in depth. To assign relative depths to different moving dots in such a display, the visual system must somehow *compare* the motions of different dots. Any such comparison must involve a computation that pulls in information about the motions of multiple dots. The question the authors address through a series of psychophysical experiments is, What are the primitive sorts of dot ensemble motions that the visual system senses in computing the curvature of the implicit surface?

Sperling and Dosher present a new model of depth perception that focuses not on the kinetic depth effect in isolation, but rather on how different cues to depth (e.g., brightness cues, stereoptic cues, and motion cues) interact to determine the perceived depth of an image component. The empirical results and the model they present have important consequences for our understanding of the kinetic depth effect. For instance, they show, among other things, that the computation of depth from two-dimensional motion does not require the prior assumption that image components are moving rigidly together in three-dimensional space. More generally, they present convincing evidence that a host of different sorts of depth cues interacts in a simple additive fashion to determine perceived depth.

Schiller's chapter (chapter 16) is concerned with the function performed by area V4 in monkey cortex. His method is to determine what deficits are produced in monkey performance on various psychophysical tasks by V4 lesions. The sorts of tasks that turn out to be most informative about V4's function are tasks in which the monkey must detect a target in a field of distractors. Although some of the stimuli Schiller uses are stimuli in which the target is defined by its motion relative to the background, V4 is not specialized for motion processing. Nor does V4 seem to be specialized for color processing, or stereopsis, or any of the functions that visual scientists typically like to allocate to separate modules in the brain. Rather, as Schiller's results dramatically show, the ablation of V4 produces a general deficit in the monkey's ability to perform the following sort of task: the selection of a target stimulus *T* from a field populated by distractors that excite low-level visual neurons more effectively than does *T*.

References

Adelson, E. H., and Bergen, J. (1985). Spatiotemporal energy models for the perception of motion. *J. Opt. Soc. Am. A 2*, 284–299.

Adelson, E. H., and Bergen, J. (1986). The extraction of spatio-temporal energy in human and machine vision. *Proc. IEEE Workshop Motion: Represent. Anal.* 151–155.

Anstis, S. M. (1970). Phi movement as a subtraction process, *Vision Res. 10*, 1411–1430.

Baker, C. L., and Braddick, O. (1982a). Does segregation of differently moving areas depend on relative or absolute displacement. *Vision Res. 22*, 851–856.

Baker, C. L., and Braddick, O. (1982b). The basis of area and dot number effects in random dot motion perception. *Vision Res. 22*, 1253–1260.

Bell, H. H., and Lappin, J. S. (1979). The detection of rotation in random dot patterns. *Percept. Psychophys. 26*, 415–417.

Braddick, O. (1973) The masking of apparent motion in random-dot patterns. *Vision Res. 13*, 355–359.

Braddick, O. (1974). A short-range process in apparent motion. *Vision Res. 14*, 519–527.

Cavanagh, P., and Mather, G. (1989). Motion: The long and the short of it. *Spatial Vision 4*, 103–129.

Cavanagh, P., Arguin, M., and von Grunau, M. (1989). Interattribute apparent motion. *Vision Res. 29(9)*, 1197–1204.

Chang, J. J., and Julesz, B. (1983a). Displacement limits, directional anisotropy and direction versus form discrimination in random dot cinematograms. *Vision Res. 23*, 639–646.

Chang, J. J., Julesz, B. (1983b). Displacement limits for spatial frequency random-dot cinematograms in apparent motion. *Vision Res. 23*, 1379–1386.

Chang, J. J., and Julesz, B. (1985). Cooperative and non-cooperative processes of apparent movement of random dot cinematograms. *Spatial Vision 1*, 39–45.

Chubb, C., and Sperling, G. (1988). Drift-balanced random stimuli: A general basis for studying non-Fourier motion perception. *J. Opt. Soc. Am. A 5*, 1986–2007.

Chubb, C., and Sperling, G. (1991). Texture quilts: Basic tools for studying motion from texture. *J. Math. Psych. 35*, 411–442.

Derrington, A. M., and Badcock, D. R. (1985). Separate detectors for simple and complex grating patterns? *Vision Res. 25*, 1869–1878.

Derrington, A. M., and Henning, G. B. (1987). Errors in direction-of-motion discrimination with complex stimuli. *Vision Res. 27*, 61–75.

van Doorn, A. J., and Koenderink, J. J. (1984). Spatiotemporal integration in the detection of coherent motion. *Vision Res. 24*, 47–54.

Fleet, D. J., and Jepson, A. D. (1985). On the hierarchical construction of orientation and velocity selective filters. University of Toronto Computer Science Department technical report RBCV-TR-85-8 on research in biological and computational vision.

Gorea, A., and Papathomas, T. V. (1989). Motion processing by chromatic and achromatic visual pathways. *J. Opt. Soc. Am. 6*, 590–602.

Gorea, A., Papathomas, T. V., and Kovacs, I. (1993). Motion perception with spatiotemporally matched chromatic and achromatic information reveals a "slow" and a "fast" motion system. *Vision Res. 33,* 2515–2534.

Green, M. (1986). What determines correspondence strength in apparent motion. *Vision Res. 26,* 599–607.

Heeger, D. J. (1987). A model for the extraction of image flow. *J. Opt. Soc. Am. A 4,* 1455–1471.

Horn, B. K. P., and Schunck, B. G. (1981). Determining optic flow. *Artificial Intelligence 17,* 185–203.

Julesz, B., and Payne, R. A. (1968). Differences between monocular and binocular stroboscopic movement perception. *Vision Res. 8,* 433–444.

Krauskopf, J., and Farell, B. (1990). Influence of color on the perception of coherent motion. *Nature (London) 348,* 328–331.

Lappin, J. S., and Bell, H. H. (1976). Perceptual differentiation of sequential visual pattern. *Percept. Psychophys. 12,* 129–134.

Lelkens, A. M. M., and Koenderink, J. J. (1984). Illusory motion in visual displays. *Vision Res. 24,* 1083–1090.

Livingstone, M. S., and Hubel, D. H. (1987). Psychophysical evidence for separate channels for perception of form, color, movement and depth. *J. Neurosci. 7,* 3416–3468.

Marr, D., and Ullman, S. (1981). Directional selectivity and its use in early visual processing. *Proc. R. Soc. London B 211,* 151–180.

Nakayama, K., and Silverman, G. (1984). Temporal and spatial characteristics of the upper displacement limit for motion in random dots. *Vision Res. 24,* 293–300.

Pantle, A., and Turano, K. (1986). Direct comparisons of apparent motions produced with luminance, contrast-modulated (CM), and texture gratings. *Invest. Ophthalmol. Visual Sci. 27,* 141.

Papathomas, T. V., Gorea, A., and Julesz, B. (1991). Two carriers for motion perception: Color and luminance. *Vision Res. 31,* 1883–1891.

Ramachandran, V. S., and Anstis, S. M. (1983). Displacement thresholds for coherent apparent motion in random dot-patterns. *Vision Res 23,* 1719–1724.

Ramachandran, V. S., and Gregory, R. L. (1978). Does color provide an input to human motion perception? *Nature (London) 275,* 55–57.

Ramachandran, V. S., Rao, V. M., and Vidyasagar, T. R. (1973). Apparent movement with subjective contours. *Vision Res. 13,* 1399–1401.

van Santen, J. P. H., and Sperling, G. (1984). A temporal covariance model of motion perception. *J. Opt. Soc. Am. A 1,* 451–473.

van Santen, J. P. H., and Sperling, G. (1985). Elaborated Reichardt detector. *J. Opt. Soc. Am. A 2,* 300–321.

Simoncelli, E. P., and Adelson, E. H. (1991). Relationship between gradient, spatiotemporal energy, and regression models for motion perception. *Invest. Ophthalmol. Visual Sci. 32,* 893.

Sperling, G. (1976). Movement perception in computer-driven visual display. *Behav. Res. Methods Instrument. 8,* 144–151.

Stromeyer, C. F., Eskew, R. T., and Kronauer, R. E. (1990). The most sensitive motion detectors in humans are spectrally opponent. *Invest. Ophthalmol. Visual Sci. (Suppl.) 31,* 240.

Turano, K., and Pantle, A. (1989). On the mechanism that encodes the movement of contrast variations: Velocity discrimination. *Vision Res. 29,* 207–221.

Victor, J. D., and Conte, M. M. (1990). Motion mechanisms have only limited access to form information. *Vision Res. 30,* 289–301.

Wallach, H., and O'Connell, D. N. (1953). The kinetic depth effect. *J. Exp. Psychol. 45,* 205–217.

Watson, A. B., and Ahumada, A. J. Jr. (1983a). A linear motion sensor. *Perception 12,* A17.

Watson, A. B., and Ahumada, A. J. Jr. (1983b). A look at motion in the frequency domain. NASA Technical Memorandum 84352.

Watson, A. B., and Ahumada, A. J. Jr. (1985). A model of human visual-motion sensing. *J. Opt. Soc. Am. A 2,* 322–342.

Watson, A. B., Ahumada, A. J. Jr. and Farrell, J. E. (1986). The window of visibility: A psychophysical theory of fidelity in time-sampled motion displays. *J. Opt. Soc. Am. A 3,* 300–307.

Zanker, J. M. (1993). Theta motion: A paradoxical stimulus to explore higher order motion extraction. *Vision Res. 33,* 553–569.

11

Is There Low-Level Motion Processing for Non-Luminance-Based Stimuli?

Patrick Cavanagh

How do we see the motion of "equiluminous" features? By equiluminous, I mean regions that have the same luminance as the background but differ in some other property such as color, texture, depth, or relative motion. The physiological literature has given ample evidence of directionally selective units at early levels of visual processing but these have been overwhelmingly tested with luminance-defined stimuli. More recent studies have revealed directionally selective responses to equiluminous color stimuli (Saito et al., 1989; Dobkins and Albright, 1993) and texture-defined stimuli (Albright, 1992) but it has been argued that these may be weak residual responses mediated by nonlinearities in the luminance pathway. In this chapter, I will examine whether there are specialized low-level motion detectors for non-luminance-based stimuli. The alternative is that the motion of non-luminance-based stimuli is detected only by a second motion system, which relies on the attentive tracking of visible features (Cavanagh, 1992). In the first series of experiments, I hunted for various types of low-level detectors by testing whether there was a common, low-level motion pathway that responded to both luminance and non-luminance-defined stimuli. In the second series of experiments, I diverted attention from moving, non-luminance-defined stimuli to see whether motion processing remained viable in the absence of attention. I am reporting only preliminary observations in the case of drifting stereo- or motion-defined structure as these patterns were created by local modulations of a static dot field. This static component may have biased the low-level motion responses. Further studies with dynamic random-dot stereograms and motion fields with short dot life times are underway to extend these preliminary observations.

Two Motion Streams

The notion of two separate motion systems was initially suggested by Julesz (1971). He claimed that the low-level movement detectors found by Hubel and Wiesel (1968) were different from higher-level movement analyzers that operate following pattern matching. Julesz described experiments on the motion of figures defined in random-dot stereograms and concluded that the motion perceived for these stimuli was mediated by a higher-order process. This early description of two motion streams was followed by similar claims by Anstis (1980) and Braddick (1974, 1980). Recently, I described these two motion streams as passive (low-level) and active (high-level) processes and considered how each of them might analyze the motion of different stimulus types (Cavanagh, 1991). Figure 11.1 shows the possible combinations of passive and active motion processes with five types of stimuli. Of these five, I have classified color and luminance as first-order stimuli and the three others as second-order stimuli (Cavanagh and Mather, 1989). These classifications are based only on stimulus structure. First-order statistics specify the frequency with which individual points in an image have specified intensity or color values. Two areas in an image differ in their first-order statistics if they have different mean luminances or spectral compositions. Motion detectors specialized for first-order patterns (or at least for luminance) therefore correspond to the extensively studied directionally selective units of the striate cortex. Recent psychophysical (Cavanagh and Anstis, 1991) and physiological studies (Dobkins and Albright, 1993) have also argued for low-level motion detectors for equiluminous color.

Two areas may have the same mean luminance and color, but differ in their spatial, temporal, or ocular distri-

Motion Process	Stimulus Factors				
	First Order		Second Order		
	Lum.	Color	Texture	Stereo	Motion
Passive					
Active					

Figure 11.1

Stimulus and process factors in motion perception. A stimulus factor divides stimulus types into first order or second order. First-order stimuli (luminance or color) can be defined at a single point. Second-order stimuli require two points, separated in space for texture, separated by eye for binocular disparity, and separated by space and time for motion. Two types of motion processes—active and passive—can respond to both of these stimulus types. Passive motion processes involve arrays of localized motion detectors that monitor all areas of the retina. Active processes involve tracking individual targets with attention as they move about the visual field. Short-range motion, as originally described by Braddick (1980) and Anstis (1980), corresponds only to the responses of passive motion processes to luminance stimuli. Long-range motion corresponds to the remaining combinations.

butions of luminance and color. The two areas are then differentiated by second-order properties such as texture, motion, or binocular disparity. The difference between first-order and second-order structure lies in the stimulus. One goal of this chapter is to determine if there are passive, low-level motion detectors for second-order stimuli defined by texture, relative motion, or binocular disparity.

In addition to the low-level, passive motion detectors there is also a second stream of motion processing that I have called active motion perception because it involves the use of attention to track moving stimuli. This attention-based motion process can obviously respond to the same stimuli (first- or second-order) that activate passive detectors; that is, as long as the stimuli are visible they can be tracked. The active/passive distinction is therefore independent of the stimuli present in the display. Compared to low-level motion processes (Braddick, 1980; Anstis, 1980), this attention-based process appears to have a limited capacity (Pylyshyn and Storm, 1988) and very different thresholds but supports more accurate velocity judgements (Cavanagh, 1992). These differences have suggested that the tracking process itself does not rely on, or at least does not require, low-level motion signals to maintain tracking of the target. For example, observers can accurately track equiluminous color targets even when their apparent velocity judged by low-level mechanisms is grossly underestimated (Cavanagh, 1992). Any given stimulus may engage either, or both, passive and active motion mechanisms and the observed performance can be interpreted meaningfully only if it is known which are involved (Cavanagh, 1991).

Julesz (1971) suggested that when cues for both motion streams are present, the low-level stream usually dominates and the operation of the higher-order mechanism is concealed. He claimed that using cyclopean stimuli avoided engaging the low-level process, allowing the higher-level one to be isolated. His conjecture will be explicitly tested in this chapter using a more general test to isolate the two motion streams. The test was developed to examine the role of low- and high-level motion in the perception of motion for color stimuli (Cavanagh and Anstis, 1991; Cavanagh, 1992). In the test, the two motion streams see opposite directions of motion and the observer can report either at will. Luminance and color gratings were superimposed and set in motion in opposite directions. Because of masking from the color grating, the bars of the luminance grating were not visible and they could not be tracked; nevertheless, their motion was visible and it determined the observed direction of rotation. This "disembodied" motion was striking because no features could be seen actually moving in the direction of the overall motion.

On the other hand, the bars of the color grating were visible and could be tracked at will by the high-level, attention-based process. The tracking of the color bars could not have been based on the motion signals from low-level detectors because the low-level motion response was dominated by the luminance grating. If the low-level signal alone were sufficient for tracking, then the luminance bars should have been tracked at least as easily as the color bars; but the luminance bars could not be tracked at all (they were not visible to the pattern pathway that supposedly mediates tracking).

In this composite stimulus, the color bars could be seen to move (in the opposite direction to the overall stimulus rotation) only when they were being tracked with attention. Evidently, the motion impressions during tracking of the color bars in this stimulus must represent the output of a distinct motion process, one that cannot be based on the motion signals from low-level detectors (these are signaling motion in the opposite direction). The results

therefore indicate that there must be two independent sources for the impressions of motion in this stimulus: one for the judgment of overall motion (passive) and a separate one for tracking (active).

The attention-based motion process might derive motion signals from position information that is read out from the focus of attention. Motion might be derived from monitoring or noticing the change in this attention-selected position signal (figure 11.2b). Alternatively, motion impressions could be based on information about the focus of attention itself, either its position or its displacement (figure 11.2c). Specifically, to perform a tracking task, some servomechanism must be comparing the position of the attentional focus to that of the tracked target and repositioning attention to follow the target. The signals from this control process, either the current position of attention or perhaps its tracking rate, would be sufficient to generate an appropriate motion impression.

Attentive tracking may be required to perceive the motion of non-luminance-based stimuli, or, to put it another way, there may be no low-level motion detectors for non-

a) Low-Level Selection

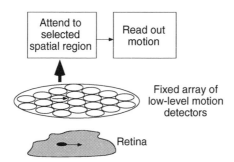

b) Retinal Position of Attended Target

c) Attention Control Signals

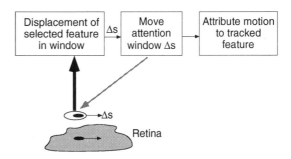

Figure 11.2
The motion sensations for an object tracked with attention could arise in a number of ways. Although they could be based on a selection from the low-level signals available in the attended region as depicted in (a), specific stimuli where this option is not available (Cavanagh, 1991) still support motion impressions independently of low-level signals. These high-level motion impressions may be derived from the position of features individuated and tracked within the focus of attention (b), or from the signals that keep the focus of attention centered over the tracked object (c).

luminance-based stimuli. If this is the case, the three top rightmost boxes of figure 11.1 would not exist. I tested for the presence of these low-level detectors by trying to get them to interact with luminance-based low-level detectors in a motion nulling task and in a plaid motion task. I also tried to divert attention from first- and second-order stimuli to see whether motion impressions and motion aftereffects could survive the removal of attention. If motion of, say, stereo-defined gratings could be perceived in the absence of attention, I would conclude that there are low-level passive motion detectors available for this attribute.

Motion Nulls between Luminance and Non-Luminance-Based Motion

If low-level detectors do operate on non-luminance-based stimuli, the different types of low-level detectors may all contribute to a common motion pathway. If this is the case, the motion of a luminance grating drifting in one direction should be able to cancel or null the motion of an oppositely moving, non-luminance-based stimulus. Nothing requires a common motion pathway for the different types of low-level detectors, so a negative outcome (e.g., if two attributes do not null) is inconclusive. On the other hand, a positive outcome (e.g., two attributes do null) does demonstrate the existence of low-level detectors for both attributes. As an example, we have been able to demonstrate motion nulling between color and luminance (Cavanagh and Anstis, 1991). When color is moving, say, to the left and luminance is moving to the right, the overall motion will appear to be in the direction of the color grating when the luminance grating has low contrast. At much higher contrasts the overall motion is in the direction of the luminance grating. At some intermediate value (between 10 and 20% contrast in our experiments), the two motions cancel and a flickering stimulus is seen. The fact that the two stimuli cancel suggests that they contribute to a common mechanism. If they did not contribute to a common mechanism, we might expect a perception of transparency with the two gratings appearing to slide through each other.

This sliding or transparency can be seen with two opposing luminance gratings if they are sufficiently separated in spatial frequency (about a factor of 4). Similarly, color and luminance gratings slide over each other if they have dissimilar spatial and temporal frequencies.

It is easy to show that the nulling of the overall motion impression between the two gratings is independent of the operation of high-level tracking processes and so re-

quires the participation of low-level processes for both the attributes being opposed. The evidence for this is that even though the overall motion of the superimposed gratings shows this nulling behavior, attentive tracking is never "nulled." The observer can switch between reporting an impression of overall motion (which shows low-level nulling) or the direction of tracking individual features. At moderate luminance contrasts (10–20%), the color bars can be tracked even though the overall motion is in the opposite direction. At higher luminance contrasts, either the color or the luminance grating can be tracked at will. These results suggest that motion nulling between two gratings of different types is a signature of a low-level detectors for both types that contribute to a common pathway. I therefore extended our first test of motion nulling for color and luminance to tests of motion nulling between luminance gratings and gratings defined by color, texture, binocular disparity, or relative motion.

Motion nulling was clear between color and luminance. It was possible to get a motion null between texture and luminance at slower speeds, although at higher speeds, they appeared to slide through each other. It was never possible to get a motion null between stereo-defined gratings and luminance or between motion-defined gratings and luminance. In both cases, the gratings appeared completely transparent and moved independently in opposite directions. These results imply that there may be a low-level motion detector responding to texture-defined gratings (see also Chubb and Sperling, 1991). The negative results for stereo-defined and motion-defined gratings may indicate that there are no low-level motion detectors for these two attributes. Contrary evidence has been reported by Patterson et al. (1993) who claim to find a motion aftereffect following adaptation to drifting stereo-defined gratings. Nishida and Sato (1993) also reported motion aftereffects following adaptation to drifting second-order stimuli.

Motion Plaids between Luminance and Non-Luminance-Based Motion

A motion plaid (Adelson and Movshon, 1982) is produced by the superposition of two gratings at different orientations. When both gratings are defined by luminance there is a range of different contrasts, speeds, and spatial frequencies of the two gratings for which they cohere and a compound pattern is seen drifting in an intermediate direction. Outside this coherence range, the two gratings appear to slide through each other. Stoner and Albright (1992) have tested gratings composed of different attributes with the assumption that coherence between different attributes shows that they activate a common motion pathway or analysis. They did find coherence between texture gratings and luminance gratings implying, as I argued above, that texture is analyzed by low-level motion detectors. I tested plaids made up of luminance gratings and either stereo-defined gratings or motion-defined gratings. It was not possible in either case to find any setting of speed or contrast that produced a coherent, compound pattern. The gratings appeared to drift over each other as if completely transparent.

Although these results are consistent with the nulling results above, other results from Krauskopf and Farell (1990) are not. These authors reported that plaids made up of color and luminance did not cohere even though, as mentioned above, we found that color and luminance would null each other (Cavanagh and Anstis, 1991) when superimposed and drifting in opposite direction. Why would the two attributes interfere when superimposed and drifting in opposite directions (let us call this a 180° plaid) but not when they were superimposed at 90°? There is no obvious answer to this discrepancy but it is possible that the results for plaid stimuli may be mediated by other processes in addition to motion (for more details, see Farell, this volume). The ability to see the two components as separate or not may also be an extension of the monocular rivalry phenomenon (Georgeson, 1984). In this stimulus, two orthogonal, superimposed gratings can be seen separately, alternating back and forth between one and the other, even though neither is moving. If this is the source of the lack of coherence for the gratings in Krauskopf and Farell's study, then these same stimuli should be easily separated when stationary as well. In this case, positive results from cross-cue plaid experiments would indicate common motion processes (e.g., texture and luminance gratings cohere, Stoner and Albright, 1992), whereas negative results (e.g., color and luminance do not cohere, Krauskopf and Farell, 1990) would not be informative.

Summary for Common Pathway Studies

Overall, we have strong evidence for low-level detectors that contribute to a common pathway for luminance-, color-, and texture-defined gratings. The lack of interaction between luminance and either stereo-defined or motion-defined gratings is clear in both the motion null and motion plaid experiments. This result might indicate that there are no low-level motion detectors for these two stimulus types but strictly speaking it may indicate only

that if these detectors are present, they do not contribute to a final pathway shared by luminance. Moreover, the lack of coherence in the moving plaids made up of luminance and either stereo- or motion-defined gratings may be a result of strong monocular rivalry. It remains to be seen whether there are low-level detectors for stereo-defined and motion-defined stimuli. The next tests considered the alternative hypothesis that the motion of these two stimulus types is mediated only by attentional processes (all five stimulus types were tested). Attention was diverted from the moving stimuli to see whether any impressions of motion would persist in the absence of attention.

Motion Perception without Attention for Non-Luminance-Based Stimuli

Gratings defined by color, texture, stereo, or relative motion can be seen to move, but all produce a degraded or slowed perception of motion. It could be argued that there are no low-level detectors for these types of stimuli and that the motion is perceived only because of the attentive tracking of the stimuli. This experiment examined the attention hypothesis by engaging attention in a secondary task (attentive tracking in an inner, counterphasing ring) and measuring the effect on motion impressions for the different stimulus types moving smoothly in an outer ring.

In the outer annulus, a grating defined by luminance, color, stereo, motion, or texture was presented rotating either CW or CCW (figure 11.3). In the inner annulus, a luminance grating was presented in counterphase flicker.

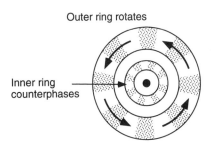

Outer ring rotates

Inner ring counterphases

Figure 11.3
A tracking task is run in the center of the display. The luminance grating is in counterphase flicker and the observer can track it either clockwise or counterclockwise. During a given trial, tracking is in one direction only. In the outer ring, a grating defined by luminance, color, texture, stereo, or motion is presented. If attention is necessary to perceive the motion of any of these stimuli, the perception of motion in the outer ring should be severely compromised, especially when its motion is in the direction opposite to the tracking direction.

The temporal frequencies of the moving and flickering gratings were the same (2 Hz). Observers were trained to track the central grating in either direction and to note the impressions of motion in the outer grating during tracking.

Observers reported clear impressions of motion in the outer grating when defined by luminance, color, or texture. It was not important whether the outer grating was moving in the same direction as the tracking for the inner grating.

Observers reported a large loss in the impressions of motion in the outer ring when the stimulus was a stereo- or motion-defined grating. The loss was not so large when the outer grating was moving in step with the tracking of the inner grating, but it was almost total when the outer grating moved in opposition to the tracking.

These results suggest that the perception of motion for stereo- and motion-defined stimuli is mediated solely by attention and that there are no low-level detectors signaling motion for these stimuli.

Motion Aftereffects for Non-Luminance-Based Stimuli

I tested for simple motion aftereffect with drifting gratings of the five stimulus types. In each case the aftereffect was verified on a static grating of the same type as the adapting grating. Aftereffects were found only for luminance and color gratings, replicating many earlier studies. Other studies have reported aftereffects for texture-defined (Nishida and Sato, 1993) and stereo-defined gratings (Patterson et al., 1993). Nishida and Sato (1993) claim that motion aftereffects can be revealed for second-order stimuli like texture if a counterphase test is used. Patterson et al. (1993) used a static luminance grating as a test so their result is quite striking. An additional difference between his studies and ours is that his stereo-defined gratings use dynamic random dots whereas ours use static random dots (modulated by disparity).

Motion Aftereffects for Luminance-Based Stimuli in the Absence of Attention

As a final test, I examined whether attention was required to produce a motion aftereffect even in the case of luminance stimuli (Chaudhuri, 1990). The double annulus stimulus shown in figure 11.3 was used with a luminance grating moving continously in the outer ring during adaptation. Observers tracked the inner ring in the direction opposite to the motion of the outer ring for about 30 sec. The motion in the outer ring was then stopped. All observers reported a motion aftereffect in the outer ring, supporting Wohlgemuth's (1911) original observations.

Conclusions

How do we see the motion of "equiluminous" features? For at least two types of non-luminance-based stimuli, color-defined and texture-defined, the evidence presented here argues that there are low-level motion detectors that signal their motion. These detectors, along with those for luminance-defined stimuli, contribute to a common motion pathway, accounting for their mutual interference in the motion nulling task. Attentive tracking would always be available to mediate the perception of motion for color and texture-defined stimuli, but motion could be seen for both even in the absence of attention.

It could be argued that the low-level responses to color and texture are due to some residual nonlinearities in luminance-based motion detectors. This possibility has been discounted for the case of color (Cavanagh and Anstis, 1991). In fact, Stromeyer et al. (1990) have shown that the threshold for drifting equiluminous gratings is as much as four times lower (in cone contrast units) than it is for a luminance grating. This finding rules out the notion that the motion response to color could be mediated by a residual distortion in the response of the luminance pathway to color. Their result has been confirmed recently by Metha et al. (1993). Chubb and Sperling (1991) have considered the nature of low-level detectors that would respond to their texture gratings and they suggest detectors with half- or full-wave rectification of image contrast. Neither of their suggested operators is present in standard motion detectors for luminance-based stimuli as contrast polarity plays a significant role in low-level motion response (Anstis and Rogers, 1975).

In each experiment, motion-defined and stereo-defined stimuli acted as if there were no low-level motion detectors specialized for these stimuli. They did not null the motion of a luminance grating moving in the opposite direction; they did not cohere with a luminance grating in a plaid; their motion was no longer seen when attention was diverted away from them.

These results would appear to validate Julesz's (1971) conjecture that the motion of cyclopean stimuli was analyzed solely by high-level mechanisms. I would add a caution, however, based on the nature of the stereo- and motion-defined stimuli used here. As mentioned in the introduction, the drifting stereo- or motion-defined structure used in these experiments was created by local modulations of a static dot field. Further studies with dynamic random-dot stereograms and motion fields with short dot life times are underway to extend these preliminary observations reported here.

Acknowledgments

This research was supported by NEI grant EY09258.

References

Adelson, E. H., and Movshon, J. A. (1982). Phenomenal coherence of moving gratings. *Nature (London) 300*, 523–525.

Albright, T. D. (1992). Form-cue invariant processing in primate visual cortex. *Science 255*, 1141–1143.

Anstis, S. M. (1970). Phi movement as a subtraction process. *Vision Res. 10*, 1411–1430.

Anstis, S. M. (1980). The perception of apparent movement. *Phil. Transact. R. Soc. London B290*, 153–168.

Anstis, S. M., and Rogers, B. J. (1975). Illusory reversal of visual depth and movement during change of contrast. *Vision Res. 15*, 957–962.

Braddick, O. (1974). A short-range process in apparent motion. *Vision Res. 25*, 839–847.

Braddick, O. (1980). Low-level and high-level processes in apparent motion. *Phil. Transact. R. Soc. London B290*, 137–151.

Cavanagh, P. (1991). Short-range vs long-range motion: Not a valid distinction. *Spatial Vision 5*, 303–309.

Cavanagh, P. (1992). Attention-based motion perception. *Science 257*, 1563–1565.

Cavanagh, P., and Anstis, S. M. (1991). The contribution of color to motion in normal and color-deficient observers. *Vision Res. 31*, 2109–2148.

Cavanagh, P., and Mather, G. (1989). Motion: the long and short of it. *Spatial Vision 4*, 103–129.

Chaudhuri, A. (1990). Modulation of the motion aftereffect by selective attention. *Nature (London) 344*, 60–62.

Chubb, C., and Sperling, G. (1991). Texture Quilts: Basic tools for studying Motion-from-Texture. *J. Math. Psychol. 35*(4), 411–442.

Dobkins, K. R., and Albright, T. D. (1993). What happens if it changes color when it moves?: The nature of chromatic input to Macaque visual area MT. *J. Neurosci.*

Georgeson, M. A. (1984). Eye movements, afterimages and monocular rivalry. *Vision Res. 24*, 1311–1319.

Hubel, D. H., and Wiesel, T. N. (1968). Receptive fields and functional architecture of monkey striate cortex. *J. Physiol. 195*, 215–243.

Julesz, B. (1971). *Foundations of Cyclopean Perception*. Chicago: University of Chicago Press.

Krauskopf, J., and Farell, B. (1990). Influence of colour on the perception of coherent motion. *Nature (London) 348*, 328–331.

Metha, A. B., Vingrys, A. J., and Badcock, D. R. (1993). Cone contrast detection and direction thresholds. *Invest. Ophthalmol. Visual Sci. 34*, 1032.

Nishida, S., and Sato, T. (1993).Two kinds of motion aftereffect reveal different types of motion processing. *Invest. Ophthalmol. Visual Sci. 34*, 1363.

Patterson, R., Bowd, C., Phinney, R., Pohndorf, R., Barton-Howard, W. J., and Angilletta, M. (1993). Properties of the stereoscopic (cyclopean) motion aftereffect. Unpublished manuscript.

Pylyshyn, Z. W., and Storm, R. W. (1988). Tracking multiple independent targets: evidence for a parallel tracking mechanism. *Spatial Vision 3*, 151–224.

Saito, H., Tanaka, K., Isono, H., Yasuda, M., and Mikami, A. (1989). Directionally selective response of cells in the middle temporal area (MT) of the macaque monkey to the movement of equiluminous opponent color stimuli. *Exp. Brain Res. 75*, 1–14.

Stoner, G. R., and Albright, T. D. (1992). Motion coherency rules are form-cue invariant. *Vision Res. 32*, 465–475.

Stromeyer, C. F. III, Eskew, R. T., and Kronauer, R. E. (1990). The most sensitive motion detectors in humans are spectrally opponent. *Invest. Ophthalmol. Visual Sci. Suppl. 31*, 241.

Wohlgemuth, J. M. (1911). On the after effect of seen motion. *Br. J. Psychol. Monogr. Suppl. 1*, 1–117.

12

Spatial Structure and the Perceived Motion of Objects of Different Colors

Bart Farell

Traditionally, visual science has taken the strategy of studying spatial vision and color vision separately. Progress has been substantial, suggesting that the visual system might engage in the analogous modular strategy of processing spatial and chromatic information separately. Yet recently there has been a good deal of interest in connections between the two realms and particularly in the contribution of chromatic channels to spatial abilities (e.g., Cavanagh, 1987; Cavanagh and Favreau, 1985; De Valois and De Valois, 1988; Krauskopf and Farell, 1990, 1991; Livingstone and Hubel, 1984; Morgan and Aiba, 1985; Mullen, 1985, 1987; Zeki, 1978). This interest expresses, in part, a desire to scrutinize modularity as the basis for understanding the functional organization of the visual system, to test its implications and limits.

Of the many possible test-beds of the modularity of color and spatial processing, the influence of stimulus color on the perception of motion has been perhaps the most extensively investigated.[1] One stage of study of this topic has largely been completed and we are now entering a second stage at something of an impasse. The initial stage, sketched out in the next section of this chapter, established that opponent-color signals do contribute effectively to the perception of motion. The second stage concerns *how* these signals contribute to motion, and specifically whether motion analysis is carried out independently on luminance and opponent-color channels (collectively, the "cardinal-axis" channels) or whether signals on these channels are combined before being fed into a common analyzer. As we will see, these two pictures—separate cardinal-axis motion channels or a common motion channel—appear incompatible, and yet each is strongly supported by a portion of the evidence.

Not yet brought fully into either picture is a consideration of the influence of the spatial properties of moving luminance and chromatic stimuli. In natural scenes the distributions of luminance and chromatic spatiotemporal variation are typically correlated, due to the presence of distinct objects. Objects in the visual field tessellate the

---

1. "Color" is to be taken broadly, encompassing both chromatic and achromatic variation.

retinal image with regions differing both in luminance and chromaticity. The experiments discussed here explore the idea that the visual system might make use of the distributional constraints that objects place on luminance and chromatic signals to guide it in describing the objects in a scene.

The experiments make use of compound gratings that have both a luminance and a chromatic modulation. Spatial factors—orientation, spatial frequency, and phase—are shown to determine whether the chromatic component is seen to move in concert with the luminance component, to move independently, or to disappear entirely. The experiments address portions of two larger issues: the organization of the multiple visual pathways within and between functionally specialized systems, such as color, stereo, texture, and motion (see Cavanagh, this volume), and the specific adaptations of the visual system to problems of object perception.

Effectiveness of Chromatic Stimuli in Motion Perception

Moving isoluminant patterns have been shown to produce perceptual effects that are qualitatively similar to those produced by moving luminance patterns: They generate motion aftereffects (Favreau, Emerson, and Corballis, 1972; Mullen and Baker, 1985), null luminance-based motion (Cavanagh and Anstis, 1991), and resolve ambiguous motion (Papathomas, Gorea, and Julesz, 1991). But these findings are inconclusive as to whether motion information is conveyed over chromatic pathways. Luminance pathways, which could have responded to nominally isoluminant stimuli by a number of means, might have been the source of effective input to the motion system (Cavanagh and Anstis, 1991).

Lingering doubts about the utility of chromatic signals to motion perception have also been sustained by anatomical and neurophysiological evidence of separate processing of chromaticity and motion (e.g., Livingstone and Hubel, 1984; Van Essen, 1985; Zeki, 1978) and by the apparent slowing, and even stopping, of motion at isoluminance (Cavanagh, Tyler, and Favreau, 1984; Mullen and Boulton, 1992; Palmer and Mobley, 1993; Ramachandran and Gregory, 1978; Teller and Lindsey, 1993).

Only quite recently has psychophysics firmly demonstrated the effectiveness of chromatic stimuli to elicit the perception of motion without the involvement of luminance pathways (Cavanagh and Anstis, 1991; Krauskopf and Farell, 1990; Krauskopf, Farell, and Movshon, 1989). In fact, at low and moderate temporal frequencies, the most sensitive motion pathway, in terms of cone activa-

tion, has opponent-color characteristics (Stromeyer et al., 1990). However, while the existence of separate luminance and chromatic pathways in the motion system seems clearly indicated by the data, one study (Krauskopf and Farell, 1990) has raised uncertainty about the organization of these pathways: Do they serve as separate inputs to a single motion mechanism or do they feed into separate motion mechanisms?

Plaids in Color Space

Krauskopf and Farell (1990) used "plaid" patterns composed of two drifting sinusoidal gratings (Adelson and Movshon, 1982). In plaids, the component gratings have different orientations and, when viewed individually, each grating drifts in a different direction. When the gratings are superimposed, however, they are perceived either as "cohering" to form a rigidly moving pattern or as "sliding" past one another without interacting, as if transparent. Gratings cohere when they are similar in

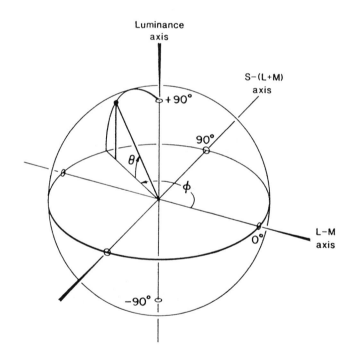

Figure 12.1
Color space. The origin of this space is an equal-energy white. There are two chromatic axes that lie within the isoluminant plane through the origin. Along one of these axes, the L-M axis, the excitation of the short-wavelength (S) cones is constant while those of the long-wavelength (L) and middle-wavelength (M) cones covary to keep luminance constant. Along the other chromatic axis, the S-(L + M) axis, only the S cone excitation varies. The third, luminance, axis is one along which the excitations of all three classes of cones vary in proportion to their values for equal-energy white. Hue varies with the azimuth (ϕ), while excursions out of the isoluminant plane are described by elevation (θ).

such properties as spatial frequency, drift rate, and contrast; they slide when they are sufficiently different.

Krauskopf and Farell's gratings varied in color. In one case the two gratings were modulated along different cardinal axes in the color space of figure 12.1 (Krauskopf, Williams, and Healy, 1982)—for example, one was an achromatic luminance grating and the other a red-green (L-M) chromatic grating. In a second case, the two gratings were modulated in different directions that were midway between pairs of cardinal axes—for example, one grating varied between light red and dark green and the other varied between dark red and light green. Spatially the gratings were as similar as possible, differing only in orientation and drift direction.

The off-axis color-space directions are related to the cardinal-axis directions by a rigid rotation. That is, off-axis and cardinal-axis gratings are represented in color space by different straight lines that pass through the central white point. This rotation through color space had a categorical influence on perceived motion. Gratings modulated on *different cardinal axes* were virtually never seen to cohere, regardless of their relative spatial frequencies, speeds, and contrasts, whereas *different off-axis* gratings nearly always cohered when their spatial frequencies, speeds, and contrasts were similar. The different perceived motions of cardinal-axis and intermediate-direction plaids reveal that color space is anisotropic with respect to motion perception.

For all pairs of cardinal axes, cardinal-axis modulations slid and off-axis modulations cohered.[2] Thus it is not just the color of the gratings but specifically their cardinal-axis composition that governs the perception of coherent motion. This can be understood by assuming multiple, independent motion analyzers, each sensitive to variation along a single cardinal axis. Gratings modulated along different cardinal axes appear to move independently because the motion of each grating is processed by a different mechanism. Off-axis gratings appear as coherent because they have the same cardinal-axis components and differ only in the relative phase of these components. To the extent that the cardinal-axis mechanisms are insensitive to phase and noncardinal mechanisms are nonexistent or weak, different off-axis gratings are, for purposes of motion perception, without effective color difference.

The data of Krauskopf and Farell constitute an existence proof of motion mechanisms tuned to the cardinal axes of color space. However, the inferred *independence* of these mechanisms has a different, and weaker, ontological status. The results show that cardinal-axis stimuli can function as independent sources of perceived motion, not that they must. The apparent independence of moving cardinal-axis stimuli could, in other words, be contingent on the stimuli or methods used. Such a contingency might explain why Krauskopf and Farell's findings do not jibe with those of others, who do find luminance-chromatic motion interactions. For example, a moving chromatic grating can null the directionally opposed motion of a luminance grating (Cavanagh and Anstis, 1991); luminance and chromatic stimuli induce cross-adaptation, each producing a motion aftereffect in the tests of the other color (Cavanagh and Favreau, 1985; Derrington and Badcock, 1985; Mullen and Baker, 1985), and observers report apparent motion between spatially separated color and luminance patches (Cavanagh, Arguin, and von Grünau, 1989; Cavanagh and Mather, 1989; Gorea, Papathomas, and Kovacs, 1993). These results suggest either a common mechanism for the processing of chromatic and luminance motion signals or an interaction between separate mechanisms (see, however, the data on color-contingent motion aftereffects of Favreau et al., 1972, and Mayhew and Anstis, 1972; also see Cavanagh, this volume, for a fuller discussion of cross-attribute motion effects). The resolute independence of Krauskopf and Farell's (1990) chromatic and luminance gratings is thus likely to be contingent on the specific spatial and color properties of these stimuli. What are those properties and why does the visual system give special treatment to them?

Spatial Influences

Let us assume that coherent motion results when at least one visual mechanism can "see" the motion of both components. Krauskopf and Farell's data imply that no such mechanism exists for components modulated along different cardinal axes. Yet these plaid components—a luminance grating and a red-green grating, say—differ not only in color, but also in their spatial properties. Minimally, they differ in orientation and in direction of motion. Thus, for cardinal-axis gratings to cohere, there would have to be a mechanism that saw the motion of

---

2. A large range of parametric variations was tried, all yielding similar results. The perceived sliding of cardinal-axis gratings was particularly robust, being immune to attempts to track the plaid's nodes and to other willful strategies aimed at inducing coherent motion. Only at long stimulus presentations were there fleeting instances of monocular rivalry (Campbell and Howell, 1972); in general both gratings were seen simultaneously as moving along separate paths.

gratings that differed in color—one lying along the luminance axis and other along the red–green axis—and spatially—in orientation and direction of motion. Stimuli that differ both in their spatial properties and in color might well fail to drive common motion mechanisms, even if neither difference alone exceeds the mechanisms' bandwidths.

Ideally, the relationship between luminance and chromatic motion signals should be examined in the absence of confounding spatial differences. One would want to look for interactions between gratings that are modulated along different cardinal axes but do not differ in orientation and direction of motion. But of course such components form a single compound grating, to which phenomena like coherence and sliding would seem not to apply. The following experiments attempt to get around this problem.

The experiments are based on the hypothesis that luminance and chromatic motion signals are combined within, not between, orientation bands. A common orientation is thus seen as a necessary (though not necessarily sufficient) condition for pooling of luminance and chromatic motion. The spatial decoupling of chromatic and luminance variation arising from a difference in orientation, as in Krauskopf and Farell's (1990) cardinal-axis plaids, is characteristic of separate objects and is perceived accordingly.

Experiment 1: Orientation and Noncardinal Sensitivity

Krauskopf and Farell (1990) presented observers with a random sequence of two types of plaids: those having different cardinal-axis gratings as components and those having different off-axis gratings as components. These plaids differ by a rotation in the color space of figure 12.1. By comparing the judged coherence of the two plaid types, Krauskopf and Farell tested the isotropy of that space and the cardinality of the luminance, L-M, and S-(L + M) axes for the analysis of motion.

The first experiment to be reported here was similar. Instead of presenting off-axis grating pairs and cardinal-axis grating pairs in a run of coherence judgments, this experiment presented off-axis grating pairs and *identically colored* grating pairs as the two stimulus classes of primary interest. An off-axis grating can be considered to be a compound of two gratings, each of which is modulated along a different cardinal axis. Off-axis gratings with identical cardinal-axis composition differ only in the phase of the modulation along these axes: a grating varying between light green and dark red and another varying between dark green and light red, for example. These off-axis gratings would be indistinguishable to a motion system of the type postulated by Krauskopf and Farell (1990), one consisting only of cardinal-axis mechanisms and insensitive to phase. To such a motion system, a plaid made up of off-axis gratings would appear as coherent as a plaid made up of identically colored grating.

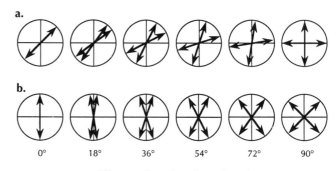

Figure 12.2
Color-space modulations of grating pairs used in experiment 1. Each double-headed arrow depicts the variation in color space across one grating cycle. Cardinal axes are represented by the vertical and horizontal lines. (*a*) Intermediate-centered grating pairs. (*b*) Axis-centered grating pairs.

Plaids were made up of drifting sinusoidal gratings and belonged to one of two conditions depending on the gratings' color. Color-space representations for the two conditions are shown in the two rows of figure 12.2. The six pairs of grating modulations on the top row are centered around a line intermediate between cardinal axes. They range from identical intermediate-direction modulations to modulations on different cardinal axes. Those in the bottom row are centered around a cardinal axis. Their range is from identical cardinal-axis modulations to different off-axis modulations. For the off-axis-centered plaids (figure 12.2a), identical modulations should cohere and, based on the results of Krauskopf and Farell (1990), modulations along different cardinal axes should slide. For cardinal-axis-centered plaids (figure 12.2b), the two modulations of each pair have identical cardinal-axis projections and should consistently cohere if motion is analyzed solely by independent cardinal-axis mechanisms.

Observers were instructed to classify the pattern as sliding if they detected relative motion between the components and as coherent otherwise. The gratings were 1 c/deg sinusoids, oriented 90° apart and drifting at 1°/sec. The direction of coherent motion was upward. The gratings appeared within a hard-edged circular window 7° in diameter. Patterns were presented for 1 sec, during which time a central fixation point remained in view. Luminance and chromatic components were set to have equal effective contrasts by a motion-coherence criterion (Farell, 1990), with luminance contrast averaging about 10% across observers. The background was an equal-energy white at 50 cd/m² , which matched each grating's average luminance.

Results

The probability of perceiving relative motion between the component compound gratings is shown for one observer in figure 12.3. These data are for modulations within the plane defined by the luminance and L-M axes; the two other cardinal-axis planes produced very similar results. The rigid motion of same-color gratings gives way to sliding as the gratings become increasingly separated in color space. In the case of off-axis-centered gratings these results are expected from Krauskopf and Farell's (1990) data. However, cardinal-axis-centered gratings are not always seen to cohere, even though their color-space representations project similarly onto the luminance and L-M axes. Different off-axis gratings, which cohered in Krauskopf and Farell's study, are ambiguous in this one. Observers classified them as slipping nearly half the time (45%). A similar percentage occurs when all the patterns of figure 12.2 appear within a run of trials.

The relative motion observed between different off-axis gratings (albeit inconsistently observed) demonstrates a

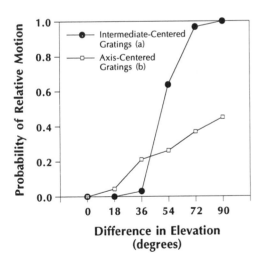

Figure 12.3
Results of experiment 1 for one observer. Probability of sliding as a function of the difference in elevation between component gratings. Gratings differing by 90° in elevation are modulated midway between the cardinal axes if they are intermediate centered, and are modulated along different cardinal axes if they are axis centered.

sensitivity to the motion of noncardinal modulations that cannot be explained by cardinal-axis mechanisms alone. This sensitivity might arise from interactions between cardinal-axis mechanisms or from separate motion mechanisms tuned to intermediate directions. In either case, the motion system's response to off-axis stimuli is relatively weak. The reason that off-axis sensitivity was apparent here and not apparent in Krauskopf and Farell's data has to do with the observer's criterion. The weakly interacting off-axis grating pairs appear to be *relatively* coherent when they are presented along with different cardinal-axis grating pairs, which cohere not at all. Conversely, they are seen as *relatively* incoherent when presented along with identically colored grating pairs, which are perceptually inseparable. For our purposes here, the important point is this relative incoherence; it indicates that perceived motion is not derived solely from independent cardinal-axis motion mechanisms.

Where are different cardinal-axis signals combined? The combination might occur in a pathway that provides input for the computation of motion, or in a stage following the separate computations of cardinal-axis grating motion. The data rule out an interaction that follows the separate computations of coherent cardinal-axis motion. This is because the cardinal-axis plaids that are contained within an off-axis plaid have the same direction of coherent motion, and yet, as shown in this experiment, the off-axis plaid itself is less coherent than single-color plaids. It is therefore likely that what is combined from the cardinal-axis components of a compound grating are either their inputs to motion analyzers or the outputs of the analysis of their separate one-dimensional motions (Adelson and Movshon, 1982).

Experiment 2: Effect of Spatial Frequency

The components of a compound grating—a luminance modulation and a red-green modulation, for example—have the same orientation, drift direction, and speed, so cohering and sliding might seem not to be applicable perceptual outcomes. Yet when viewed in isolation, a luminance and a chromatic grating often appear to move at quite different speeds, whereas the compound grating made from these components has a single perceived speed, a weighted average (Cavanagh and Favreau, 1985; Cavanagh et al., 1984; Smith and Edgar, 1991). More interesting still are the possible outcomes of combining a compound grating with a simple cardinal-axis grating at a different orientation, to form a plaid. An example is a compound light-red/dark-green grating oriented at 45°

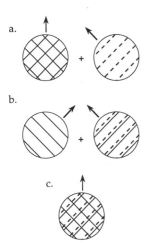

Figure 12.4
Possible outcomes of experiment 2. Solid and dashed lines represent components modulated along different cardinal axes. Arrows represent perceived drift directions. Patterns with different drift directions are spatially segregated here for clarity. (*a*) Grouping by color. (*b*) Grouping by orientation. (*c*) Grouping by color and orientation.

with a "northwest" drift direction that is paired with a simple red-green grating oriented at 135° with a "northeast" drift direction. Three outcomes make sense in light of what is already known.

Grouping by Color

A coherent plaid of one color moves transparently with respect to the simple grating of the other color. This grouping-by-color outcome, schematized in figure 12.4a, is expected from independent cardinal-axis motion mechanisms.

Grouping by Orientation

Here the compound grating slides with respect to the simple grating, i.e., gratings that differ in orientation are seen to move independently (figure 12.4b). Note that the sliding of gratings with different orientations implies that the components of the compound grating are cohering: If these two components were *not* cohering, then one of them would cohere with the component having the same color and different orientation, as it does when *these* are the only components in view.

Grouping by Color and Orientation

All three gratings move together coherently (figure 12.4c). In this case, as in the previous one, there is coherence across different cardinal axes.

There are several advantages in using compound gratings to examine the color modularity of motion per-

ception. For one, they eliminate the confounding of differences in stimulus color and differences in orientation and drift direction. This allows the influence of other spatiotemporal variables, such as spatial frequency, to be studied in isolation. This was done here. The spatial frequency of chromatic components, in both simple and compound gratings, was 1 c/deg, and that of luminance components ranged from 0.25 to 4.0 c/deg. The gratings drifted at a speed of 1 deg/sec. The compound grating contained luminance and red—green components and was oriented 45° to one or the other side of vertical. The simple grating was either a luminance grating or a red-green grating and was orthogonal in orientation to the compound grating. In other details the method paralleled that of the first experiment.

Results

Of the three possible outcomes described in figure 12.4, one of them, grouping by orientation, was never observed. Instead, motion segregated by color—an upward-drifting plaid moved transparently across a simple grating moving off to the side by 45° (figure 12.4a)—or all components cohered into a rigidly moving multicolored plaid (figure 12.4c).

The proportion of trials on which the components of the compound grating were seen as sliding (i.e., not part of a multicolored plaid) is plotted in figure 12.5 as a function of the luminance-chromatic spatial frequency ratio. Data are plotted separately for patterns in which the sim-

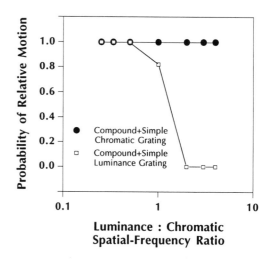

Figure 12.5
Results of experiment 2 for one observer. Probability of sliding as a function of the ratio of the spatial frequencies of the luminance and chromatic components. Results are plotted separately for the pairing of compound gratings with simple luminance gratings and with simple chromatic gratings.

ple grating was a luminance modulation and for patterns in which it was a chromatic modulation.

Adding a simple chromatic grating to a luminance-chromatic compound grating (filled symbols in figure 12.5) dissociates the compound grating into its components (figure 12.4a). The luminance component is seen to move in the direction of its spatial modulation, e.g., to the "northwest." The chromatic component combines with the simple grating to form a coherent red–green plaid drifting due "north." The two resulting patterns—a luminance grating and a chromatic plaid—are seen as sliding transparently across each other. Their motions were independent; direction matching showed that each pattern moved as it does in isolation. As seen in figure 12.5, the ratio of the spatial frequencies of the luminance and chromatic modulations did not affect perceived motion over a 16-fold range (4:1 to 1:4).

Changing the color of the simple grating to black–white from red–green has a profound effect. The perceived motion now depends strongly on the relative spatial frequencies of the luminance and chromatic components, as seen by open symbols in figure 12.5. When the luminance components have the lower frequency, $F_l < F_c$, the compound grating separates into its components, and a red-green grating is seen to slide transparently across a luminance plaid. However, when $F_l > F_c$, no relative motion is seen. Instead, all three components fuse into a multicolored plaid.

This perceptual switch—from motion segregated by color to coherent motion between cardinal-axis components—occurs within a fairly narrow range of spatial-frequency ratios, centered roughly on a ratio of 1.0. The first of these outcomes is expected if motion signals from different cardinal axes were analyzed separately. The second outcome is expected if motion signals were analyzed without regard to their source in color space.

The way in which luminance and chromatic motion signals contribute to a final motion percept is shown here to vary with the spatial parameters of the stimuli. Similarity of orientation is one important spatial requirement for the combining of these signals. Without common orientations, patterns drawn from different cardinal axes are seen as moving independently (Krauskopf and Farell, 1990). More surprising is the effect of relative spatial frequency. Luminance and chromatic signals appear to interact not within a spatial-frequency band, but across bands. Frequency doubling of the chromatic signal (Derrington, Krauskopf, and Lennie, 1984) appears not to be a factor, for motion percept is unchanged whether the ratio is 2:1 or 4:1.

Experiment 3: The Uses of Luminance Edges

The previous experiments showed that motion interactions across the cardinal axes vary with the spatial properties of the stimuli, in particular with their relative orientations and spatial frequencies. If we knew the extent to which these interactions are spatially localized, the role of spatial variables would be clarified. One way to investigate this is to look at the effect of shifting the relative spatial phase of the luminance and chromatic stimuli.

Because of their spatial frequency difference, the compound grating components that cohered in the previous study are not entirely appropriate for this experiment, so the luminance components were modified, as shown in figure 12.6. Instead of sinusoids, fluted luminance square waves were used: The fundamental frequency was removed from luminance square waves of 0.5 c/deg. Two drifting fluted luminance square waves, oriented 90° apart, were summed. The red-green grating was, as before, sinusoidal; its frequency matched that of the luminance fundamental and it had the same orientation as one of the luminance gratings and moved at the same speed and direction. This arrangement maintains the $F_l > F_c$ relation in spatial frequency and introduces a luminance profile having a wide period, a desirable property for a high-frequency pattern used to examine the effect of relative phase. Figure 12.6 shows the profiles of the parallel red-green and luminance gratings; the luminance edges coincided either with chromatic zero-crossings (in phase) or with chromatic peaks (90° phase shift).

Results

Observers saw all components of the pattern moving coherently as a rigid multicolored plaid on every trial in the

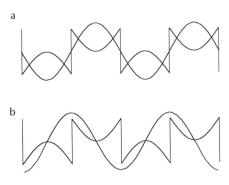

Figure 12.6
Compound grating profiles used in experiment 3. Luminance varies as a missing-fundamental square-wave grating; red-green variation has a sinusoidal profile. (*a*) In-phase. (*b*) 90° relative phase.

in-phase condition. This result is expected from the previous experiment. Shifting the relative phase by 90° produced no change in motion. Instead, it led to a change in the perceived color of the pattern. The first trial began with the luminance and chromatic components in the 90° phase-shift condition appearing to move coherently upward. The chromatic component then faded from view, leaving a moving achromatic plaid. The initial fading took several (1–3) seconds, which could extend over several successive presentations of the pattern (interstimulus interval ≈ 2 sec). Thereafter, stimulus onset restored at most a hint of color. After the color had vanished, saccades of around 2° or more would bring it back before it again rapidly faded. Small saccades had no effect.

Shifting the relative phase of luminance and chromatic grating components did have an effect, suggesting spatially local interactions, but it did not have the expected effect of decoupling the gratings' motions. Instead, the chromatic component became invisible. This is quite remarkable, for a low spatial- and temporal-frequency, high-contrast red-green grating is normally a maximally visible chromatic stimulus. If the chromatic signals between luminance edges were integrated or averaged, one would expect achromacy in the 90° phase-shift condition and a sparing of red-green contrast in the in-phase condition, as was observed. Direction matching data support the view that the visual system used chromatic information to "fill-in" a moving surface demarcated by luminance edges: The amount of chromatic contrast had no effect on the direction of the plaid.[3]

Discussion

Perception of the spatiotemporal properties of objects has traditionally been explained in terms of the processing of spatiotemporal luminance information. Chromatic content has seemed largely inessential to the process; old movies gain little from being colorized. However, we see from the experiments reported here that color can have dramatic effects on the perceived motion of a pattern and that these effects depend on how chromatic and luminance contrasts are distributed across the pattern's spatial features. The results offer a glimpse into the visual system's construction of objects.

Previous data are split over the question of whether the luminance and chromatic components of a scene are analyzed by common motion mechanisms or by independent mechanisms that partition the motion of a scene into separate streams. Physiologically, either alternative seems possible. Parallel magnocellular and parvocellular pathways have been suggested as a substrate for the separate processing of luminance and chromatic information (Livingstone and Hubel, 1987). In particular, the broadband magnocellular pathway provides much of the input to neurons in area MT, which are known to be involved in motion processing (De Yoe and van Essen, 1988). Complicating matters is the magnocellular response to isoluminant stimuli (Schiller and Colby, 1983; Derrington, Krauskopf, and Lennie, 1984) and the partial convergence of magno and parvo pathways (Ts'o and Gilbert, 1988). The parvo stream likewise provides input for motion analysis (Merigan and Maunsell, 1990; Schiller, Logothetis, and Charles, 1989), though with a temporal frequency tuning and contrast response that differ from those of the magno stream. The parvo contribution might also, like the magno contribution, be mediated in part by cells in area MT (Saito et al., 1989). Whether parvocellular luminance and chromatic signals are processed separately, in MT or elsewhere, and how they might combine with the magno input, is unclear. But the potential for interaction is there; the present data suggest that finding such an interaction might require choosing stimuli with an eye out for the luminance and chromatic spatial parameters that characterize objects.

Conditions for Independence and Interaction

The experiments used compound gratings to show, first, that the visual system can combine the motions of stimuli drawn from the colors of different cardinal axes, but appears to do so only within orientation bands. This combination precedes the site at which the motions of stimuli of different orientations, modulated along a single cardinal axis, are combined. The second experiment showed that, for the particular stimuli used, luminance–chromatic interactions occur across spatial frequency bands and are dominated by the motion of relatively high-frequency luminance components. As shown by a third experiment, phase matters; a balanced red-green modulation lying be-

3. Motion capture is related to filling-in and shows an asymmetry between luminance and chromaticity akin to that of experiment 2. Ramachandran (1986, 1987) found that moving luminance contours impart motion on a stationary chromatic stimulus, but a movement of chromatic contours did not affect stationary luminance stimuli; however, it was uncertain how well, if at all, the physically moving chromatic stimulus had been seen to move. Ramachandran

assumed that chromatic *borders* were captured by luminance borders, contrary to the indications of the data here. Also, the *lower* the spatial frequency of a drifting achromatic grating, the more effectively it captures superimposed achromatic randomly moving dots (Ramachandran and Cavanagh, 1987; Ramachandran and Inada, 1985), very different from the spatial-frequency relation observed in the present data (also see Yo and Wilson, 1992).

tween luminance edges is suppressed, possibly because of chromatic integration.

The experiments support a generality, to which prior data also conform: Stimuli modulated along different cardinal axes are perceived as moving independently when their orientations differ. Orientation differences produce no comparable impediment to motion interactions *within* cardinal axes, as witnessed by the coherent motion of gratings of the same color. Shared orientation is not a sufficient condition for luminance-chromatic interactions. Other spatial factors, such as relative frequency and phase, appear to play a catalytic role. The specific spatial conditions that promote the interaction of luminance and chromatic motion signals—shared orientations, $F_l > F_c$—are not typical of gratings but can be found in natural objects, if one looks selectively at chromatic surfaces and the luminance edges that frame them. Near threshold contrast, at least, visual sensitivity is tuned to the corresponding frequencies, displaying a low-pass profile for chromatic variation and a band-pass profile for luminance (Kelly, 1983; Mullen, 1985).

The visual system might differentially use the spatial features of luminance and chromatic variation in order to cut down on redundant processing—i.e., by a division of processing labor between luminance and chromatic mechanisms. This would also contribute to the perceptual coherence of objects. For example, the spatial parameters of shadow would tend not to involve it in luminance-chromatic interactions. The occasional disappearance of chromatic modulations would be have to be counted among the inevitable costs of such processing strategies.

Color, Space, and Objects

The visual system must somehow integrate information across parallel pathways. It is usually assumed that the intended outcome is a percept that veridically represents the combination of properties belonging to external objects. But visual psychophysicists rarely design displays in which information integration can fail in telling ways; narrow-bandwidth stimuli and isolated channels are *de rigueur* (though there are exceptions: Julesz, 1971, 1980, 1981). As a result, there is little consensus about the definition of objects or about their computational status in visual processing.

Intuitively, we might expect two pathways to contribute to the perception of a single object if the activity in both pathways is consistent with the same shape in the

same location moving at the same speed and in the same direction. Remarkably, this intuition does not hold up; in a perceptual tug-of-war, pathways responding to a difference in color can override those responding to shared spatiotemporal features. As seen in this chapter, a stimulus that varies sinusoidally between dark red and light green is not processed by the motion system as a unitary stimulus. Rather, it is processed as separable red-green and luminance modulations, even though these modulations may be *spatiotemporally identical*. Adding a simple grating of differing orientation and drift direction can split the red-green and luminance components between two distinct objects—a plaid and a simple grating—that are segregated by color.[4] The potency of color in determining what objects are seen is one of two points demonstrated in the present studies.

The second point demonstrated here is that color and spatial variables do not affect motion perception independently. Their interactions are complex. Perceived motion depends on the specific distribution of luminance and chromatic variation across the spatial frequency components and orientations of the display. Chromatic- and luminance-derived motion signals are processed both independently and interactively; apparent inconsistencies in the experimental literature simply reflect variations in the spatial parameters that govern interactions across color space. It is suggested that these interactions have a functional role as specializations for the perception of objects and may be regarded as the visual system's attempt to exploit the correlation between luminance and chromatic spatial distributions that it expects in a world of objects.

Acknowledgment

Preparation of this chapter was supported by NEI grant EY09872.

References

Adelson, E. H., and Movshon, J. A. (1982). Phenomenal coherence of moving visual patterns. *Nature (London) 300*, 523–525.

Campbell, F. W., and Howell, E. R. (1972). Monocular alternation: A method for the investigation of pattern vision. *J. Physiol. 225*, 19–21P.

Cavanagh, P. (1987). Reconstructing the third dimension: Interactions between color, texture, motion, binocular disparity, and shape. *Comput. Vision Graphics Image Process. 37*, 171–195.

4. It would be interesting to see if a similar dissociation could be induced (at higher spatial frequencies than used here) between a chromatic stimulus and the luminance signal it generates because of chromatic aberration.

Cavanagh, P., and Anstis, S. (1991). The contribution of color to motion in normal and color-deficient observers. *Vision Res. 31*, 2109–2148.

Cavanagh, P., and Favreau, O. E. (1985). Color and luminance share a common motion pathway. *Vision Res. 25*, 1595–1601.

Cavanagh, P., and Mather, G. (1989). Motion: The long and short of it. *Spatial Vision 4*, 103–129.

Cavanagh, P., Tyler, C. W., and Favreau, O. E. (1984). Perceived velocity of moving chromatic gratings. *J. Opt. Soc. Am. A 1*, 893–899.

Cavanagh, P., Arguin, M., and von Grünau, M. (1989). Interattribute apparent motion. *Vision Res. 29*, 1197–1204.

Derrington, A. M., and Badcock, D. R. (1985). The low level motion system has both chromatic and luminance inputs. *Vision Res. 25*, 1879–1884.

Derrington, A. M., Krauskopf, J., and Lennie, P. (1984). Chromatic mechanisms in lateral geniculate nucleus of macaque. *J. Physiol. 357*, 241–265.

De Yoe, E. A., and Van Essen, D. C. (1988). Concurrent processing streams in monkey visual cortex. *Trends in Neurosci. 11*, 219–226.

De Valois, R. L., and De Valois, K. K. (1988). *Spatial Vision*. New York: Oxford University Press.

Farell, B. (1990). When chromatic and luminance gratings cohere. *Invest. Ophthalmol. Visual Sci. (Suppl.), 31*, 518.

Favreau, O. E., Emerson, V. F., and Corballis, M. C. (1972). Motion perception: A color-contingent aftereffect. *Science 212*, 831–832.

Gorea, A., Papathomas, T. V., and Kovacs, I. (1993). Motion perception with spatiotemporally matched chromatic and achromatic information reveals a "slow" and a "fast" motion system. *Vision Res. 33*, 2515–2534.

Julesz, B. (1971). *Foundations of Cyclopian Perception*. Chicago: University of Chicago Press.

Julesz, B. (1980). Spatial frequency channels in one-, two-, and three dimensional vision: Variations on a theme by Bekesy. In C. S. Harris (Ed.), *Visual Coding and Adaptability* (pp. 263–316). Hillside, NJ: Erlbaum.

Julesz, B. (1981). Textons, the elements of texture perception, and their interactions. *Nature (London) 290*, 91–97.

Kelly, D. H. (1983). Spatiotemporal variation of chromatic and achromatic contrast thresholds. *J. Opt. Soc. Am. A 73*, 742–750.

Krauskopf, J., and Farell, B. (1990). Influence of colour on the perception of coherent motion. *Nature (London) 348*, 328–331.

Krauskopf, J., and Farell, B. (1991). Vernier acuity: Effects of chromatic content, blur and contrast. *Vision Res. 31*, 735–749.

Krauskopf, J., Williams, D. R., and Healy, D. W. (1982). Cardinal directions of color space. *Vision Res. 22*, 1123–1131.

Krauskopf, J., Farell, B., and Movshon, J. A. (1989). Phenomenal coherence of moving chromatic gratings. *Invest. Ophthalmol. Visual Science* (Suppl.) 30, 389.

Livingstone, M. S., and Hubel, D. H. (1984). Anatomy and physiology of a color system in primate primary visual cortex. *J. Neurosci. 4*, 309–356.

Livingstone, M. S., and Hubel, D. H. (1987). Psychophysical evidence for separate channels for perception of form, color, movement and depth. *J. Neurosci. 7*, 3416–3468.

Mayhew, J. E. W., and Anstis, S. M. (1972). Movement aftereffects contingent on colour, intensity and pattern. *Vision Res. 12*, 77–85.

Merigan, W. H., and Maunsell, J. H. R. (1990). Macaque vision after magnocellular lateral geniculate lesions. *Visual Neurosci 5*, 347–352.

Morgan, M. J., and Aiba, T. S. (1985). Positional acuity with chromatic stimuli. *Vision Res. 25*, 689–695.

Mullen, K. T. (1985). The contrast sensitivity of human colour vision to red-green and blue-yellow chromatic gratings. *J. Physiol. 359*, 381–400.

Mullen, K. T. (1987). Spatial influences on colour opponent contributions to pattern detection. *Vision Res. 27*, 829–839.

Mullen, K. T., and Baker, C. L. (1985). A motion aftereffect from an isoluminant stimulus. *Vision Res. 25*, 685–688.

Mullen, K. T., and Boulton, J. C. (1992). Absence of smooth motion perception in color vision. *Vision Res. 32*, 483–488.

Palmer, J., and Mobley, L. A. (1993). Motion at isoluminance: discrimination/detection ratios and the summation of luminance and chromatic signals. *J. Opt. Soc. Am. A 10*, 1353–1362.

Papathomas, T. V., Gorea, A., and Julesz, B. (1991). Two carriers for motion perception: Color and luminance. *Vision Res. 31*, 1883–1891.

Ramachandran, V. S. (1986). Capture of stereopsis and apparent motion by illusory contours. *Percept. Psychophys. 39*, 361–373.

Ramachandran, V. S. (1987). Interaction between colour and motion in human vision. *Nature (London) 328*, 645–647.

Ramachandran, V. S., and Cavanagh, P. (1987). Motion capture anisotropy. *Vision Res. 27*, 97–106.

Ramachandran, V. S., and Gregory, R. L. (1978). Does colour provide an input to human motion perception? *Nature (London) 275*, 55–57.

Ramachandran, V. S., and Inada, V. (1985). Spatial phase and frequency in motion capture of random dot patterns. *Spatial Vision 1*, 57–67.

Saito, H., Tanaka, K., Isono, H., Yasuda, M., and Mikami, A. (1989). Directionally selective response of cells in the middle temporal area (MT) of the macaque monkey to the movement of equiluminous opponent color stimuli. *Exp. Brain Res. 75*, 1–14.

Schiller, P. H., and Colby, C. L. (1983). The responses of single cells in the lateral geniculate nucleus of the rhesus monkey to color and luminance contrast. *Vision Res. 23*, 1631–1641.

Schiller, P. H., Logothetis, N. K., and Charles, E. R. (1989). Functions of the colour-opponent and broad-band channels of the visual system. *Nature (London) 343*, 68–70.

Smith, A. T., and Edgar, G. K. (1991). Perceived speed and direction of complex gratings and plaids. *J. Opt. Soc. Am. A 8*, 1161–1171.

Stromeyer, C. F., Eskew, R. T., and Kronauer, R. E. (1990). The most sensitive motion detectors in humans are spectrally-opponent. *Invest. Ophthalmol. Visual Sci. (Suppl.) 31*, 240.

Teller, D. Y., and Lindsey, D. T. (1993). Motion at isoluminance: motion dead zones in three-dimensional color space. *J. Opt. Soc. Am. A 10*, 1324–1331.

Ts'o, D. Y., and Gilbert, C. D. (1988). The organization of chromatic and spatial interactions in the primate striate cortex. *J. Neurophysiol. 8,* 1712–1727.

Van Essen, D. C. (1985). Functional organization of the primate visual cortex. In A. Peters and E. G. Jones (Eds.), *Cerebral Cortex* (Vol. 3). New York: Plenum.

Yo, C., and Wilson, H. R. (1992). Moving two-dimensional patterns can capture the perceived directions of lower or higher spatial frequency gratings. *Vision Res. 32,* 1263–1269.

Zeki, S. M. (1978). Functional specialization in the visual cortex of the rhesus monkey. *Nature (London): 274,* 423–428.

13

Depth from Motion

George Sperling and Barbara Anne Dosher

Overview

This chapter is concerned with the perception of object depth and object structure that results from monocular viewing as distinct from stereoptic depth that results from binocular viewing. Two successive views of a rotating object contain precisely the same kind of information as the two views from different eyes. As an object rotates, there is a continuum of views. Therefore, there is no physical reason why the depth that is perceived in viewing a rotating object might not appear to be even more realistic and more depthful than stereoptic depth.

We will demonstrate here that it is the motion flow field that contains the information that is used to extract perceived depth from dynamic monocular displays. Once a display is perceived as having three-dimensional (3D) depth, its apparent rigidity—or lack thereof—is a property derived from the successive 3D structures over time, rather than vice versa, as would be suggested by algorithms that use rigidity itself to extract the depth structure (e.g., Gryzwacz and Hildreth, 1987; Grywacz et al., 1988; Hildreth et al., 1990; Bennett et al., 1989; Koenderink and van Doorn, 1986; Longuet-Higgins and Prazdny, 1980; Ullman, 1984). In other words, we hypothesize that the sequence of perceptual computations is first *depth from motion*, then *structure from depth*.

Motion-Depth-Sign Ambiguity

The computation of depth from object motion is inherently ambiguous with respect to the sign of the depth (the *motion-depth-sign*). Without an additional cue (such as knowledge of the self-motion that produced the motion flow field), a particular motion flow field supports two plausible depth isomers, with depth relations that are mirror reflections of each other (e.g., Ullman, 1979). A first step in computing depth from motion is the choice of one of these two possible depth isomers. For example, when self-motion produces the object motion (motion parallax), the perceptual motion–depth computation is immediately disambiguated (Ono and Steinbach, 1990; Ono, Rivest, and Ono, 1986). Many cues can exert a powerful influence on the motion-depth-sign. The decision mechanism for determining the motion-depth-sign is like a balance scale that tilts in either one of two directions. We will show that cues favoring one depth isomer versus another exert their influence by combining additively, just like weights in the two pans of the balance scale.

The potency of a depth-disambiguation cue is greatest during the very first instant of viewing a dynamic display. Once a particular motion-depth isomer is perceived, it is quite stable and resistant to change. This path dependence is characteristic of winner-take-all cooperation–competition neural networks (e.g., Sperling, 1970) and also of systems of dipoles such as those responsible for the magnetic properties of metals (Julesz, 1971). Some of the consequences of this kind of computation are considered below.

Size Indeterminacy of Monocular Vision

Because the distance between the eyes is known, stereopsis can give absolute depth information; for example, we can use stereopsis to thread a needle. Monocular vision without head or body movements, and neglecting accommodation, is geometrically excluded from yielding absolute size information. A firefly in front of the eye and a cataclysmic solar event could cast identical retinal images.

Depth-Scale Indeterminacy of Instantaneous Flow Fields

Indeed, the *instantaneous* motion flow field fails not only to yield absolute size, but also to yield the depth scale of a shape: An instantaneous flow field could have been generated by a very small movement of a very depthful object, or a larger movement of a relatively flatter object (cf. Adelson, 1985). However, under ordinary circumstances, two different flow fields suffice to yield the depth scale. That is, once the angle of object rotation around an axis perpendicular to the line of sight is greater than zero (in a noiseless system), depth-scale ambiguity is optically resolvable. When the angle of rotation reaches 90°, the object that was initially viewed end-on has rotated to appear sideways, and the 90° image provides perfect shape resolution. The minimum angle of rotation required for perceptual resolution of depth-scale ambiguity depends, of course, on the shape of the object and the quality of the image.

Processing Architecture: Common Depth Channel

The perception of depth from 2D projections without stereo, shading, or parallax is the *kinetic depth effect* or KDE (Wallach and O'Connell, 1953). When one views KDE stimuli such as rotating Necker cubes, especially in a setting that removes incidental cues to the depth of the display screen on which they are represented, the sense of depth organization for the perceived object is quite vivid —as vivid as the depth organization supported by stereopsis. That perceived depth from kinetic cues can be as realistic as perceived depth from stereopsis suggests that both sources of information feed into a *common depth channel*.

A proposed architecture for the relations and interactions between the various cues to depth and shape is indicated in figure 13.1. The top channel of figure 13.1 indicates a motion signal (a motion flow field) being processed to extract depth from motion. The sign ($+$ or $-$) of the extracted depth is indeterminate and this indeterminacy is resolved by a *bistable motion–depth inverter* that multiplies the extracted depth-from-motion relations by either $+1$ or -1.

Depth from stereopsis is computed in parallel with depth from motion. The depth values computed by stereopsis influence the bistable motion-depth inverter, and, together with other influences, determine the sign (-1 or $+1$) of the inverter.

Luminance-contrast also influences the bistable motion-depth inverter: High-contrast objects and regions tend to be perceived as being closer than low-contrast objects. The influences from stereo and from luminance add linearly to produce a net influence (e.g., Dosher, Sperling, and Wurst, 1986). Together, motion and stereo depth signals determine a *joint depth map*. This is an assignment of a depth value to each point in the cyclopean x, y image. Just how the depth information from motion and from stereo jointly determine the joint depth map is an interesting, not fully resolved problem.

Depth information also is potentially available from texture, from shading, and from other kinds of inputs. Whether these sources of depth information influence the bistable motion–depth inverter is not yet known. On the other hand, they apparently do influence the joint depth map—at least, that is one way to interpret the findings of Maloney and Landy (1989), who studied the apparent shape of surfaces defined by various combinations of these cues.

A depth map is merely an input to higher perceptual processes, it does not produce any output directly to effectors. The particular higher perceptual process of concern here is object perception, represented in figure 13.1 as an object module that derives object structure from its various inputs. Information encoding at the level of object module is not in terms of an x, y, z, t depth map but in

FORM OF REPRESENTATION

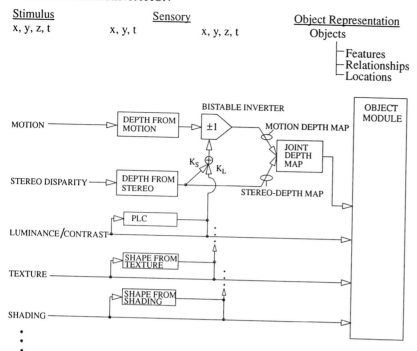

Figure 13.1

Flow chart for the computations of depth recovery from sensory cues and for its relation to the representation of features in an object-memory. External visual stimuli (neglecting color) are represented by their luminance as a function of space x, y, z, (z is the depth dimension) and time t. On the retina, a stimulus is merely a function of x, y, t. For a stationary observer, estimates of the lost dimension z are produced by the depth-from-motion and depth-from-stereo computations. The depth ambiguity of the depth-from-motion computation is resolved by the bistable depth inverter module, which receives additive inputs from stereo disparity, from luminance-contrast computations (proximity luminance covariance, PLC), and perhaps from other cues to produce a joint depth map. Objects are represented as lists of features, relationships, and location; cues (such as motion) are represented here directly in the object module as an object feature, in addition to any depth values that may have been computed from it. It is hypothesized that object rigidity is first computed at this stage.

terms of object components (e.g., geons or volumetric units, Biederman, 1987; Pentland, 1989; Pentland and Sclaroff, 1991) in which depth relations are represented as the shapes of object components (features) rather than as x, y properties of the object as a whole.

Undoubtedly, there is feedback from the object module back to the computations that provide the inputs. For example, the perceived depth isomer of ambiguous objects tends to alternate (Cornwell, 1976; Orbach, Ehrlich, and Heath, 1963; Spitz and Lipman, 1962) and, in our architecture, this would most naturally be implemented by feedback from the object module to the bistable motion–depth inverter.

Finally, it should be noted that in addition to their contribution to a depth computation, motion, texture, shading, and other inputs are represented directly as attributes or features of objects.

We now consider some of the properties and psychophysics of perceptual shape recovery from dynamic visual displays—evidence for the assertions made above.

The Linear Addition of Cue Strengths

The Multistable Perceptions of Necker Cubes

The 3D object interpretation resulting from a 2D projection of 3D rigid-object motion is generally ambiguous, corresponding to two stable perceptual depth isomers. We illustrate this with a Necker cube, a wire object that can be perceived as either one of two depth isomers. The probability of seeing a simple wire Necker cube as one versus the other isomer reflects biases and incidental cues. Among the cues that can disambiguate depth ordering, stereopsis is one of the strongest. Self-motion (motion parallax) also provides a powerful disambiguating cue. A third cue that is sufficient to affect the determination of a depth isomer is luminance contrast: regions of high contrast tend to be perceived as in front of low-contrast regions.

The above cues to depth work about equally well to determine the perceptual depth isomer of a Necker cube whether it is displayed with orthographic (parallel) projection or perspective projection. In orthographic projection, the two depth isomers are mirror equivalent, so there is no intrinsic reason to choose one over the other. However, when a Necker cube is displayed in perspective transformation (or when a real Necker cube subtends a greater-than-zero visual angle), the two depth isomers are not the same shape: one is a rigidly rotating cube and the other is a nonrigid truncated pyramid, the degree of nonrigidity being proportional to the degree of perspective. The remarkable fact about the perceptual bistability of such rotating Necker cubes is that rigidity per se has little effect on the probability of perceiving one depth isomer versus another. For example, in experiments of Schwartz and Sperling (1983) that used rotating Necker cubes viewed in perspective projection, the probabilities of perceiving the rigid and nonrigid depth isomers were about equal (in uniform-contrast displays). While rigidity had a too-small-to-measure influence on the sign of motion-depth, a minor cue, such as contrast, was highly potent. In these rotating Necker cube displays, differential contrast induced the high-contrast-forward depth isomer in 95% of presentations, for all subjects, whether it was the rigid depth isomer or not.

Jointly Independent Cues to Depth

An objective method for comparing the strengths of the various cues to depth in KDE displays was developed by Dosher, Sperling, and Wurst (1986), who first proposed that multiple cues to depth combine linearly. These investigators studied kinetic depth involving the collateral cues of stereopsis and what they called "proximity-luminance covariation" (see figure 13.2). They presented perspective Necker cubes rotating around a vertical axis to subjects who were asked to report on the direction of rotation (front to the right or front to the left). In such displays, the direction of rotation is apparent immediately at the onset of rotation, and it is perfectly coupled with the either the rigid or the nonrigid perceptual mode.

The two collateral cues to depth organization are schematically illustrated in figure 13.2. The contrast manipulation (proximity luminance covariation) changed the intensity $I(j)$ of the line j in the Necker cube according to several different front-to-rear luminance-falloff schemes. When contrast falls off from front to rear (figure 13.2b), it favors perceiving a rigid cube; when contrast falls off from rear to front (figure 13.2c), it favors perceiving a truncated pyramid. The second cue was rotational stereo, illustrated in figure 13.2e. Stereo disparity could either agree with the generating Necker cube (the rigid isomer) or with the nonrigid truncated pyramid.

A Thurstone Case 5 Model for Predicting Perceptual Mode

Dosher et al. (1986) found that the probability of perceiving the rigid cube isomer was jointly determined by the two cues, and could be accounted for by an additive model that is equivalent to Thurstone's (1947) Case 5 (figure 13.2g–k). Let p be the probability of perceiving the rigid depth isomer. In the absence of any cue, p is assumed to be determined by an individual bias and by internal noise. Internal noise is the standard against which all cues are measured and it is assumed to be normally distributed around zero with unit variance. Positive values correspond to the rigid perception and negative values to the nonrigid perception. Individual bias corresponds to a shift of the noise distribution, corresponding to a tendency to perceive either the rotating cube as rigid or nonrigid in the absence of any other cue. The strengths of the stereo cue and the contrast cue are then estimated in isolation for seven different levels of each, in terms of how far they shift the noise distribution (figure 13.2j). According to the model, when the stereo and contrast cues are now combined in the 7×7 different combinations, their strengths simply add, whether the cues be in concert or in opposition. In fact, this additive strength model provided essentially perfect predictions of the probability of perceiving the rigid cube versus the truncated pyramid for the 7×7 cue combinations.

Why Does an Additive Cue-Strength Model Work so Well?

One way to conceptualize the two stable perceptual states (rigid, nonrigid) for a perspective Necker cube is in terms of an energy map (Sperling, 1970; Sperling and Dosher, 1987). The energy map in figure 13.2k represents the perceived nonrigidity under rotation of all the perceptual 3D reconstructions—rigid and nonrigid—of the Necker cube as indexed by their perceived front-to-rear depth. The minima (energy wells) represent the two rigid depth isomers under parallel projection. Assume that at the instant a display depicting a rotating cue is turned on, the perceived front-to-rear distance is zero. This perceptually flat Necker cube would appear to be highly nonrigid under rotation. The high degree of nonrigidity is represented by the high ridge between the two energy wells. A marble represents the current state of the system; at the onset, it is delicately perched on the ridge dividing the two energy wells. At this instant, the system is in highly unstable equilibrium. Cues are represented as forces acting to push the marble in one direction or the other. Forces combine linearly, but once the marble is in

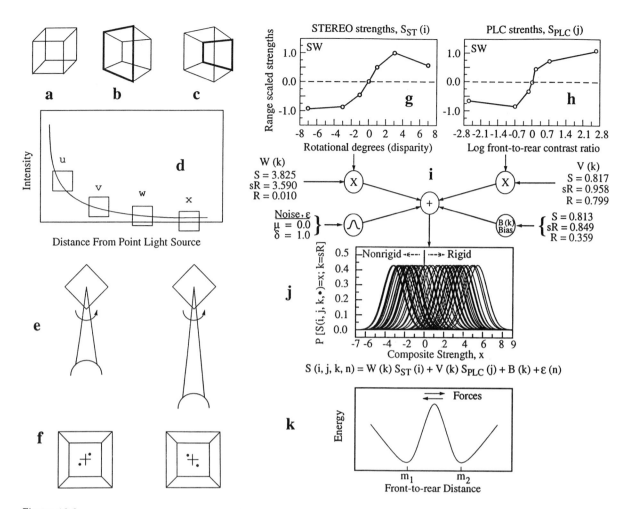

Figure 13.2

The perceived depth isomer of a Necker cube is predicted by a model of additive cue integration. (*a–c*) Necker cubes: (*a*) has neither perspective not contrast cues; (*b*) contrast agrees with perspective; (*c*) contrast opposes perspective. When (*c*) rotates in 3D, the dominant percept is a nonrigid truncated pyramid. (*d*) A diagram to indicate how intensity (or contrast) would fall off from the front to the rear of a self-luminous Necker cube at various distances. Within (*d*), the strength of contrast cue is (*u*) > (*v*) > (*w*) > (*x*). (*e*) illustrates two simulated extents of stereo; large stereo disparity on the left, and smaller disparity on the right. In inverted stereo, the left and right eye's views are switched, favoring perception of a nonrigid, truncated pyramid. (*f*) Left and right eye views showing the arrangement of the fixation cross and dots. A trial began only after the subject simultaneously perceived all four dots. (*g–j*) Illustration of an application of the *linear cue integration model* to the data of subject SW. (*g*) Weight of strength favoring the rigid depth isomer as a function of stereo disparity (in degrees of rotation between left- and right-eye images). (*h*) Weight of strength favoring the rigid depth isomer as a function of the log (base 10) of the ratio: (contrast of front)/(contrast of rear). (*i*) The model. Contrast strength W(k), disparity strength V(k), a (usually very small) rigidity bias B(k), and random noise ε are added; k indicates condition. A sum greater than 0 corresponds to the rigid Necker isomer being perceived; otherwise, the nonrigid isomer is perceived. (*j*) The result of the addition, illustrated for all 7 × 7 combinations of stereo (*g*) and front/rear contrast (*h*) cue values. (*k*) An energy map of perceived nonrigidity versus perceived structure illustrating two stable states of depth from motion (corresponding to the two perceptual depth isomers, m_1 and m_2). When a display is first turned on, a marble representing the current depth state is momentarily at the ridge between m_1, m_2, and moves according to a vertical force (gravity) and horizontal forces (generated by stereo and contrast cues) into one or the other energy well.

one of the energy wells, the lateral forces exerted by the steep walls (representing rapid loss of perceived rigidity away from the minimum) overwhelm the cue forces. The energy wells provide stable percepts even in the face of contradictory evidence.

This model offers a succinct representation of the fact that a quick acting force (such as line contrast) can exert a greater effect than stereopsis when displays move immediately on presentation, and why stereopsis is relatively much more effective when Necker cubes are first shown in a static (pre)view and only begin moving a second later. Stereopsis, which is perceived more slowly but which is a more powerful cue than the line contrast, wins when it is given ample time to exert itself in the static preview, but loses when line contrast tips the marble into a stable state before stereopsis can be effective.

Additive-Cue Models for the Perceived Depth of Surfaces

The additive framework has subsequently been applied by Johnston, Cumming, and Parker, (1993), Landy et al. (1991b), and Maloney and Landy (1989) to the problem of how the *shape* of recovered depth depends on various cues (stereo and texture, stereo and motion, texture and motion), which differ in depicted depths by small amounts. Although there are some anomalies in these data, it appears that the additive cue integration framework can account not just for the relative dominance of multistable percepts, but the depths recovered from nonambiguous displays. In the context of an energy-surface conceptualization, these multiple cues combine with the motion cue to determine not just which minimum along an energy surface is selected, but some details of the shape of the energy surface as well.

Determining the Essential Stimulus Elements for Human Depth-from-Motion Processing

Experimental Methods in the Study of Depth-from-Motion

Introspection

Motion perception has played an important role in the history of psychology, especially among the Gestalt psychologists. They were much concerned with pure "phi motion"—a perception of motion between two briefly flashed bars that seemed to exist independently of any moving object. The introspective tradition continued with the discovery of the KDE by Wallach and O'Connell (1953), in the sense that emphasis was placed on introspective observations, such as judgments of amount of perceived depth, apparent coherence of moving points (resulting in one or more moving objects), apparent rigidity, and overall judgments of the quality of perceived depth. Two things were implicitly assumed in early KDE studies (i.e., Green, 1961): first, that kinetic depth is a unitary phenomenon so that any depth indicator would be sufficient as a yardstick and, second, that introspective judgments captured the essential features of the perception of depth from motion.

Objective Performance Tasks

With respect to the various measures of the kinetic depth effect, our own observations demonstrated that depthfulness, coherence, rigidity, and other properties were far from perfectly correlated, and no single such dependent variable could serve alone as an indicator of KDE (Dosher, Landy, and Sperling, 1989a). However, a more serious problem with introspective approaches is that they do not deal with the evolutionary purposes for which the ability to perceive depth from motion evolved. Evolution did not develop the systems subserving the recovery of 3D depth from 2D images in order to yield perceptions of rigidity or coherence or depthfulness, but in order to give organisms the ability to function in movement and action in the real world—to identify and discriminate shapes and surfaces in depth. For the study of KDE, it seemed to us essential to develop an objective task in which to study the capacity of depth-from-motion processes (Sperling et al., 1989, 1990). In our experiments, subjects are presented with kinetic depth displays, and asked to identify the shape from a lexicon of 55 similar shapes (figure 13.3).

What Can be Learned from Experiments with Feedback?

Given that objective measures of performance rather than introspection are used to study KDE, there remains the critical question of whether to provide to subjects feedback about the correctness or incorrectness of their responses. Feedback critically distinguishes what can be learned from experiments (Sperling et al., 1990): Experiments without feedback study the generalization of subjects' past experiences to the present experimental situation. In other words, experiments without feedback measure *achievement*; experiments with feedback can measure aptitude or ultimate *capacity* (Sperling et al., 1990). Aptitude and ultimate capacity are the words used to describe the asymptotic limit of a subject's performance (e.g., in a KDE shape identification task) after training with feedback.

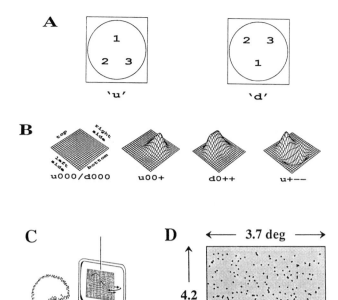

Figure 13.3
A 3D shape identification task. Subjects must indicate which shape they perceive from a 53-element lexicon of shapes built on splined bumps and depressions at three locations in one of the two configurations shown in (*A*). (*B*) Four sample shapes. (*C*) Random points on the surfaces of these shapes are projected and displayed undergoing sinusoidal rotation around a top-to-bottom axis (*B*). (*D*) A single freeze-frame of the projected points.

To prove that subjects require a particular cue (such as a motion flowfield) and cannot use other cues to solve a KDE shape-discrimination task, both an objective method and feedback are required. For example, when, in Sperling et al.'s (1989) procedure, subjects could not learn to use a texture density cue to solve the shape task, we know this failure represents an inherent biological limitation because subjects were given ample opportunity to learn.

Unfortunately, there is a hazard in experiments with feedback: subjects can use the feedback to learn to use incidental or artifactual cues (Braunstein and Todd, 1990). The solution to this potential problem is to refine the experimental procedure. Experiments with feedback intrinsically require more attention to detail and more experimenter work than experiments without feedback (Sperling et al., 1990).

Relative Depth Is Recovered from Motion Flow Fields

What is the evidence that relative depth information in kinetic depth displays is recovered from the motion flow field versus from a geometric calculation based on the 2D trajectories of identifiable features? To investigate the visual processes leading to recovery of 3D object depth, Dosher, Landy, and Sperling (1989b) began with kinetic depth displays and the objective shape identification task outlined in figure 13.3. 3D surfaces defined by dots were rocked back and forth 20° around a vertical axis. Dot density and contrast of the standard displays were set so as to yield shape identification performance in the high 90% range for most observers.

Changing 2D Dot Density—A Potential Confound

In a rigid object defined by dots painted on its surface, the 2D density of dots increases when the surface normal departs from the line of sight. In such surfaces, dot density is a cue to slant and thereby to depth. The density cue is eliminated by randomly adding or subtracting dots from any small area in which 2D dot density changes as a consequence of 3D motion so as to maintain locally uniform dot density. For motion confined to rocking of ±20° around the line of sight, the elimination and addition of dots to maintain constant dot density involve about 5% of the dots per new frame. This percent of dots is small enough so the scintillation effect of adding and removing dots does not impair performance. On the other hand, when the density cue alone is presented in displays with motion cues removed, only one of three observers could use dot density to identify the shapes, and performance was 30%, compared to 90% performance with motion cues.

Dot Lifetimes Discriminate Flow Fields from Feature Tracking

To demonstrate that the necessary cue in their KDE displays was indeed motion and not the tracking of specific dots or groups of dots, Dosher et al. (1989b) used a dot lifetime manipulation in which each individual dot survived only for two frames (two frames is the minimum to define motion) and it was then replaced with another dot at a new location, which also survived for only two frames. On each frame (8 frames/sec), half the dots were replaced. The two-frame dot lifetime manipulation introduces an enormous amount of scintillation noise into the display plus much spurious motion "noise" produced by accidental apparent motion between unrelated dots. Nevertheless, KDE shape identification performance survives 2-frame lifetimes remarkably well. This result was confirmed by Todd and Bressan (1990) in subsequent, similar observations.

The 2-frame lifetime displays exemplify motion flow fields: they are devoid of larger features and even the microfeatures (hundreds of tiny dots) persist only for about 1/10 sec. The relatively good shape-identification performance in 2-frame lifetime displays demonstrates that the tracking of individual dots or groups of dots is not necessary for the perceptual recovery of depth from motion.

What Kind of Flowfield Is Necessary to Recover Depth-from-Motion?

First-Order Motion

A great deal is now known about visual motion analyzers as they apply to planar motion stimuli (van Santen and Sperling, 1984; Adelson and Bergen, 1985; Watson and Ahumada, 1985). It is quite well established experimentally that early motion analysis reflects a so-called first-order analysis of the stimulus—a computation based on the space–time Fourier motion components of the stimulus (van Santen and Sperling, 1984, 1985; Watson, Ahumada, and Farrell, 1986).

Second-Order Motion

In addition to the first-order analysis, the visual system is capable of detecting motion via a second-order analysis that requires initial space-time filtering followed by full-wave rectification prior to motion analysis (Chubb and Sperling, 1988, 1991). The evidence for second-order motion detection is the ability of subjects to detect motion in many kinds of displays that would be invisible to all the proposed first-order motion analyzers, the ability of subjects to perceive simultaneously first- and second-order motion embedded in the same display in opposite directions (Chubb and Sperling, 1989b; Solomon and Sperling, 1993), and the ability of subjects to discriminate the direction of first-order motion in the presence of strong second-order masking and vice versa (i.e., if there were only one system, the masking would destroy the ability of that system to perceive motion, Solomon and Sperling, 1994). Does the first- or second-order motion system subserve depth from motion?

Displays That Selectively Stimulate First- and Second-Order Motion-Analysis Systems

To study the dependence of depth from motion on first- and second-order motion detection mechanisms, Dosher, Landy, and Sperling (1989b) and Landy et al. (1991a) varied various aspects of KDE stimuli to make them rela-

tively more or less useful to each of the motion detection systems. For example, normally all dots that define a surface were painted as white dots on a gray background. In alternating-polarity displays, the color of a moving dot alternated from white to black to white and so on in successive frames. Alternating polarity destroys the first-order motion signal but leaves the second-order signal completely intact. Alternating polarity was found to destroy subjects' ability to identify shape from motion in the displays, suggesting that first-order motion signals were necessary to solve the shape discrimination task.

In control experiments, subjects were required to judge the direction of motion of normal and alternating polarity displays. Even when normal and alternating-polarity stimuli were matched in this control task, the alternating-polarity stimuli failed to support depth from motion while the normal stimuli succeeded (Dosher et al., 1989b). Therefore, the failure of second-order stimuli to support depth from motion is not due to their inability to convey motion; it is a specific deficiency of second-order stimuli for a shape-identification task.

In another control experiment, subjects searched 3 × 3 arrays in which eight areas were defined by motion in one direction and one area was defined by motion in the opposite direction. Performance with second-order stimuli suffered as much in the search task as in the depth-from-motion task (Dosher et al., 1989b). However, in the search task, the origin of the problem was determined to be that subjects could search only one or two locations successfully for second-order motion. This is related to the more general observation that spatial resolution for second-order motion is much coarser in peripheral vision than in central vision (Solomon and Sperling, 1995); and since resolution is already poor in central vision, not enough remains to support performance in either depth from motion or in search tasks. While it is not obvious at how many locations and with what accuracy the motion flow-field needs to be sampled in order to solve the shape-from-motion task, it is obvious that the resolution of the second-order motion system was completely insufficient for Sperling et al.'s (1989) shape identification task.

Net Directional First-Order Motion Power (DP)

Alternating polarity is merely one of many stimulus transformations that selectively affect first-order versus second-order motion strength. Other transformations included alternating contrast strength in successive frames, interposing blank frames, replacing dots with other tokens (disks, lines, alternating-polarity point clusters), etc. The effects of all such stimulus transformations on

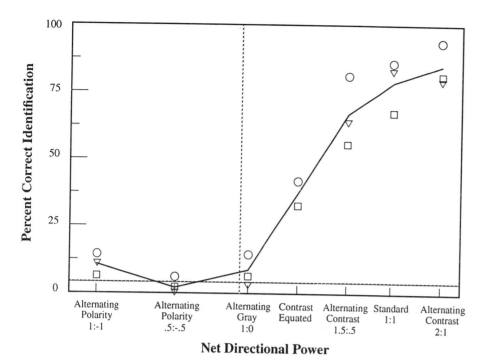

Figure 13.4

3D shape identification accuracy as a function of the *net directional power* (DP) of various stimulus types. Data are shown for three subjects. DP is computed from the Fourier amplitude transform of a stimu-

lus trajectory (see text); it is the power of Fourier components above a threshold ε within a "window of visibility" (30 Hz × 30 c/deg).

subjects' accuracy in the shape-from-motion task are summarized in a single computation: net directional power. To derive directional power, Dosher et al. (1989b) compute the 2D Fourier power spectrum of the trajectory of a single dot. Following Watson, Ahumada and Farrell (1986), the analysis is confined to a window of visibility bounded by 30 cycles/degree and 30 Hz. Within this window, all Fourier components above a small threshold ε are given equal weight. Net directional power is simply the power of components in the intended direction minus the power in the opposite direction. Figure 13.4 shows that the proportion of correct shape-from-motion responses ranged from chance to very high levels in direct, monotonic relation to the directional power. In other words, the quality of the first-order motion signal directly predicts success in the shape-from-motion task.

Conclusions

1. The recovery of 3D depth from motion in monocular 2D displays reflects the output of a common depth channel that also records stereopsis.

2. The linear combination of cues to depth from motion is consistent with the computation of a bistable $(-1, +1)$

motion–depth–sign; the computation can be represented by an energy surface with two minima. The initial state is at the ridge separating the minima; conflicting cues represent forces directed towards opposite minima.

3. The sufficient cue to depth is the 2D motion flow field; subjects fail to derive depth from a changing texture-density cue nor do they require information derived from tracking specific dots or features.

4. Performance in 3D shape identification varies monotonically with the *net directional first-order motion power* contained in the stimulus.

Acknowledgments

This work was supported by ONR, Perceptual Sciences Program, grant N00014-88-K-0569 and by AFOSR, Visual Information Processing Program, grant 91-0178.

References

Adelson, E. H. (1985). Rigid objects that appear highly non-rigid. *Suppl. Invest. Ophthalmol. Visual Sci. 26,* 56.

Adelson, E. H., and Bergen, J. R. (1985). Spatiotemporal energy models for the perception of motion. *J. Opt. Soc. Am. A 2,* 284–299.

Bennett, B. M., Hoffman, D. D., Nicola, J. E., and Prakash, C. (1989). Structure from two orthographic views of rigid motion. *J. Opt. Soc. Am A 6*, 1052–1069.

Biederman, I. (1987) Recognition-by-components: A theory of human image understanding. *Psychol. Rev 94*, 115–117.

Braunstein, M. L., and Todd, J. T. (1990). On the distinction between artifacts and information. *J. Exp. Psychol. Human Percept. Perform. 16*, 211–216.

Chubb, C., and Sperling, G. (1988). Drift-balanced random stimuli: A general basis for studying non-Fourier motion perception. *J. Opt. Soc. Am. A Opt. Image Sci. 5*, 1986–2006.

Chubb, C., and Sperling, G. (1989a). Second-order motion perception: Space-time separable mechanisms. In *Proceedings: Workshop on Visual Motion* (March 20–22, 1989, Irvine, California) (pp. 126–138). Washington, D.C.: IEEE Computer Society Press.

Chubb, C., and Sperling, G. (1989b). Two motion perception mechanisms revealed by distance-driven reversal of apparent motion. *Proc. Natl. Acad. Sci. U.S.A. 86*, 2985–2989.

Chubb, C., and Sperling, G. (1991). Texture quilts: Basic tools for studying motion-from-texture. *J. Math. Psychol. 35*, 411–442.

Cornwell, H. G. (1976). Necker cube reversal: sensory or psychological satiation? *Percept. Motor Skills 43*, 3–10.

Dosher, B. A., Sperling, G., and Wurst, S. (1986). Tradeoffs between stereopsis and proximity luminance covariance. *Vision Res. 26*, 973–990.

Dosher, B. A., Landy, M. S., and Sperling, G. (1989a). Ratings of kinetic depth in multi-dot displays. *J. Exp. Psychol. Human Percept. Perform. 15*, 816–825.

Dosher, B. A., Landy, M. S., and Sperling, G. (1989b). Kinetic depth effect and optic flow: I. 3D shape from Fourier motion. *Vision Res. 29*, 1789–1813.

Green, B. F. (1961). Figure coherence in the kinetic depth effect. *J. Exp. Psychol. 62*, 272–282.

Grzywacz, N. M., and Hildreth, E. C. (1987). The incremental rigidity scheme for recovering structure from motion: Position vs. velocity based formulations. *J. Opt. Soc. Am. A 4*, 503–518.

Grzywacz, N. M., Hildreth, E., C., Inada, B. K., and Adelson, E. H. (1988). The temporal integration of 3-D structure from motion: A computational and psychopysical study. In W. von Seelen, G. Shaw, and U. M. Leinhos (Eds.), *Organization of Neural Networks: Structure and Models* (pp. 239–259). Weinhein, Germany: VCH.

Hildreth, E. C., Grzywacz, N. M., Adelson, E. H., and Inada, V. K. (1990). The perceptual buildup of three-dimensional structure from motion. *Percept. Psychophys. 48*, 19–36.

Johnston, E. B., Cumming, B. G., and Parker, A. J. (1993). Integration of depth modules: Stereopsis and texture. *Vision Res. 33*, 813–826.

Julesz, B. (1971). *Foundations of Cyclopian Perception*. Chicago: University of Chicago Press.

Koenderink, J. J., and van Doorn, A. J. (1986). Depth and shape from differential perspective in the presence of bending deformations. *J. Opt. Soc. Am. A 3*, 242–249.

Landy, M. S., Dosher, B. A., Sperling, G., and Perkins, M. E. (1991a). The kinetic depth effect and optic flow: II. First- and second-order motion. *Vision Res. 31*, 859–876.

Landy, M. S., Maloney, L. T., Johnston, E. B., and Young, M. (1991b). Measurement and modeling of depth cue combination: In defense of weak fusion. Mathematical studies in perception and cognition, 91–3. New York University Technical Report.

Longuet-Higgins, H. C., and Prazdny, K. (1980). The interpretation of a moving retinal image. *Proc. R. Soc. London B 208*, 385–397.

Loomis, J. M., and Eby, D. W. (1987). Perceiving 3-D structure from motion: Importance of axis of rotation. *Suppl. Invest. Opthalmol. Visual Sci. 28*, 234.

Maloney, L. T., and Landy, M. S. (1989). Psychophysical estimation of the human depth combination rule. In W. A. Perlman (Ed.), *Visual Communication and Image Processing IV, Proceedings of the SPIE, 1199*, 1154–1163.

Ono, H., and Steinbach, M. (1990). Monocular stereopsis with and without head movement. *Percept. Psychophys. 48*, 179–187.

Ono, M. E., Rivest, J., and Ono, H. (1986). Depth perception as a function of motion parallax and absolute-distance information. *J. Exp. Psychol. Human Percept. Perform. 12*, 331–337.

Orbach, J., Ehrlich, D., and Heath, H. (1963). A. Reversibility of the "Necker cube": I. An examination of the concept of "satiation of orientation." *Percept. Motor Skills 17*, 439–458.

Pentland, A. (1989). Part segmentation for object recognition. *Neural Comp. 1*, 82–91.

Pentland, A., and Sclaroff, S. (1991). Close form solutions for physically based shape modelling and recognition. *IEEE Transact. Pattern Anal. Machine Intelligence 13*, 715–729.

Schwartz, B. J., and Sperling, G. (1983). Luminance controls the perceived 3D structure of dynamic 2D displays. *Bull. Psychon. Soc. 21*, 456–458.

Solomon, J. A., and Sperling, G. (1994). Fullwave and halfwave rectification in motion perception. *Vision Res. 34*, 2239–2257.

Solomon, J. A., and Sperling, G. (1995). 1st- and 2nd-order motion and texture resolution in central and peripheral vision. *Vision Research, 35* (1). (In press.)

Sperling, G. (1970). Binocular vision: a physical and a neural theory. *Am. J. Psychol. 83*, 461–534.

Sperling, G., and Dosher, B. (1987). Predicting rigid and nonrigid perceptions. *Suppl. Invest. Ophthalmol. Visual Sci. 28(3)*, 362.

Sperling, G., Dosher, B., and Landy, M. S. (1990). How to study the kinetic depth effect experimentally. *J. Exp. Psychol. Human Percept. Perform. 16*, 445–450.

Sperling, G., Landy, M. S., Dosher, B., and Perkins, M. (1989). The kinetic depth effect and identification of shape. *J. Exp. Psychol. Human Percept. Perform. 15*, 826–840.

Spitz, H. H., and Lipman, R. S. (1962). Some factors affecting necker cube reversal rate. *Percept. Motor Skills 15*, 611–625.

Thurstone, L. L. (1947). *Multiple-Factor Analysis: A Development and Expansion of the Vectors of Mind*. Chicago: University of Chicago Press.

Todd, J. T., and Bressan, P. (1990). The perception of 3-dimensional affine structure from minimal apparent motion sequences. *Percept. Psychophys. 48,* 419–430.

Ullman, S. (1979). *The Interpretation of Visual Motion.* Cambridge, MA: MIT Press.

Ullman, S. (1984). Maximizing rigidity: The incremental recovery of 3-D structure from rigid and non-rigid motion. *Perception 13,* 225–274.

van Santen, J., and Sperling, G. (1984). A temporal covariance model of motion perception. *J. Opt. Soc. Am. A 1,* 451–473.

van Santen, J., and Sperling, G. (1985). Elaborated Reichardt detectors. *J. Opt. Soc. Am. A 2,* 300–321.

Wallach, H., and O'Connell, D. N. (1953). The kinetic depth effect. *J. Exp. Psychol. 45,* 205–217.

Watson, A. B., and Ahumada, A. J. (1985). Model of human visual-motion sensing. *J. Opt. Soc. Am. A 1,* 322–342.

Watson, A. B., Ahumada, A. J., and Farrell, J. E. (1986). Window of visibility: A psychophysical theory of fidelity in time-sampled visual motion displays. *J. Opt. Soc. Am. A 3,* 300–307.

14

Spatial Primitives for Seeing Three-Dimensional Shape from Motion

Joseph S. Lappin, Ulf B. Ahlström,
Warren D. Craft, and
Steven T. Tschantz

The Nature of Spatial Primitives in Motion Perception

When a solid object rotates in depth relative to an observer, its image deforms, and these image deformations constitute information about the shape of the object. Considerable psychophysical evidence indicates that biological vision is highly sensitive to this information. The specific image properties that carry this information have not been clearly identified, however.

Motion involves a change relative to a spatial reference system, and different frames of reference provide different descriptions of motion. In vision, several forms of image motion are potentially relevant, defined by reference to different spatial structures. The goal of this study was to characterize the primitive structures and motions that carry visible information about shape.

Representing the primitive spatial relations detected by early vision is fundamental for theories of the mechanisms that process this input information: Vision involves a transformation of input into output; representing the input and output defines the computational problem, and constrains the processes that can accomplish this transformation. Assumptions about the input primitives are implicit in virtually all theories of spatial vision and motion perception, but have received surprisingly little direct investigation.

A principal exception to the tendency to take this issue for granted is Julesz's program of research on stereopsis (e.g., Julesz, 1960, 1964, 1971), motion (e.g., Chang and Julesz, 1983), and especially on spatial primitives in texture segregation (e.g., Julesz, Gilbert, and Victor, 1978; Caelli and Julesz, 1978; Caelli, Julesz, and Gilbert, 1978; Julesz, 1981, 1984). The primary goal of the present study was the same as in much of Julesz's research—to identify spatial primitives.

Several frameworks might be used to describe spatial structure. One approach is the statistical geometry developed by Julesz and his colleagues to describe texture, based on spatial relations among n points—e.g., dipoles and other *n-gons*. A related approach involves spatial derivatives of a two-dimensional (2D) Gaussian (cf. Koenderink and van Doorn, 1992a,b; Adelson and Bergen, 1991). These two frameworks are related: The n-gons can be regarded as primitive spatial elements of the optical pattern, and the differential structure might describe the spatial organization of neural operators as well as that of the optical patterns. The differential order corresponds to the number of zero-crossings between oppositely weighted neighboring regions of the operator. Individual points in the *n-gon* can be regarded as located within these separate regions of the receptive field of a neural operator. Thus, the differential order is one less than the number of points in the *n-gon*.

Optical patterns in the present experiments consisted of five bright dots arranged in a cross-like pattern. The center dot is taken as the origin or reference point for describing changes in the surrounding neighborhod, represented by relative displacements of the other four dots. Although the present experiments examined only these simple patterns with binary luminance values, these patterns are tentatively taken to represent a larger class of patterns that may be continuous in space and time.

Five hypotheses about the complexity of such spatial primitives are the following:

1. *Zero-order*: Spatial structure may be described by positions of individual points—by reference to an extrinsic coordinate system. Measures of retinal velocity implicitly rely on such an extrinsic coordinate system. Simpson's (1993) review of literature on computing and perceiving depth from optic flow uses this representation.

2. *First-order*: Spatial patterns may be described by relations among pairs of points—by the dipole statistics or Fourier power spectrum. First- (and higher) order differential structure is *intrinsic* to the optical pattern, independent of location on the retinal coordinate system. Contemporary models of spatial vision based on both electrophysiology and psychophysics (e.g., De Valois and De Valois, 1988) often emphasize the first-order representation.

3. *Second-order*: *second derivatives in one dimension*: Relative distances among three collinear points correspond to second spatial derivatives.

4. *Second-order*: *first derivatives in two dimensions*: This second-order structure corresponds to a triangular shape of three points. Deformations of such structure provide information about the tilt and slant of a local surface patch and, therefore, might constitute primitives for seeing structure from motion (Koenderink and van Doorn, 1976). A special case of such deformations is a shearing motion that alters the collinearity of three points. The informativeness of this deformation has been demonstrated both psychophysically and computationally (Cornilleau-Pérès and Droulez, 1989; Weinshall, 1991). Moreover, Julesz and his colleagues have found quasi-collinearity to be a spatial primitive in texture discrimination (Caelli and Julesz, 1978; Caelli et al., 1978; Julesz, 1980).

5. *Fourth-order*: *second derivatives in two dimensions*: This spatial structure may be described by relations among five points in a cross-like pattern, with two orthogonal sets of three approximately collinear points, oriented so that one is parallel and the other perpendicular to the direction of motion, and intersecting at a common center point. (A general-purpose operator with orientation independent of the optic flow would require such second-order measures in at least three directions. See Koenderink and van Doorn, 1992b.) Schematic illustrations are shown in figure 14.1.

A principal motivation for considering this fourth-order structure as a primitive for shape from motion is that deformations of this structure specify local surface shape (cf. Koenderink and van Doorn, 1992b). Second-order deformations (Hypothesis 4) provide information about local surface orientation, but this varies with the object's position relative to the observer. Fourth-order structure, however, describes local surface shape invariant

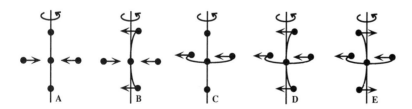

Figure 14.1
Five different deformation patterns of local fourth-order differential structure associated with depth-rotations of qualitatively different shapes of a local surface patch around a vertical axis. (*A*) Associated with a planar patch, (*B*) a horizontally oriented parabolic (cylindrical) patch, (*C*) a vertical parabolic patch, (*D*) an elliptic (ellipsoidal) patch, and (*E*) a hyperbolic (saddle-shaped) patch. The local shape of any smooth surface is one of these five types, characterized by the relative curvature in two orthogonal directions.

under changes in the observer's position. The local shape of any smooth surface is one of four types: *planar, parabolic* (curved in one direction), *elliptic* (curved in two dimensions, with the same sign of curvature in both directions), or *hyperbolic* (curved in two directions, with opposite signs of curvature). As illustrated in figure 14.1, each of these types yields a qualitatively different pattern of relative motion. These image deformations are sufficient to specify qualitative local surface shape. Two second-order components involve (1) shearing deformations that alter collinearity, as in hypothesis 4, associated with a surface curvature perpendicular to the direction of image motion, and (2) differential compression, as in hypothesis 3, associated with a surface curvature parallel to the image motion.

This study sought to determine whether any of these second- or fourth-order image deformations are directly visible or is derived from lower-order properties.

Visibilities of the two second-order deformations were independently evaluated. Simple five-dot patterns were globally jittered, with the component dots displaced as if attached to a surface rotating rigidly in depth by small random amounts. The observer's task was to detect second-order deformations. Visual information from lower order relationships was controlled by adding independent random perturbations of the lower order but not second-order relationships.

Experiment 1: Detectabilities of Second-Order Deformations

Visibilities of these two forms of second-order deformation were evaluated in two different psychophysical tasks: In the *Collinearity Task*, observers detected shearing deformations that altered the collinearity of the three vertically aligned dots in the canonical five-dot patterns shown in figure 14.1. Two alternative patterns were generated by shifting the five dots as if attached to either a horizontally oriented cylinder (figure 14.1B) or a plane (figure 14.1A) rotated by small amounts around the vertical axis—where rotations of the cylinder altered collinearity and rotations of the plane did not.

In the *Bisection Task*, observers detected deformations that altered the equal spacing among the three horizontally aligned dots. The two alternative patterns were generated by shifting the five dots as if attached to either a vertically oriented cylinder (figure 14.1C) or a plane (figure 14.1A) rotated around the vertical axis. Rotations of the cylinder altered the symmetry of the horizontal dots, while rotations of the plane did not.

(The deformations of these simple five-point patterns were not sufficient to produce perceptions of surfaces rotating rigidly in depth. The shearing motions in the Collinearity Task often did produce subjective impressions of motion in depth, but the image deformations in the Bisection Task rarely produced any impression of motion in depth. Thus, observers simply tried to detect the specified deformation rather than to discriminate perceived surfaces.)

The deformations in these two tasks also involve both zero- and first-order changes. The signal-to-noise ratio of the lower-order motions was reduced by adding random perturbations of lower-order structure in both of the cylinder and plane patterns.

Two qualitatively different effects of this added zero- and first-order noise might be expected:

1. If second-order structure is obtained by subtracting visually independent measures of lower order relations, then discriminations of second-order structure should be hindered by the added variability and similarity in lower-order structure of the cylinder and plane. This conception is implicit in the belief that measures of differential structure are vulnerable to noise and error (cf. Simpson, 1993).

2. If visual measures of lower-order relations are correlated rather than independent, then difference measures may suppress the effects of correlated noise in the lower order structure, yielding coherent higher-order structure.

Method

Five-dot patterns were rigidly and randomly jittered by selecting spatial positions independently in successive frames. The observer's task was to discriminate two alternative structures defined by the relative motions of these randomly jittering dots. This method is an extension of one we have used previously to investigate the perception of coherent structure and motion (Lappin et al., 1991; Mowafy et al., 1990).

Detectability of each of the two forms of second-order deformations was evaluated in six conditions—two different magnitudes of second-order motion each combined with three different magnitudes of first-order motion. The first-order motions were added as independent random vectors to both the plane and cylinder patterns, thereby lowering the signal-to-noise ratio of the first-order information.

Additionally, independent zero-order motions were added by randomly jittering the whole pattern rigidly in the horizontal direction with displacements comparable to those for the first- and second-order motions. Since the zero-, first-, and second-order motions were all added as independent random horizontal displacements, this zero-order noise had the effect of requiring that reliable discriminations were based on deformations of higher order structure rather than simple horizontal motions of individual dots.

Optical Patterns

Five dots were arranged in a cross-like pattern, similar to the schematic illustrations in figure 14.1A–C. Prior to rotation in depth, the upper, lower, left, and right dots were all 30 min arc (1 cm) from the center dot. In each discrimination task, two alternative patterns were produced by projecting the five dots onto either a plane or a cylinder. Before rotation in depth, the images of both plane and cylinder were identical, though on the horizontal cylinder the upper and lower dots had greater depth, and on the vertical cylinder the left and right dots had greater depth. For each of these surfaces, five different images corresponded to rotations of the surface either $0°$, $\pm 15°$, or $\pm 30°$ from the center position, and these images were selected independently with equal probability in a sequence of 40 frames, each 50 msec in duration. Table 14.1 lists quantitative characteristics of the spatial positions and motions produced by the three independent random variables associated with (1) rotations in depth,

(2) first-order 2D rotations or expansions, and (3) zero-order horizontal translations. The sequential positions of each dot were given by the sums of these three independent random variables.

As illustrated in figure 14.1A, rotation of the planar shape around the vertical axis produced symmetric contractions of the left and right dots toward the center dot, and no motion at all of the top, bottom, and center dots.

In the Collinearity Task, this planar pattern was discriminated from one produced by depth rotation of a horizontal cylinder, which differed from the planar pattern by horizontal motions of the top and bottom dots, altering the collinearity of the three vertically aligned dots, as illustrated in figure 14.1B. The depths of the top and bottom dots were both either 0.0375 or 0.075 cm, where greater depth produced greater shearing motion.

In the Bisection Task, the planar pattern was discriminated from a vertical cylinder, which differed from the planar pattern by asymmetrical motions of the left and right dots that altered the center dot's bisection of distance between the left and right dots, as illustrated in figure 14.1C. The depths of the left and right dots were both either 0.075 or 0.15 cm, with greater depth producing greater differential motion.

For the horizontal cylinder in the Collinearity Task, the magnitude of second-order deformation is given by the

Table 14.1
Horizontal image displacements (min arc) for the surfaces and transformations in experiment 1

Transformation	Five alternative displacements from untransformed position					Frame-to-frame motions			
						Mean	SD	RMS	Max
Plane (left and right)	−4.02	−1.02	0.0	−1.02	−4.02	1.77	1.62	2.37	4.02
Horizontal cylinder ($z = .0375$)	−0.56	−0.29	0.0	0.29	0.56	0.45	0.35	0.57	1.12
Horizontal cylinder ($z = .075$)	−1.13	−0.58	0.0	0.58	1.13	0.91	0.69	1.13	2.25
Vertical cylinder ($z = .075$)	−5.15	−1.60	0.0	−0.44	−2.89	2.04	1.69	2.63	5.14
Second-order	−2.25	−1.16	0.0	1.16	2.25	1.81	1.39	2.27	4.50
Vertical cylinder ($z = .15$)	−6.27	−2.19	0.0	0.14	−1.77	2.40	2.28	3.28	6.41
Second-order	−4.50	−2.33	0.0	2.33	4.50	3.62	2.78	4.53	9.00
2D Rotation ($1.07°$)	−0.56	−0.28	0.0	0.28	0.56	0.45	0.34	0.56	1.12
2D Rotation ($3.21°$)	−1.68	−0.84	0.0	0.84	1.68	1.34	1.03	1.68	3.36
Expansion (8%)	−2.40	−1.20	0.0	1.20	2.40	1.92	1.47	2.40	4.80
Expansion (12%)	−3.60	−1.80	0.0	1.80	3.60	2.88	2.20	3.60	7.20
Horizontal translation	−2.40	−1.20	0.0	1.20	2.40	1.92	1.47	2.40	4.80

Note: Each transformation had five equiprobable alternative values, designated by the horizontal shift from the untransformed position away from the center dot (negative numbers are toward the center dot). The frame-to-frame horizontal motions were computed from the 25 equiprobable combinations of the five alternative image positions. The resulting image position of each dot in each frame was determined by the vector sum of three independent random transformations: depth rotation around the vertical axis of the surface (plane, horizontal cylinder, or vertical cylinder) + zero-order horizontal translation + first-order 2D rotation or expansion.

range of horizontal motions of the top and bottom dots. For the vertical cylinder in the Bisection Task, the magnitude of the second-order deformation is given by the difference in distances of the left and right dots from the center dot. In both cases, differential motion is proportional to depth: For the horizontal cylinder the shearing displacement is $z \sin \alpha$, where z is the relative depth and α is the angle of rotation from the central position; for the vertical cylinder the differential compression is $2 z \sin \alpha$.

To reduce the discriminability of the plane and cylinder patterns based on zero- and first-order motions, zero- and first-order noise was added to both of these patterns. Five equally likely alternative values of both the zero- and first-order motions were added as independent random vectors to the displacements produced by rotations in depth. Since all the relevant motions were horizontal, the random zero-order translations were only horizontal. The zero-order translations were somewhat larger than those produced by depth rotations of the plane or cylinder.

In the Collinearity Task, depth rotations of the cylinder altered orientations of the imaginary line segments from the center dot to the top and bottom dots. To mask this first-order information, random rigid 2D rotations around the center dot were added to both the planar and horizontal cylinder patterns. Three magnitudes of rotation were used: $0°$, $\pm 1.07°$, and $\pm 3.21°$. The range of horizontal motion produced by the $\pm 1.07°$ rotation was essentially the same as that produced by depth rotation of the less curved cylinder; and the motion produced by the $\pm 3.21°$ rotation was greater than that produced by the more curved cylinder. Thus, two cylinder depths were combined with three magnitudes of 2D rotation to form six conditions, run in separate blocks of trials.

In the Bisection Task, depth rotations of both the plane and cylinder patterns altered the distances of the left and right dots from the center dot. To reduce this first-order information, random global expansions of the positions of the four outside dots were added to both the planar and vertical cylinder patterns in the Bisection Task. The magnitude was either 0%, $\pm 8\%$ (± 2.40 min arc) or $\pm 12\%$. Thus, two cylinder depths were combined with three magnitudes of expansion to form six conditions, run in separate blocks of trials.

These patterns were displayed on point-plot CRTs (Tektronix 608), with P-31 phosphor, controlled by a Macintosh IIx computer with a D/A interface with 16-bit resolution in the horizontal and vertical axes. The size of each dot was approximately 45 sec arc (0.25 mm). The displays were binocularly viewed in a dimly lit room from a distance of 115 cm.

Procedure

Two observers each completed 200 trials in each of the 12 conditions. Both observers completed the Bisection Task before the Collinearity Task. Four sessions were devoted to each task, each session consisting of six blocks of 50 trials plus four practice trials, one block for each of the six conditions for that task. Two successive blocks of trials were for each level of first-order motion, one block for each cylinder depth; and the easier discrimination (greater depth and deformation) always preceded the more difficult. The order of the three first-order noise conditions within each condition was approximately counterbalanced over sessions and observers. Both observers participated in two or more practice sessions for each task prior to collecting the reported data, sufficient to achieve asymptotic performance.

Both tasks were conducted as yes/no detection tasks— with either plane or cylinder presented on each trial and two corresponding alternative responses. Only two alternative patterns were presented in a given block of trials, and the observers were familiar with these two patterns. Auditory feedback was given for correct responses. The duration of each display was 2 sec or terminated by the observer's response.

The two observers were coauthors of this paper.

Results

Figure 14.2 shows the detection accuracy in each of the 12 conditions as a function of the range of second-order image motion for each task. The lower left graph gives the average accuracy of the two observers expressed in terms of the signal detection measure, d', which may be regarded as the output signal-to-noise ratio. The joint dependence of these discriminations on the second-order deformation signal and first-order noise provides evidence about the visual influence of these two types of motion.

In the Collinearity Task, discriminations were only slightly affected by random first-shorter rotations. With no first-order noise, the cylinder with depth less than 0.04 cm yielded 71% correct discriminations ($d' = 1.11$) from the plane. The maximum differential motion was 1.12 min arc, which occurred on only 8% of the frame-to-frame displacements, and the root mean square (RMS) motion was just 0.57 min arc. Recall that these differential motions were added to random zero-order horizontal translations of the whole patterns with an RMS value of 2.4 min arc and a maximum of 4.8 min arc. When the relative depth and differential motion were doubled, then

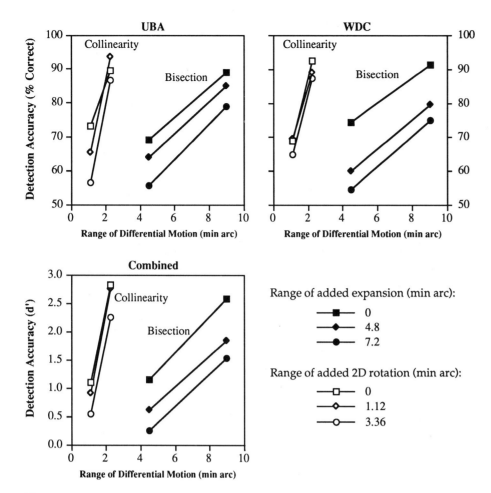

Figure 14.2

The results of experiment 1 for each condition and observer. Results for each of the two observers are given in the two upper graphs, and the combined results for both observers are given in the lower graph.

Note that the dependent measure of accuracy has been changed from percentage correct in the upper graphs to the signal detection measure, d', in the lower graph.

detectability improved by a factor greater than two, to $d' = 2.83$ (91% correct).

These discriminations must not have derived simply from the zero-order horizontal translations of individual dots, say by comparing the motions of the upper or lower dot with the center dot: For an ideal observer who perfectly integrated independent observations of the successive frame-to-frame displacements of each dot and then made detection decisions based on the difference in total motion of the center dot and one of the outside dots, the predicted detectabilities would have been $d' = 1.18$ and 2.36 for the two cylinders, as compared to obtained values of $d' = 1.11$ and 2.83.

The small decrements produced by first-order rotations also indicate that this visual information did not derive from the first-order changes in orientation. If the signal-to-noise ratio were based on this first-order information, then the slope of the psychometric function (d' as a func-

tion of the range of differential motion) would decrease in inverse proportion to the noise. As illustrated in figure 14.2, this did not occur. The slopes were 1.53, 1.64, and 1.51 d' per min arc for the three conditions with RMS first-order noise equal to 0.0, 0.56, and 1.38 min arc, respectively. The corresponding 75% correct ($d' = 1.35$) "thresholds" for these three conditions were 1.28, 1.39, and 1.65 min arc range of differential shear. Thus, visibility of these deformations was approximately independent of the first-order changes in orientation, and was based mainly on the second-order changes in collinearity (hypothesis 4).

Results for the Bisection Task were different. The asymmetrical compressions for the vertical cylinder were certainly visible and discriminable from the symmetrical motions for the plane, but these differential motions usually appeared as two spatially disconnected motions rather than rigid motions of a single object. The poorer detectability of the differential compressions relative to the shearing motions may have been associated with greater first-order similarity of the plane and cylinder in this task: Depth rotations produced zero- and first-order motions for both plane and cylinder in the Bisection Task, but in the Collinearity Task zero- and first-order motions of the top and bottom dots occurred only for the cylinder.

First-order noise also had a greater adverse effect in the Bisection than in the Collinearity Task. Although this first-order noise affected mainly the intercepts rather than the slopes of the psychometric functions, these slopes were smaller in this task—0.32, 0.27, and 0.28 *d'* per min arc deformation for RMS added expansions of 0.0, 2.4, and 3.6 min arc, respectively. The 75% thresholds for these three conditions were 5.09, 7.16, and 8.37 min arc range of differential compression. As will be seen below, these slopes were small and the thresholds were large compared to those for the first-order compressions and expansions. Thus, the perception of differential compressions in the Bisection Task was evidently derived from differences in the perceived first-order changes in length (Hypothesis 2).

Experiment 2: Detection of First-order Motions

The purpose of this supplementary experiment was to determine the relative visibility of the two forms of first-order motion involved in experiment 1. If perceptions of the second-order motions were derived from primitive first-order motions, then first-order motions may be more detectable than second-order motions.

Method

The optical displays, experimental procedures, and observers were the same as in the main experiment, with the following exceptions: The motions applied to these five-dot spatial patterns were either *2D rotations*—±0.5° (0.26 min arc) or ±1.0° (0.52 min arc)—or *expansions*—±1.4% (0.42 min arc) or ±2.1% (0.63 min arc)—plus independent random translations—±2.4 min arc in both horizontal and vertical directions. These values of rotation and expansion were chosen on the basis of pilot observations to yield an appropriate range of detectability.

This detection task involved discriminations between random 2D translations alone or the same 2D translations plus either 2D rotations or expansions, depending on the particular condition.

The same two observers each performed 200 trials for each of the two ranges of motion in both the Rotation and Expansion Tasks. Each observer participated in four experimental sessions—two sessions for each task. Each session consisted of four blocks of 50 trials plus four practice trials, with two blocks in each session devoted to each of the two ranges of motion in counterbalanced order. The two sessions for each task were completed before beginning the other task, and the order of these two tasks was different for the two observers.

Results

Figure 14.3 shows the detection accuracies for each of the four conditions as a function of the range of image motion. As may be seen, rotations were more detectable than expansions. The psychometric functions had similar

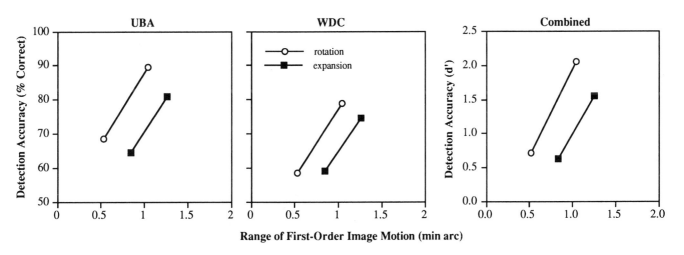

Figure 14.3
The results of experiment 2 for each condition and observer. Data for the two observers are given in the two graphs on the left, and the combined results for both observers are given in the graph on the right. Note that the dependent measure has been changed for the combined data.

Lappin et al.: Primitives for Structure from Motion

slopes but the function for the expansions is shifted to the right. The slopes were 2.55 and 2.19 d' per min arc for the rotations and expansions, respectively. The 75% correct thresholds for the two motions were 0.77 and 1.17 min arc.

Both of these first-order motions were more easily detected than the second-order motions in experiment 1, but the difference was not great between the 2D rotations and the shearing motions examined in the Collinearity Task. Both of the latter had similar intercepts on the horizontal axis, approximately 1/4 min arc in both cases, but the slope was lower for the Collinearity Task—approximately 1.5 d' per min arc as compared to about 2.5 d' per min arc for the rotations.

The difference was much greater between the differential motions in the Bisection Task and the expansions in the present experiment. The difference was mainly between the slopes rather than the intercepts of the psychometric functions—with the slope for the first-order expansions being steeper by a factor of about 6.9 than that for the second-order differential motions.

General Discussion

Results for the two forms of second-order image deformation were qualitatively different and suggest different conclusions about whether these constitute primitives detected by early vision. Accurate performance in the Collinearity Task suggests that perception of this shearing motion was detected as a primitive image property rather than derived as a difference between two first-order orientations. Moreover, these patterns usually appeared subjectively as a single rigid object moving in depth.

Julesz's studies of texture segregation provide additional evidence that such second-order spatial structure is a visual primitive. Spatial differences in *quasi-collinearity* are known to produce spontaneous texture discrimination (Caelli and Julesz, 1978)—one of the first discoveries that spontaneous texture discrimination does not require differences in dipole statistics.

In contrast, discriminations of symmetrical vs. asymmetrical compressions in the Bisection Task suggest that information about these second-order deformations was probably derived from differences between perceived first-order motions: Observers were relatively insensitive to the second-order as compared to the first-order motions, and detectability of the second-order deformations was hindered by first-order noise. These image motions also appeared subjectively as two disconnected motions rather than as attached to a single rigid object.

The superior visibility of shearing deformations relative to differential compressions has also been found in previous experiments (Braunstein and Andersen, 1984; Cornilleau-Pérès and Droulez, 1989; Nakayama et al., 1985; Norman and Lappin, 1992; Rogers and Graham, 1983). More densely dotted surfaces were used in these other experiments, indicating that the difference in detectability in the present experiment was not an artifact of the simplified patterns we used. The new evidence in the present study is that differential shearing motion serves as a visual primitive while differential compression seems to be derived from first-order expansions.

If the perception of these two deformations were derived from primitive zero-order retinal velocities, then such differences in detectability would not be expected to result from differences in relative location of the motions. Similarly, the relative difficulties of the Collinearity and Bisection Tasks would not be expected from the visibilities of the first-order rotations and expansions: The results of Lappin et al. (1991) and of experiment 2 indicate little difference in visibility of rotations and expansions. Thus, the difference in performance of the Collinearity and Bisection Tasks must involve differences in visibility of second-order motions.

Although the second-order differential expansions in the present study apparently were not directly visible as primitive motions, surfaces curved only in the direction of rotation can produce compelling impressions of rigid rotation in depth when the dot density and depth are sufficient. Diagonally aligned dots in such patterns, however, also undergo shearing deformations. Perceived structure and motion in depth might well be entirely attributable to these shearing deformations and not at all to the second-order differential compressions (Cornilleau-Pérès and Droulez, 1989; Norman and Lappin, 1992; Weinshall, 1991).

If cross-like patterns similar to those in figure 14.1 contained more collinear dots, providing added redundant differential expansions, might these second-order differential compressions be more directly visible? We explored this question with 13-point patterns containing two perpendicular collinear arrays of seven dots. These patterns still produced no subjective impressions of rigid structure and motion in depth nor any obvious improvement in detecting differential compression.

The results of this study support hypothesis 4, that vision is directly sensitive to second-order shearing deformations that alter the collinearity of three or more points. These shearing deformations probably constitute visual primitives for seeing the qualitative curvature of surfaces rotating in depth.

Acknowledgment

This research was supported in part by NIH Research grants EY05926 and P30EY08126.

References

Adelson, E. H., and Bergen, J. R. (1991). The plenoptic function and the elements of early vision. In M. S. Landy and J. A. Movshon (Eds.), *Computational Models of Visual Processing* (pp. 3–20). Cambridge, MA: MIT Press.

Braunstein, M. L., and Andersen, G. J. (1984). Shape and depth perception from parallel projections of three-dimensional motion. *J. Exp. Psychol. Human Percept. Perform. 10,* 749–760.

Caelli, T., and Julesz, B. (1978). On perceptual analyzers underlying visual texture discrimination: Part I. *Biol. Cybern. 28,* 167–175.

Caelli, T., Julesz, B., and Gilbert, E. (1978). On perceptual analyzers underlying visual texture discrimination: Part II. *Biol. Cybern. 29,* 201–214.

Chang, J. J., and Julesz, B. (1983). Displacement limits for spatial frequency filtered random-dot cinematograms in apparent motion. *Vision Res. 23,* 1379–1385.

Cornilleau-Pérès, V., and Droulez, J. (1989). Visual perception of surface curvature: Psychophysics of curvature detection induced by motion parallax. *Percept. Psychophys. 46,* 351–364.

De Valois, R. L., and De Valois, K. K. (1988). *Spatial Vision.* New York: Oxford University Press.

Julesz, B. (1960). Binocular depth perception of computer-generated patterns. *Bell Syst. Tech. J. 39,* 1125–1162.

Julesz, B. (1964). Binocular depth perception without familiarity cues. *Science 145,* 356–362.

Julesz, B. (1971). *Foundations of Cyclopean Perception.* Chicago: University of Chicago Press.

Julesz, B. (1980). Spatial-frequency channels in one-, two-, and three-dimensional vision: Variations on an auditory theme by Bekesy. In C. S. Harris (Ed.), *Visual Coding and Adaptability* (pp. 263–316). Hillsdale, NJ: Lawrence Erlbaum.

Julesz, B. (1981). Textons, the elements of texture perception, and their interactions. *Nature (London) 290,* 91–97.

Julesz, B. (1984). Toward an axiomatic theory of preattentive vision. In G. M. Edelman, W. E. Gall, and W. M. Cowan (Eds.), *Dynamic Aspects of Neocortical Function* (pp. 585–612). New York: Wiley-Interscience.

Julesz, B., Gilbert, E. N., and Victor, J. D. (1978). Visual discrimination of textures with identical third-order statistics. *Biol. Cybern. 31,* 137–140.

Koenderink, J. J., and van Doorn, A. J. (1976). Local structure of movement parallax of the plane. *J. Opt. Soc. Am. 66,* 717–723.

Koenderink, J. J., and van Doorn, A. J. (1992a). Generic neighborhood operators. *IEEE Transact. Pattern Anal. Machine Intelligence 14,* 597–605.

Koenderink, J. J., and van Doorn, A. J. (1992b). Second-order optic flow. *J. Opt. Soc. Am. A 9,* 530–538.

Lappin, J. S., Norman, J. F., and Mowafy, L. (1991). The detectability of geometric structure in rapidly changing optical patterns. *Perception 20,* 513–528.

Mowafy, L., Blake, R., and Lappin, J. S. (1990). Detection and discrimination of coherent motion. *Percept. Psychophys. 48,* 583–592.

Nakayama, K., Silverman, G. H., MacLeod, D. I., and Mulligan, J. (1985). Sensitivity to shearing and compressive motion in random dots. *Perception 14,* 225–238.

Norman, J. F., and Lappin, J. S. (1992). The detection of surface curvatures defined by optical motion. *Percept. Psychophys. 51,* 386–396.

Rogers, B. J., and Graham, M. E. (1983). Anisotropies in the perception of three-dimensional surfaces. *Science 221,* 1409–1411.

Simpson, W. A. (1993). Optic flow and depth perception. *Spatial Vision 7,* 35–75.

Weinshall, D. (1991). Direct computation of qualitative 3-D shape and motion invariants. *IEEE Transact. Pattern Anal. Machine Intelligence 13,* 1236–1240.

15

Of Models and Men: Mechanisms of Human Motion Perception

Johannes M. Zanker

Whenever we move our body, head, or eyes, or whenever any object is moving through our surroundings, or even changes its shape over time, the image on the retina is not static but dominated by a multitude of displacements. Because, in reverse, the two-dimensional retinal map of motion signals conveys most fundamental information about the dynamic three-dimensional structure of the external world, evolution has developed highly specialized eyes and brains throughout the animal kingdom that cope with moving images so well and easily that we are not even aware of the incredible information-processing capacity underlying this performance. The most obvious behavior that relies on motion detection is the control of eye, head, and body movements in order to stabilize gaze (Miles and Kawano, 1987; Egelhaaf et al., 1988; Dieringer, 1991). In addition to its role in this "optomotor response," motion detection is critically involved in visual control of limbs or tools, as well as in tracking moving or static objects such as prey or mating partners (Rossel, 1980; Poggio and Reichardt, 1981; Collewijn, Curio, and Grüsser, 1982). Furthermore, the depth structure of the three-dimensional outside world can be extracted in so-called flowfield analysis (Gibson, 1979; Koenderink, 1986; Regan, 1985; Warren and Hannon, 1988) from the two-dimensional retinal images by exploiting motion parallax, i.e., the geometric fact that closer objects move faster across the retina than more distant objects. Relative motion is a strong cue for breaking camouflage; the detection of an object hidden in a background of the same intensity, color, and texture is called "figure-ground discrimination" (Reichardt and Poggio, 1979; Regan, 1989; Reichardt, 1990). The three-dimensional structure of a rigid object also can be derived from the spatial distribution of the motion signal, usually referred to as "structure from motion" (Ullman, 1979; Dick, Ullman, and Sagi, 1991). When observing the parts of nonrigid objects moving relative to each other, motion information can be used for object recognition. In so-called biological motion paradigms, for instance, a walking human body is recognized in the dark on the basis of a few light points attached to the major joints (Johansson, 1975; Bertenthal et al., 1985).

Besides looking at the performance of the complete system on the behavioral level, there are many efforts to understand the underlying mechanisms by breaking down complex tasks into more comprehensible experimental questions. In psychophysics this approach has led to the formulation of a growing sample of motion processing problems, such as the "correspondence problem" or the "aperture problem" (Ullman and Hildreth, 1983; Hildreth and Koch, 1987; Nakayama and Silverman, 1988) or experimental paradigms, such as "motion capture" or "moving plaids" (Ramachandran and Cavanagh, 1987; Adelson and Movshon, 1982; Yo and Wilson, 1992). Other considerations were guided by theoretical concepts, such as "apparent and real motion" or "optic flow" (Anstis, 1978; Burr, Ross, and Morrone, 1986; Koenderink, 1986). A promising attempt to bind together all these threads of thought to a unified view of human motion processing can be pursued in a computational approach. When algorithmic models are formulated beyond merely sketching information flow in schematic block diagrams, human performance can be compared directly to that of the models. By means of computer simulations it can be tested whether—and within what range of parameters— the proposed models predict the percepts observed in the psychophysical experiments. Following this approach, model responses to classic and recently developed motion stimuli are used to consider how perception can be accounted for by assuming that elementary detectors of the correlation type provide the local motion information that is fed into further processing steps with integrating or differentiating properties, thus opening the perspective on "higher" perceptual performance.

Basic Models

It should be very easy to extract the motion of an object by relating the changes in position to the time used in making such changes. Because this requires that certain objects or features be identified explicitly and matched with the corresponding targets in succeeding images, this mechanism is referred to as "token matching" (Ullman and Hildreth, 1983; Nagel, 1988). However, token matching is not always a simple task; in so-called bistable motion displays the percept can switch between two interpretations, for instance. When an object is presented in alternation with two objects at two positions in space, one of which has the same shape but a different brightness, the other the same brightness but a different shape, an oscillation could be perceived between the objects of corresponding shape or of corresponding brightness (cf.

Ramachandran and Anstis, 1986), but usually the brightness overrules the shape effect. In random-dot kinematograms (RDKs) objects become easily visible within a pattern of randomly distributed black and white dots by the coherent displacement of a group of such dots, although the identification of individual dots would be extremely difficult. In RDKs motion perception breaks down above a certain displacement limit, d_{max}, which depends on the angular displacement rather than on the number of dots by which the patterns are displaced, when dot size is varied (Braddick, 1974, 1980). All this indicates that the information from two spatially fixed inputs is compared in order to detect motion, instead of tracking individual dots. Thus an intensity-based motion detection mechanism was suggested that precedes object discrimination (and therefore cannot be object based), which immediately operates on the spatiotemporal intensity distribution. Since d_{max}, as measured with RDKs, is much smaller than the displacement limit known for apparent motion stimuli with single objects, this "short-range" motion detecting system was suggested to complement the "long-range" system relying on object identification and matching in successive presentations (Anstis, 1980; Braddick, 1980; Prazdny, 1986).

A classic intensity-based model that was originally proposed to account for the optomotor behavior of insects is the elementary motion detector (EMD) of the correlation type (Hassenstein and Reichardt, 1956; Reichardt and Varju, 1959; Reichardt, 1961, 1987). In a simple form (see figure 15.1a), such an EMD consists of two input elements, or receptors, each feeding into a temporal low-pass filter and two nonlinear operators in which the direct input from one receptor interacts with the temporally filtered signal from the other receptor, for instance in a multiplicative way. The directional selectivity of an EMD is enhanced considerably by taking the difference of the outputs of two such antisymmetrical subunits (for review, see Borst and Egelhaaf, 1989). How this rather simple model can account for many psychophysical observations is exemplified in figure 15.1d for the perception of apparent motion, which was often juxtaposed to real motion (Anstis, 1980, 1978; Gregory and Harris, 1984). An apparent motion stimulus with five displacement steps of a bright object in front of a dark background (first to the right and then to the left) is shown in the upper space-time diagram. In such diagrams moving objects lead to contours with oblique orientation, and the mechanism of motion detection can be interpreted correspondingly as a spatiotemporally oriented (nonlinear) filter operating on the spatial and temporal intensity distribution. The output of an array of EMDs is displayed in

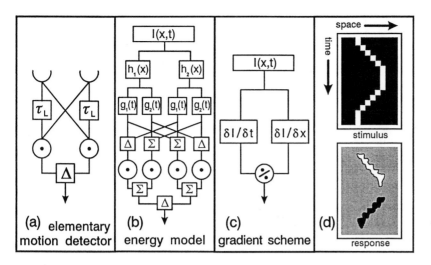

Figure 15.1
Motion detector models, simplified for only one spatial dimension. (*a*) The elementary motion detector (EMD) of the correlation type consists in a simple form of two input elements (receptors indicated by half circles) followed by two temporal filters (first order low-pass with time constant τ_L) and two nonlinear operators (multiplication indicated by dot) combining the direct input from one receptor with the filtered input from the other. The outputs of two such mirror-symmetric subunits are subtracted (Δ) to provide the final detector output. (*b*) In the energy model (Adelson and Bergen, 1985) linear spatial and temporal filters [$h(x)$ and $g(t)$] are combined (by subtraction Δ and summation $\sum$) to construct spatiotemporally inseparable filters that are oriented in the space-time domain. Squaring (circle with multiplication sign) the outputs and summing quadrature pairs (90° out of phase) leads to phase- and intensity-sign-independent extraction of motion energy from the input intensity distribution $I(x, t)$. (*c*) The gradient scheme is a formal computation of the pattern velocity by extracting the ratio (circle with division sign) of the temporal and spatial derivative ($\delta I/\delta t$ and $\delta I/\delta x$) of the input intensity distribution $I(x, t)$. (*d*) Computer simulation of the response (lower panel) of a one-dimensional network of EMDs (as sketched in *a*) to an apparent motion stimulus (upper panel). In the space–time diagram the history of a horizontal section through the stimulus is plotted vertically; regions of positive response (i.e., motion to the right) are indicated by white color, whereas black color indicates negative response (leftward motion).

the lower space-time diagram, with white and black areas indicating regions of positive and negative local detector responses, respectively. It is immediately clear from this simulation that the EMD output unambiguously reflects apparent motion direction. Similar results are obtained for many other motion stimuli, suggesting that there is no immediate need to assume different mechanisms operating at different spatial scales (see Zanker, 1994). A set of EMDs with a variety of receptor separations can account for the various phenomena observed with variable discrete or continuous object displacements. This is by no means an exotic proposal in light of the substantial evidence that the human visual system applies motion detectors at various spatial scales (Chang and Julesz, 1983; van de Grind, Koenderink, and van Doorn, 1986; Snowden and Braddick, 1989; Morgan and Fahle, 1992). Indeed in a comprehensive review of the recent literature on human motion processing (Cavanagh and Mather, 1989) the distinction between short-range and long-range mechanisms was actually challenged, arguing that the spatial scale should not be confused with the type of mechanism underlying a given motion percept. Keeping these aspects in mind, EMDs of the correlation type will be used here as a basis to discuss human motion perception, because

on the one hand they are simple to simulate without the necessity for additional assumptions, and on the other hand they are very powerful in predicting various psychophysical phenomena.

There are quite a few alternatives to the basic model that are extensively discussed in the literature. A prominent type of mechanism to account for the detection of motion is the so-called energy model, which applies spatial and temporal filters to extract oriented spatiotemporal energy, as illustrated in the space-time diagrams (Adelson and Bergen, 1985; Watson and Ahumada, 1985; Watson, 1990). Usually the output of linear spatiotemporal filters that are oriented in the space-time domain are squared, and a quadrature pair (i.e., being 90° out of phase) is summed to give a measure of motion energy. As in the EMD, a subtraction stage of two opponent units enhances directional selectivity (see figure 15.1b). This model basically can be transformed into a version formally equivalent to the correlation detector (Adelson and Bergen, 1985; van Santen and Sperling, 1985). Within the group of intensity-based schemes the correlation type detector is often opposed to the so-called gradient scheme, which originates from computer vision (Fennema and Thompson, 1975; Limb and Murphy, 1975; Ullman, 1981; Marr and Ullman, 1981). This model in a purely formal sense derives the velocity from the ratio between the spatial and the temporal derivative of the input distribution (see figure 15.1c). These operations have to be translated into realistic filter elements (Feijin and Srinivasan, 1990; Srinivasan, 1990). For instance, the spatial and temporal derivative could be approximated by corresponding high-pass filters, and the division was even proposed to be interpreted in terms of neural inhibition. It always has to be avoided by some additional assumptions that the denominator of the division approaches zero. When implementing such restricted versions of the gradient scheme, it may resemble formally the correlation detector (Hildreth and Koch, 1987; Borst and Egelhaaf, 1993).

Nonlinear Preprocessing

So far, this chapter has exclusively dealt with motion stimuli in which moving objects are characterized in a visual scenery by intensity contrast, such as a dark bar displaced in front of a bright background, or black and white dots shifted in a RDK. Moving contours between regions of different color can in principle be perceived in the same manner, although the relative importance of color information for motion perception is still debated (Ramachandran and Gregory, 1978; Livingstone and Hubel, 1987; Derrington and Badcock, 1985a; Gorea and Papathomas, 1989; Papathomas, Gorea, and Julesz, 1991) (cf. Farell, this volume). Since the spatiotemporal Fourier analysis of a shift of the intensity profile leads to a systematic distribution of the Fourier components along an oblique line in frequency space (Fahle and Poggio, 1981), such stimuli are usually called Fourier motion (Sperling, 1989; Chubb and Sperling, 1988). Motion-specific spatiotemporal Fourier components (motion energy) correspond to the oblique lines in the space-time diagrams that are due to the displaced intensity profiles (cf. figure 15.1d, for instance). Accordingly, such motion is extracted by means of EMDs with appropriate spatial and temporal front-end filters (i.e., tuned to the corresponding motion energy). In recent years however, stimuli without coherent shift of the intensity profile were introduced in various forms (for review, see Cavanagh and Mather, 1989). Following a proposal of Chubb and Sperling (1988), they are often called non-Fourier or drift-balanced motion, because local shifts of intensity contours are randomly distributed and thus on average lead to zero motion energy.

In an early version (Petersik, Hicks, and Pantle, 1978), the class of non-Fourier motion stimuli appeared as a Ternus display (three dots are alternating between two locations in space such that two dots always appear at the same positions [Ternus, 1926]; human observers either perceive three dots jumping to and fro as a group, or one dot jumping from one side of two static dots to the other). Flickering bars were generated in a random-dot pattern by statistically independent replacement of all dots within a certain region in front of a static background. Two such flickering bars are alternating between two positions in space, with one of the bars always appearing at the same center position. Although no dots are displaced coherently, human observers perceive motion in a bistable manner, just as in the intensity-defined classic Ternus display: either one bar is experienced jumping around a static one in the middle, or two bars are perceived oscillating in synchrony. A multiframe non-Fourier stimulus was produced by Lelkens and Koenderink (1984), which they called μ-motion, with a flickering bar moving through several steps in apparent motion. Conventional EMDs are not able to extract the direction of bar motion from such stimuli, so they proposed an appropriate mechanism employing flicker detectors as input elements of a correlation-type motion detector. It is immediately evident that such a model should be able to detect the movement of a flickering bar, while a higher order nonlinearity is introduced as compared to the basic EMD. The distinction between Fourier and non-Fourier, or drift-balanced, motion, which is based on the systematic theoretical treatment of a variety of motion stimulus configurations (Chubb and Sperling, 1988, 1989), gives rise to a family of possible stimuli: In a very simple case, only a border between two static patterns is shifted across space, in more elaborate stimuli the borders between areas of different spatial or temporal pattern characteristics might be moved. Or it is simply the shift of the spatial function modulating the local contrast of a pattern that leads to a vivid motion sensation. The latter effect is easily generated by superimposing two sinewave gratings with slightly different frequencies. When one of them is drifting, it looks like a low-frequency sinewave contrast modulation function being shifted across a high-frequency sinewave carrier intensity distribution (Derrington and Badcock, 1985b; Henning and Derrington, 1988; Turano and Pantle, 1989). It has to be noted, however, that such moving "beat patterns" contain minor Fourier motion components in opposite direction to the traveling modulation function (Badcock and Derrington, 1989), and thus cannot be regarded as perfect case of non-Fourier stimuli.

As Chubb and Sperling (1988) showed theoretically, an additional nonlinearity is necessary prior to a correlation-type motion detector for all such stimuli, in order to extract the movement. In contrast to the earlier proposal

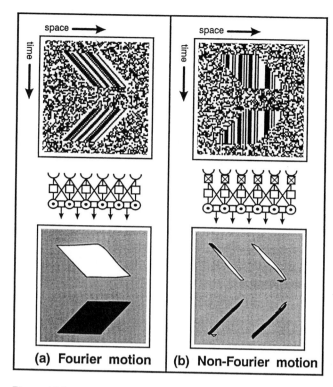

(a) Fourier motion   **(b) Non-Fourier motion**

Figure 15.2

Simulation of Fourier and non-Fourier motion detection. Conventions as in figure 15.1d. (*a*) In the Fourier motion stimulus (space-time diagram in top panel), a group of random dots is displaced coherently (leading to oblique black and white stripes) in front of a dynamic noise background generated by black and white dots, which are replaced independently from each other in space and time (randomly distributed black and white dots in the space–time diagram). The response (bottom panel) of an array of simple EMDs (the schematic sketch in the middle is not scaled with respect to the space-time diagrams) clearly reflects the movement to the right and to the left (white and black regions indicating positive and negative response, respectively). The clear responses presented here are partially due to vertical pooling across several rows of EMDs, which are not represented in the space-time diagrams; due to the erratic intensity changes within RDKs, the response of a single EMD would be superimposed by a considerable amount of irregular fluctuations. The clear result shown here comes with spatial integration along the vertical spatial axis (by averaging several simulation sweeps), which cannot be displayed in the space-time diagrams. (*b*) In the non-Fourier motion stimulus (space-time diagram in top panel), a region is shifted within the dynamic noise background, which displays static black and white dots (leading to oblique parallelograms of vertical black and white stripes). The response (bottom panel) of an array of EMDs with nonlinear preprocessing (schematic sketch in the middle, the crosses in the input box indicate a fullwave rectification) reflects the movement to the right and to the left (white and black regions indicating positive and negative response, respectively) at the object boundaries.

invoking flicker detectors as front-end filters (see above), however, they demonstrated that a squaring nonlinearity, or even a mere fullwave or halfwave rectification suffices to make an EMD sensitive to many sorts of drift-balanced motion stimuli. The action of this model elaboration is illustrated by the computer simulations depicted in figure 15.2 (cf. Zanker, 1993). The output of a network of simple EMDs reflects the diretion of object motion in a Fourier motion stimulus in which a group of dots is moving coherently in front of a dynamic noise pattern in the background (see figure 15.2a). The output of the same model to a corresponding drift-balanced stimulus in which the dots inside the object area are static (cf. stimulus diagram in figure 15.2b) consists of tiny, randomly distributed areas of small positive or negative outputs (response not shown). However, when the EMD is equipped with a full-wave rectification in the input lines, the model provides an output signal which indeed reflects the direction of object motion (lower panel of figure 15.2b). A temporal high-pass filter was introduced into the model preceding the rectification operator, in order to provide it with positive and negative deviations from average intensity instead of positive intensity values only. It can be demonstrated correspondingly, that the perception of other drift-balanced motion stimuli can be accounted for by the average output of EMDs with various sorts of nonlinear preprocessing, but non-Fourier motion cannot be extracted by EMDs with purely linear front-end filters.

A Two-Layer Model

In the two classes of stimuli discussed so far, either the dots on the surface of an object were moving in the same direction as the object itself, or else they were static. However, when the dots move in the direction opposite that of the object, a paradoxical stimulus is generated. The stimulus motion energy, corresponding to the shift of the moving intensity contours, is in the direction opposite from the object's displacement. In figure 15.3 (top panel) it is shown how such a "theta motion" stimulus (Zanker, 1990, 1993) looks in the space-time diagram. The oblique stripes to the left are orthogonal to the oblique borders of the object to the right, in contrast to the parallel stripes and borders of the object in Fourier motion (cf. figure 15.2a, top panel). It is obvious that in this stimulus configuration EMDs, being sensitive to oriented stripes, should detect the dot motion. A mechanism that goes beyond extracting motion energy is required to detect the movement of the motion signal. It was shown in various psychophysical experiments that this kind of motion is actually perceived by human subjects. The perception of

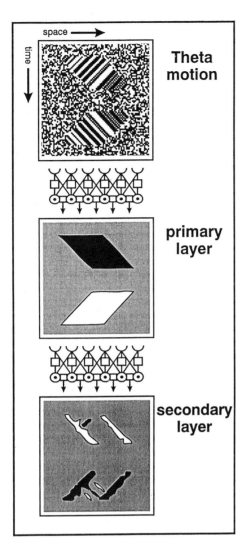

Figure 15.3
Simulation of theta motion processing. Conventions as in figure 15.2.
Theta motion stimulus (*top*): in front of a dynamic noise background an
object region is shifted that displays black and white dots moving in
the direction opposite to the object itself, leading to oblique parallelograms of perpendicularily oblique black and white stripes in the space-
time diagram. The response (*bottom*) of an array of simple EMDs
(upper model sketch) clearly reflects the movement of the dots within
the object boundaries to the left and to right (black and white regions
indicating negative and positive response, respectively). When this
response is fed into a second layer of EMDs (lower model sketch,
spatial low-pass filtering not indicated) the motion direction of the
object itself is reflected by the model output (white and black regions
indicating positive and negative response, respectively). As a result of
the specific simulation parameters, as in the case of non-Fourier motion
(cf. figure 15.2b) the response is limited to the object boundaries; minor
response components with opposite sign can still be observed in
neighboring regions.

theta motion can be elicited within a large range of stimulus conditions, and the sensitivity, as measured by noise
thresholds, can be very similar for Fourier, drift-balanced,
and theta motion stimuli (Zanker, 1990; Hüpgens and
Zanker, 1992; Zanker, 1993). The dependence of theta
motion perception on various stimulus variables, like displacement amplitude and stimulus geometry, has been
investigated experimentally so far, whereas many other
questions, such as those concerning the range and the
optimum of spatiotemporal parameters appropriate to
elicit the percept or the influence of training, remain to be
answered.

Computer simulations of a model responding to theta
motion are shown in figure 15.3. As expected for a mechanism extracting motion energy, an array of simple EMDs
of the correlation type detects the direction of dot motion
in the theta motion stimulus but does not give any hint at
the direction of object motion (middle panel of the figure):
the response in the first part of the stimulus cycle is black,
indicating leftward motion, whereas in the second part it
is white, indicating rightward motion. The same result is
achieved with elaborated versions of the EMD assuming
some sort of nonlinear preprocessing (data not shown, for
details of these simulations, see Zanker, 1993). Thus the
models discussed so far do not account for the psychophysical results, as would be expected from the motion
energy contained in the theta stimulus. If the EMD outputs represented by the oblique black and white areas are
fed into a second array of EMDs, however, they should
give a response depending on the movement direction of
the motion signal, irrespective of the sign of the primary
motion signal (just as the motion direction of a bright or
dark spot should be detected irrespective of the sign of
intensity contrast). The bottom panel of figure 15.3 confirms this expectation that a model with two consecutive
layers of EMDs is able to extract the movement direction
of an object exclusively defined by motion. The second
layer of EMDs detects the displacement of the motion
signal, irrespective of the sign of the signal itself, which is
detected by the first layer of EMDs. The second-layer
response is most prominent on the object borders because
in these regions the decisive displacement of the motion
border is fed into the second layer, whereas within the
motion-defined object there is no coherent spatiotemporal signal modulation of the first-layer output. This
corresponds to the experimental observation that the extraction of object motion from a theta stimulus critically
depends on the stimulus geometry. Whereas the basic
structure of this two-layer model is straightforward, some
issues should be mentioned. First of all, the spatial layout
of the second layer is different from that of the first layer.

To produce a smooth and reliable result, spatial integration is necessary at the input elements that reduces the local fluctuations of the first layer output, which are due to the erratic intensity changes in RDKs. The corresponding reduction of the spatial resolution for theta motion perception can indeed be observed in psychophysical experiments using grating versions of paradoxical motion stimuli (Zanker, 1992). Furthermore, the possibility of extracting the movement of the motion signal by the second layer does not depend critically on the type of preprocessing of the first layer. Assuming nonlinear preprocessing in the first layer and appropriate spatiotemporal layout of the second layer, the two-layer model can be tailored such that it actually predicts the results of psychophysical experiments quantitatively (Zanker, 1994).

Conclusions

In the previous sections it was shown, in a few examples, how highly artificial motion stimuli are used to test spe-

cific hypotheses about mechanisms underlying human motion perception. Starting from very basic apparent motion stimuli, random-dot kinematograms of increasing complexity were introduced (Fourier, drift-balanced, theta-motion) that challenge the perceptual capabilities, as well as our understanding, of the visual system. On the other hand, models of motion processing were considered that get more complex in parallel to the stimuli. Two questions will now be adressed to clarify how this approach helps to understand human brain function: (1) Can the models be integrated into some systematic order and related to physiology? (2) Can any behavioral significance be attributed to these mechanisms?

A comprehensive list of possible multi-input nonlinear interactions, and a graphic notation of such systems, was proposed by Poggio and Reichardt (1973, 1980) and is illustrated in figure 15.4. For comparison, the model sketches used here to account for the detection of Fourier, drift-balanced, and theta motion (shaded boxes in top row of the figure) are transposed into the graphical notation of Poggio and Reichardt (middle row), and the other way

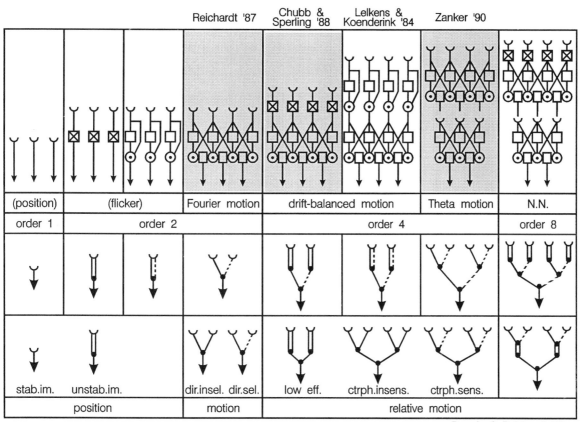

Figure 15.4
Systematic list of possible multiinput nonlinear interaction models. Details in text.

around. In the top row the models are sketched as flow diagrams with various inputs (symbolized by semicircles) connected to linear and nonlinear processing stages that are symbolized by open boxes (temporal filters or subtractions), crossed boxes (nonlinear transfer functions), and circles with dots (multiplications). Simple input lines would provide the visual system with a mere position signal for stabilized images (first column), whereas some nonlinear operation would lead to flicker sensitivity supporting position sensing in unstabilized images (next two columns). In the graphs of Poggio and Reichardt (bottom, for details see original paper), nonlinear one-input systems are symbolized by a single dot of nonlinear interaction combining two input lines from one receptor (in the asymmetrical case one input is connected by a broken line). It is trivial that the EMD used here for the detection of Fourier motion appears in their list as direction-selective motion detector; the model sketch used here (top row of column 4) translates into the symbolic graph with asymmetrical nonlinear interaction between two inputs (middle row). Higher-order nonlinear interactions, using two (bottom row of column 5) or four separate inputs in space (bottom row of columns 6 and 7), were proposed by Poggio and Reichardt in different versions, in order to account for figure-ground discrimination with low (2 inputs) or high efficiency (4 inputs), and being insensitive (column 6, symmetrical nonlinear interaction) or sensitive (column 7, asymmetrical nonlinear interaction) to counterphase motion of figure and background. However, these proposals, only by virtue of the number of inputs and nonlinear steps, but not in the construction details, correspond to the graphic translations of the models discussed here to account for detection of drift-balanced and theta motion (top and middle row of columns 5–7). Especially, Poggio and Reichardt did not include a graph in which the second nonlinear interaction is asymmetric, as is required for the models for detecting the movement of a flicker or motion signal. Finally, in the last column, a two-layer model is sketched with additional nonlinear preprocessing (top row), which is not analyzed experimentally with appropriate stimuli ("N.N.") so far. Such a model, which actually can account for the extraction of Fourier, drift-balanced, and theta motion at the same time (Zanker, 1994), could be loosely related to a graph of Poggio and Reichardt with four inputs and three nonlinear processing steps (bottom row).

As can be seen in figure 15.4, the performance of a given system depends on the number of inputs, the symmetry properties, and the order of nonlinearity. Beyond the impression of similarity and increasing complexity, there are two points to note about this model zoo. (1) The order of nonlinearity of a given system is defined by the highest exponent of the Volterra series describing its transfer function (for details, see Poggio and Reichardt, 1980). This order, given by the essential nonlinearities of a system, may differ considerably from the order of its actual implementation, because any nonessential nonlinearity will make the exponents grow without necessarily affecting the model performance observed under standard experimental conditions. Here not only physiologically plausible nonlinearities such as thresholds or saturations have to be considered, but also implicit nonlinear operators that often are not obvious, such as hidden in orientation selective input filters. (2) Already for a basic EMD just accounting for the detection of Fourier motion, the order of nonlinearity is two; it is four when minimum models accounting for the detection of drift-balanced and theta motion are considered, although qualitatively different model structures have to be assumed. Therefore, terms like "first-order" and "second-order" processing referring to the "order" of a model's nonlinearity can be misleading. Since two steps of specific motion processing are involved in the extraction of object motion in a theta stimulus, it could be called "secondary" instead. On the other hand, "primary" processing of Fourier or drift-balanced motion stimuli requires only one step of motion detection, but may depend on an EMD with linear or nonlinear preprocessing. This notation is less sensitive to problems originating from specific assumptions about the preprocessing or even the neural implementation, but it slightly differs from the "first-" and "second-order" classification used by other authors (Cavanagh and Mather, 1989; Sperling, 1989) who distinguish direct intensity or color inputs to a motion detector from all types of nonlinear preprocessing, such as flicker, stereo, or motion.

Thinking of the implementation of such a model structure in the architecture of real brains (cf. Schiller, this volume), it is very tempting to expect the two layers of motion processing to be localized in distinct anatomical layers or regions, despite the incredibly complex wiring scheme of the visual brain regions (Van Essen, Anderson, and Felleman, 1992). There is some electrophysiological evidence from primates that directional selective neurons in area V2 not only process Fourier but also non-Fourier motion (Albright, 1992). However, no electrophysiological data are available for stimulation with primary and secondary motion signals in opposite directions. There are attempts to localize specific motion processing by means of recording slow cortical potentials in humans observing the three classes of motion stimuli. Interestingly, no motion-specific responses can be found over the occipital recording sites, which correspond to the cortical input regions, but specific responses can be found at the parietal recording sites, which reflect the direction of a moving object irrespective of the direction of dot motion defining the object (Patzwahl, Zanker, and Altenmüller, 1993). Since these recording sites lie above higher cortical areas, which may be related to the human analogue of monkey area MT (Zeki et al., 1991; Zihl, von Cramon, and Mai, 1983), this type of experiment might help to trace a possible hierarchical organization of motion processing in the human cortex.

What could be the functional significance of all these peculiar motion-processing mechanisms? In a very general sense, secondary motion processing could be valuable in increasing signal-to-noise ratios in difficult perceptual environments, for instance, when a flying bird has to be detected between foliage driven by the wind (Sperling, 1989). However, the key role of higher order motion processing in the figure-ground discrimination task, as discussed together with figure 15.4, leads to a more specific viewpoint. Secondary motion processing is important when differential information about motion has to be extracted by some sort of comparison of the local information (cf. Lappin et al., this volume). This could be achieved linearly, for instance, when some sort of motion-contrast enhancement is realized by a subtractive center-surround organization of perceptive fields (Regan and Beverley, 1984; Nakayama et al., 1985). On the other hand, there is psychophysical evidence for cooperative, nonlinear interactions between neighboring regions of motion (Chang and Julesz, 1984; Williams and Phillips, 1987; Nawrot and Sekuler, 1990). Relating the motion information from neighboring areas to each other is important not only in figure-ground discrimination. The reconstruction of the three-dimensional structure from the local distribution of motion signals, for instance, depends on comparison of neighboring motion signals (Ullman, 1979; Grzywacz and Hildreth, 1987). Furthermore, the analysis of the retinal flow, which is important for controlling and guiding body movements in three-dimensional space, essentially relies on the comparison of motion signals (Nakayama, 1985; Regan, 1985). For example, the pole of a flowfield generated by egomotion, which is characterized by the absence of local image motion, indicates the heading angle (Warren and Hannon, 1988). Therefore a system that detects the movement of such a pole would be very useful. This is actually a secondary processing task. Whereas primary and secondary processing in the context of egomotion control by means of flowfield analysis may act on a very coarse scale, the structure-from-motion task requires a rather scrutinized knowledge about differences in the local motion signals.

Thus further research in human motion processing may be directed to the spatial layout of the basic motion-detecting mechanisms, the integration stages, and the differential operators involved in secondary motion processing (Braddick, 1993). The two-layer model originally introduced to account for the detection of theta motion could thus play an important role in the context of understanding the first steps of higher-order motion processing necessary for many visual processing tasks.

Acknowledgments

I thank A. Borst, V. Braitenberg, M. Egelhaaf, and M. Fahle for their critical comments on earlier versions of this manuscript. Financial support came from the Max-Planck-Gesellschaft and the DFG (Zr 1/9-1).

References

Adelson, E. H., and Bergen, J. R. (1985). Spatiotemporal energy models for the perception of motion. *J. Opt. Soc. Am. A 2*, 284–299.

Adelson, E. H., and Movshon, J. A. (1982). Phenomenal coherence of moving visual patterns. *Nature (London) 300*, 523–525.

Albright, T. D. (1992). Form-cue invariant motion processing in primate visual cortex. *Science 255*, 1141–1143.

Anstis, S. M. (1978). Apparent movement. In R. Held, H. W. Leibowitz, and H. L. Teuber (Eds.), *Handbook of Sensory Physiology VIII* (pp. 655–673). Berlin: Springer.

Anstis, S. M. (1980). The perception of apparent movement. *Phil. Trans. R. Soc. B 290*, 153–168.

Badcock, D. R., and Derrington, A. M. (1989). Detecting the displacements of spatial beats: no role for distortion products. *Vision Res. 29*, 731–739.

Bertenthal, B. I., Proffitt, D. R., Spetner, N. B., and Thomas, M. A. (1985). The development of infant sensitivity to biomechanical motions. *Child Dev. 56*, 531–543.

Borst, A., and Egelhaaf, M. (1989). Principles of visual motion detection. *Trends Neurosci. 12*, 297–306.

Borst, A., and Egelhaaf, M. (1993). Detecting visual motion: Theory and models. In F. A. Miles, and J. Wallman, (Eds.), *Visual Motion and Its Role in the Stabilization of Gaze* (pp. 3–27). Amsterdam: Elsevier.

Braddick, O. J. (1974). A short-range process in apparent motion. *Vision Res. 14*, 519–527.

Braddick, O. J. (1980). Low-level and high-level processes in apparent motion. *Phil. Trans. R. Soc. London B290*, 137–151.

Braddick, O. J. (1993). Segmentation versus integration in visual motion processing. *Trends Neurosci. 16*, 263–268.

Burr, D. C., Ross, J., and Morrone, M. C. (1986). Smooth and sampled motion. *Vision Res. 26*, 643–652.

Cavanagh, P., and Mather, G. (1989). Motion: The long and short of it. *Spatial Vision 4*, 103–129.

Chang, J. J., and Julesz, B. (1983). Displacement limits for spatial frequency filtered random-dot cinematograms in apparent motion. *Vision Res. 23*, 1379–1385.

Chang, J. J., and Julesz, B. (1984). Cooperative phenomena in apparent movement perception of random-dot cinematograms. *Vision Res. 24*, 1781–1788.

Chubb, C., and Sperling, G. (1988). Drift-balanced random stimuli: a general basis for studying non-Fourier motion perception. *J. Opt. Soc. Am. A5*, 1986–2006.

Chubb, C., and Sperling, G. (1989). Two motion perception mechanisms revealed through distance-driven reversal of apparent motion. *Proc. Natl. Acad. Sci. USA 86*, 2985–2989.

Collewijn, H., Curio, G., and Grüsser, O. J. (1982). Spatially selective visual attention and generation of eye pursuit movements. *Human Neurobiol. 1*, 129–139.

Derrington, A. M., and Badcock, D. R. (1985a). The low level motion system has both chromatic and luminance inputs. *Vision Res. 25*, 1879–1884.

Derrington, A. M., and Badcock, D. R. (1985b). Separate detectors for simple and complex grating patterns? *Vision Res. 25*, 1869–1878.

Dick, M., Ullman, S., and Sagi, D. (1991). Short- and long-range processes in structure-from-motion. *Vision Res. 31*, 2025–2028.

Dieringer, N. (1991). Comparative aspects of gaze stabilization in vertebrates. *Zool. Jb. Physiol. 95*, 369–377.

Egelhaaf, M., Hausen, K., Reichardt, W., and Wehrhahn, C. (1988). Visual course control in flies relies on neuronal computation of object and background motion. *Trends Neurosci. 11*, 351–358.

Fahle, M., and Poggio, T. (1981). Visual hyperacuity: spatiotemporal interpolation in human vision. *Proc. R. Soc. London B 213*, 451–477.

Feijin, Z., and Srinivasan, M. V. (1990). Neural gradient models for the measurement of image velocity. *Vision Neurosci. 5*, 261–271.

Fennema, C. L., and Thompson, W. B. (1975). Velocity determination in scenes containing several moving objects. *Comput. Graph. Image Proc. 9*, 301–315.

Gibson, J. J. (1979). *The Ecological Approach to Visual Perception*. Hillsdale, NJ: Lawrence Erlbaum.

Gorea, A., and Papathomas, V. (1989). Motion processing by chromatic and achromatic visual pathways. *J. Opt. Soc. Am. A6*, 590–602.

Gregory, R. L., and Harris, J. P. (1984). Real and apparent movement nulled. *Nature (London) 307*, 729–730.

Grzywacz, N. M., and Hildreth, E.-C. (1987). Incremental rigidity scheme for recovering structure from motion: Position-based versus velocity-based formulations. *J. Opt. Soc. Am. A 4*, 503–518.

Hassenstein, B., and Reichardt, W. (1956). Systemtheoretische Analyse der Zeit-, Reihenfolgen- und Vorzeichenauswertung bei der Bewegungsperzeption des Rüsselkafers Chlorophanus. *Z. Naturforsch. 11b*, 513–524.

Henning, G. B., and Derrington, A. M. (1988). Direction-of-motion discrimination with complex patterns: Further observations. *J. Opt. Soc. Am. A5*, 1759–1766.

Hildreth, E.-C., and Koch, C. (1987). The analysis of visual motion: From computational theory to neuronal mechanisms. *Ann. Rev. Neurosci. 10*, 477–533.

Hüpgens, I. S., and Zanker, J. M. (1992). Human sensitivity to paradox motion stimuli (theta-motion). In N. Elsner, and D. W. Richter (Eds.), *Rhythmogenesis in Neurons and Networks* (pp. 341). Stuttgart: Georg Thieme Verlag.

Johansson, G. (1975). Visual motion perception. *Sci. Am. 232*, 76–88.

Koenderink, J. J. (1986). Optic flow. *Vision Res. 26*, 161–180.

Lelkens, A. M. M., and Koenderink, J. J. (1984). Illusory motion in visual displays. *Vision Res. 24*, 1083–1090.

Limb, J. O., and Murphy, J. A. (1975). Estimating the velocity of moving images in television signals. *Comput. Graph. Image Proc. 4*, 311–327.

Livingstone, M. S., and Hubel, D. H. (1987). Psychophysical evidence for separate channels for the perception of form, color, movement, and depth. *J. Neurosci. 7*, 3416–3468.

Marr, D., and Ullman, S. (1981). Directional selectivity and its use in early visual processing. *Proc. R. Soc. London B211*, 151–180.

Miles, F. A., and Kawano, K. (1987). Visual stabilization of the eyes. *Trends Neurosci. 10*(4), 153–158.

Morgan, M. J., and Fahle, M. (1992). Effects of pattern element density upon displacement limits for motion detection in random binary luminance patterns. *Proc. R. Soc. London [Biol.] 248*, 189–198.

Nagel, H.-H. (1988). From image sequences towards conceptual descriptions. *Image Vision Comput. 6*, 59–74.

Nakayama, K. (1985). Biological image motion processing: a review. *Vision Res. 25*, 625–660.

Nakayama, K., and Silverman, G. H. (1988). The aperture problem—II—Spatial integration of velocity information along contours. *Vision Res. 28*, 747–753.

Nakayama, K., Silverman, G. H., MacLeod, D. I. A., and Mulligan, J. B. (1985). Sensitivity to shearing and compressive motion in random dots. *Perception 14*, 225–238.

Nawrot, M., and Sekuler, R. (1990). Assimilation and contrast in motion perception: Explorations in cooperativity. *Vision Res. 30*, 1439–1451.

Papathomas, V., Gorea, A., and Julesz, B. (1991). Two carriers for motion perception: Color and luminance. *Vision Res. 31*, 1883–1891.

Patzwahl, D., Zanker, J. M., and Altenmüller, E. (1993). Cortical potentials in humans reflecting the direction of object motion. *NeuroRep 4*(4), 379–882.

Petersik, J. T., Hicks, K. I., and Pantle, A. (1978). Apparent movement of successively generated subjective figures. *Perception 7*, 371–383.

Poggio, T., and Reichardt, W. (1973). Considerations on models of movement detection. *Kybern. 13*, 223–227.

Poggio, T., and Reichardt, W. (1980). On the representation of multiinput systems: Computational properties of polynomal algorithms. *Biol. Cybern. 37*, 167–186.

Poggio, T., and Reichardt, W. (1981). Visual fixation and tracking by flies: Mathematical properties of simple control systems. *Biol. Cybern. 40*, 101–112.

Prazdny, K. (1986). What variables control (long-range) apparent motion? *Perception 15*, 37–40.

Ramachandran, V. S., and Anstis, S. M. (1986). The perception of apparent motion. *Sci. Am. 254* (6), 102–109.

Ramachandran, V. S., and Cavanagh, P. (1987). Motion capture anisotropy. *Vision Res. 27*, 97–106.

Ramachandran, V. S., and Gregory, R. L. (1978). Does colour provide an input to human motion perception? *Nature (London) 275*, 55–56.

Regan, D. (1985). Visual flow and direction of locomotion. *Science 227*, 1063–1065.

Regan, D. (1989). Orientation discrimination for objects defined by relative motion and objects defined by luminance contrast. *Vision Res. 29*, 1389–1400.

Regan, D., and Beverley, K. (1984). Figure-ground segregation by motion contrast and by luminance contrast. *J. Opt. Soc. Am. A1*, 433–442.

Reichardt, W. (1961). Autocorrelation, a principle for the evaluation of sensory information by the central nervous system. In W. A. Rosenblith (Ed.), *Sensory Communication* (pp. 303–317). Cambridge, MA: MIT Press.

Reichardt, W. (1987). Evaluation of optical motion information by movement detectors. *J. Comp. Physiol. A161*, 533–547.

Reichardt, W. (1990). Movement Detection and Figure-Ground Discrimination. In L. Deecke, J. C. Eccles, and V. B. Mountcastle (Eds.), *From Neuron to Action* (pp. 267–276). Berlin: Springer-Verlag.

Reichardt, W., and Poggio, T. (1979). Figure-ground discrimination by relative movement in the visual system of the fly. *Biol. Cybern. 35*, 81–100.

Reichardt, W., and Varju, D. (1959). Übertragungseigenschaften im Auswertesystem für das Bewegungssehen. *Z. Naturforsch. 14b*, 674–689.

Rossel, S. (1980). Foveal fixation and tracking in the praying mantis. *J. Comp. Physiol. 139*, 307–331.

Snowden, R. J., and Braddick, O. J. (1989). Extension of displacement limits in multiple-exposure sequences of apparent motion. *Vision Res. 29*, 1777–1787.

Sperling, G. (1989). Three stages and two systems of visual processing. *Spatial Vision 4*, 183–207.

Srinivasan, M. V. (1990). Generalized gradient schemes for the measurement of two-dimensional image motion. *Biol. Cybern. 63*, 421–431.

Ternus, J. (1926). Experimentelle Untersuchungen über phenomenale Identität. *Psychol. Forschg. 7*, 81–136.

Turano, K., and Pantle, A. (1989). On the mechanism that encodes the movement of contrast variations: velocity discrimination. *Vision Res. 29*, 207–221.

Ullman, S. (1979). The interpretation of structure from motion. *Proc. R. Soc. London B 203*, 405–426.

Ullman, S. (1981). Analysis of visual motion by biological and computer systems. *Computer Aug 1981*, 57–69.

Ullman, S., and Hildreth, E.-C. (1983). The measurement of visual motion. In O. J. Braddick, and A. C. Sleigh (Eds.), *Physical and Biological Processing of Images* (pp. 154–176). New York: Springer.

van de Grind, W. A., Koenderink, J. J., and van Doorn, A. J. (1986). The distribution of human motion detector properties in the monocular visual field. *Vision Res. 26*, 797–810.

Van Essen, D. C., Anderson, C. H., and Felleman, D. J. (1992). Information processing in the primate visual system: An integrated systems perspective. *Science 255*, 419–423.

van Santen, J. P. H., and Sperling, G. (1985). Elaborated Reichardt detectors. *J. Opt. Soc. Am. A 2*, 300–321.

Warren, W. H., and Hannon, D. J. (1988). Direction of self-motion is perceived from optical flow. *Nature (London) 336*, 162–163.

Watson, A. B. (1990). Optimal displacement in apparent motion and quadrature models of motion sensing. *Vision Res. 30*, 1389–1393.

Watson, A. B., and Ahumada, A. J. (1985). Model of human visual-motion sensing. *J. Opt. Soc. Am. A 2*, 322–342.

Williams, D. W., and Phillips, G. (1987). Cooperative phenomena in the perception of motion direction. *J. Opt. Soc. Am. A 4*, 878–885.

Yo, C., and Wilson, H. R. (1992). Perceived direction of moving two-dimensional patterns depends on duration, contrast and eccentricity. *Vision Res. 32*, 135–147.

Zanker, J. M. (1990). Theta motion: A new psychophysical paradigm indicating two levels of visual motion perception. *Naturwissenschaften 77*, 243–246.

Zanker, J. M. (1992). Paradoxical motion stimuli (theta-motion) realized as periodic gratings. *Perception 21*, A 45.

Zanker, J. M. (1993). Theta motion: A paradoxical stimulus to explore higher order motion extraction. *Vision Res. 33*, 553–569.

Zanker, J. M. (1994a). Modelling human motion perception. I. Classical stimuli. *Naturwissenschaften 81*, 156–163.

Zanker, J. M. (1994b). Modelling human motion perception. II. Beyond Fourier motion stimuli. *Naturwissenschaften 81*, 200–209.

Zeki, S. M., Watson, J. D. G., Lueck, C. J., Friston, K. J., Kennard, C., and Frackowiak, R. S. J. (1991). A direct demonstration of functional specialization in human visual cortex. *J. Neurosci. 11*, 641–649.

Zihl, J., von Cramon, D., and Mai, N. (1983). Selective disturbance of movement vision after bilateral brain damage. *Brain 106*, 313–340.

16

Visual Processing in the Primate Extrastriate Cortex

Peter H. Schiller

It has been known for nearly a hundred years that there are several distinct visual areas in the posterior cortex of the primate (Brodmann, 1909). Having histologically differentiated areas 17, 18, and 19, Brodmann proposed that each has a distinct visual function. This idea gained momentum after the discoveries made by Hubel and Wiesel (1962, 1965, 1970) and subsequently by Semir Zeki (1973, 1974, 1980) when they examined the response characteristics of single neurons in various parts of visual cortex. On the basis of this work they suggested that area V2 (Brodmann's area 18) is devoted to the analysis of stereoscopic depth perception, whereas area V4 is devoted to the analysis of color and the middle temporal area (MT) to the analysis of motion. This formulation has often been referred to as the "one area one function" hypothesis.

During the past 25 years, as a result of systematic exploration of posterior cortex, many additional visual areas have been identified (Felleman and Van Essen, 1991). Anatomical, physiological, and lesion studies culminated in a hypothesis according to which visual information is processed along two major streams that emanate from the striate cortex (Ungerleider and Mishkin, 1982). It was proposed that the first stream, which receives its input from the midget system that originates in the retina, makes its way to the striate cortex through the parvocellular portions of the lateral geniculate nucleus and courses toward the temporal lobe via area V4. This first stream is involved in the analysis of color and form. The second stream, which is driven selectively by the parasol system of the retina and makes its way to cortex through the magnocellular portions of the lateral geniculate nucleus, courses toward the parietal lobe via area MT. This second stream is involved in the analysis of space, motion, and depth (Livingstone and Hubel, 1987, 1988; Newsome and Wurtz, 1988).

Several current lines of work raise questions about these hypotheses. More than 30 visual areas have been identified which make more than 300 interconnections. Many of these visual cortical areas are not homogeneous; instead, they appear to be modular; within each module single cells have different, if somewhat overlapping receptive-field properties (Livingstone and Hubel, 1988;

Felleman and Van Essen, 1991). Especially notable in this respect is area V2, which at one time had been thought to be a homogeneous area involved in the processing of stereopsis (Hubel and Wiesel, 1970). Subsequently it was shown that (1) cells processing stereopsis by virtue of retinal disparity are already present in the striate cortex (see chapter by Poggio, this volume) and (2) area V2 is modular and that the cells within the various modules have different receptive field organization and receive selective input from either the midget or the parasol systems (Poggio and Poggio, 1984; Livingstone and Hubel, 1988).

The hypothesis that area MT receives its input predominantly from the parasol system and area V4 from the midget system of the retina has been put to direct test recently. While recording the responses of single cells in these two areas Maunsell and his collaborators have reversibly inactivated either the parvocellular or magnocellular portions of the lateral geniculate nucleus, thereby temporarily blocking either the parasol or midget systems (Ferrera et al., 1992; Maunsell et al., 1990). When they did this they found that area MT does indeed receive its main input from the parasol system. However, area V4 was found to get inputs equally from both systems. In an earlier study it was shown, using similar methods, that already in the striate cortex some neurons receive convergent input from these two systems (Malpeli et al., 1981).

Single-cell recordings also raise questions about the hypothesis that there is neat specialization of function in the extrastriate cortex. While there seems to be rather good agreement to the effect that area MT and the areas to which it projects contain cells that are especially sensitive to moving stimuli, recordings in area V4 do not uniformly support the contention that this is a color area. Cells sensitive to form and orientation are plentiful in area V4 and direction specific cells are not uncommon (Desimone et al., 1985; Schein and Desimone, 1990). Recordings in trained, alert monkeys, furthermore, have shown that the responses of single cells in area V4 are modulated by such factors as stimulus relevance and attention (Moran and Desimone, 1985; Haenny and Schiller, 1988; Haenny et al., 1988). The chapter by Gallant, Van Essen, and Nothdurft in this volume provides more detail on the response characteristics of V4 neurons to visual stimuli.

In an attempt to gain a better understanding of the roles of various extrastriate cortical areas in visual information processing, a number of laboratories have recently undertaken to study the effects of selective lesions on the visual capacities in the rhesus monkey (Dean, 1979; Heywood and Cowey, 1987; Schiller, 1993). In the work

we have been carrying out we made restricted lesions in areas V4 and MT. The lesions affected only portions of the visual field representation in each area. Procedures were therefore devised that allowed us to confine visual stimuli to selected portions of the visual field. The animals were trained to fixate and to make saccadic eye movements to selected targets. Eye-movement recordings assured us of doing this successfully. Such procedures have one very important advantage: data can be collected concurrently in intact and in lesioned portions of the visual field representation. The resultant comparisons therefore have high reliability. Both percent correct and saccadic reaction time data were obtained. The results and conclusions are based on 9 V4 and 4 MT lesions. In two animals combined V4 and MT lesions were made. For detailed account of the procedures and the histology see Schiller (1993).

During the experimental sessions monkeys were seated in a primate chair facing a color monitor; to assure accurate eye-movement recordings, their heads were secured. Two basic testing paradigms were used: detection and discrimination. In the detection paradigm, after the fixation of a small central fixation spot, a single target stimulus was presented randomly in one of several preselected visual-field locations. The animal's task was to make a single saccadic eye movement to the target within a time period set by the experimenter. In the discrimination paradigm several stimuli appeared following the presentation and foveation of the fixation spot. Most commonly eight stimuli were used, seven of which were identical and were called the comparison stimuli. The eighth stimulus, the target, was different from the comparison stimuli on any one of several dimensions. The task for the animal was to make a saccadic eye movement to the target stimulus. The discrimination task used is similar to the so-called oddity task employed in classic behavioral experiments. Figure 16.1 shows examples of the stimulus configurations used.

Since considerable uncertainty exists as to the role of the various extrastriate visual areas in vision, our strategy was to test animals on a broad range of visual capacities that included assessment of luminance and color-contrast sensitivity, color discrimination, shape, pattern, and texture perception, stereopsis, motion, and flicker perception. Here I will concentrate on those aspects of vision with which Bela Julesz has been extensively concerned in his research: stereopsis, form, color, motion, attention, and perceptual learning.

The perception of color: To study color vision we used the discrimination task extensively. The comparison stim-

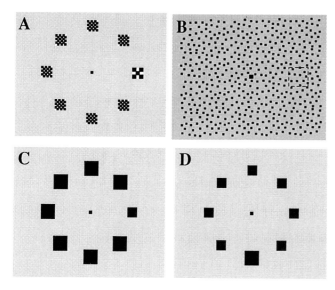

Figure 16.1
Examples of the kinds of stimuli used in assessing various visual capacities. (*A*) A test for form perception using checkerboard stimuli. The target has a different spatial frequency than the comparison stimuli. (*B*) A test for motion perception. Following the appearance of the dot array within a small area, as marked by the rectangle, the dots begin to move; this is the target region to which the animal has to make a saccadic eye movement to be rewarded. (*C, D*) The oddity task using target and comparison stimuli that differ in size. In (*C*) the target is smaller than the comparison stimuli and in (*D*) the target is larger.

uli were identical in shape, color, and luminance. The target stimulus, to which the animal had to make a saccadic eye movement to be rewarded, was of a different color. The difference between the target and comparison stimuli was varied systematically to generate psychometric functions by varying either color saturation or color angle (Derrington et al., 1984). The stimuli were generally set to be isoluminant or were varied in luminance from trial to trial. The location of the target and comparison stimuli was randomized by trial.

The perception of form: Several tests were devised to study shape, pattern, size, and texture perception. For the study of pattern high-contrast checkerboards were used with the discrimination paradigm in which the target had a different spatial-frequency checkerboard than the comparison stimuli. Figure 16.1A shows an example of checkerboard stimuli used in the discrimination task.

The perception of stereoscopic depth: Stereopsis was tested using three different methods: (1) Static random-dot stereograms: two stereograms appeared on the color monitor that were viewed by the animal through a stereoscope. In the case of detection, following fixation, the stereograms appeared with a small square area having the dots horizontally displaced in one of the stereograms; conse-

quently this area appeared at a different depth from the background. In the case of discrimination four to eight stimuli appeared, one of which had a greater disparity from that of the others. The spatial frequency, contrast, color, and degree of disparity (to create different perceptions of depth) could be systematically varied. (2) Low spatial-frequency stereopsis: through the same stereoscope the animal viewed eight disks with Gaussian luminance profiles that were equidistant from each other and from the fixation spot. Disparity was introduced by displacing corresponding disks relative to each other. (3) Dynamic stereo: 32 random-dot stereograms were created and were stored in the memory of the image-processing system. During stimulus presentation the frame buffer window was scrolled over the 32 memory locations resulting in animated random motion of the individual dots. Monocular viewing provided no information about the location of the square that appeared in depth under binocular viewing. Under monocular viewing conditions, in fact, the animals were unable to perform at all on these stereo tasks.

The perception of motion: Both the detection and the discrimination paradigms were used. Following fixation a random-dot array appeared on the monitor screen. In the case of detection, in one small area the dots began to move coherently and the task was to make a saccadic eye movement to this location. The size, contrast, numerosity of the dots, and their motion velocity could be systematically varied. The luminance of the stationary and moving dots was the same. In the case of discrimination, either a different rate of movement or a different direction of movement was introduced for one of the four to eight stimuli presented. This was the target stimulus to which the animal had to make a saccadic eye movement in order to receive a reward. Figure 16.1B provides an example of the stimulus display used for the study of motion.

The selection of "greater" and "lesser" stimuli in the oddity task: In the discrimination task the target and comparison stimuli can be presented in two ways. If the target and comparison stimuli form two sets called A and B, the target can be either A or B, with the comparisons being the other. In the case of size discrimination, for example, the target can be either larger or smaller than the comparison stimuli. Figure 16.1C and D are examples of this task. In these experiments, during any given session, the target and comparison stimuli were purposefully not randomly interchanged as is typically done in the classic oddity task. Thus when monkeys were tested for brightness discrimination, for example, for one set of trials the target was always the bright stimulus in the array while the

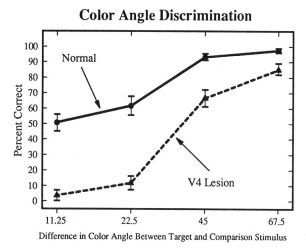

Color Angle Discrimination

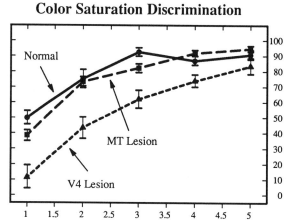

Color Saturation Discrimination

Figure 16.2

The effects of V4 and MT lesions on the perception of color. *Color-angle discrimination*: Target and comparison stimuli have the same color contrast (6%) around the color circle but have different color angle values for the comparison stimuli as shown on the abscissa. The color angle of the target was constant at 0° (CIE: $x = 0.355$, $y = 0.300$). The color angles of the comparison stimuli were 11.25° (CIE: $x = 0.342$,

$y = 0.282$), 22.5° (CIE: $x = 0.330$, $y = 0.266$), 45° (CIE: $x = 0.306$, $y = 0.245$), and 67.5° (CIE: $x = 0.284$, $y = 0.236$). Percent correct data are shown for one animal. *Color-saturation discrimination*: The same 6% color contrast target stimulus is used. The color saturation of the comparison stimuli varies from 0.5 to 5% at the 0 color axis. The data shown are from another animal.

brightness of the comparison stimuli was collectively varied. After obtaining such data, in some later session, the procedure could be reversed so that now the target was the dim stimulus and the comparison stimuli were all brighter, with the brightness difference between the target and comparison stimuli varied randomly by trial. This approach led to one of our major findings showing that the selection of "lesser" stimuli was greatly impaired by V4 but not by MT lesions. The following greater and lesser stimulus arrangements were studied using the discrimination paradigm: greater and lesser contrast, larger and smaller stimulus size, larger and smaller stereoscopic stimulus disparity, and faster and slower stimulus motion. Here only data pertaining to size differences will be shown.

The procedures and the stimuli used for assessing visual functions have been described in greater detail in previous publications (Schiller, 1993; Schiller at al., 1990).

Visual learning: Visual learning was assessed simply by plotting percent correct and reaction time performance over a period of days during the learning of a new task. Performance was plotted separately for conditions under which the target stimulus appeared in the intact portions of the visual field and for conditions under which the target appeared in portions of the visual field affected by the lesions.

The results of this work are summarized under seven headings.

The Perception of Color

Color-contrast sensitivity and the ability to make various discriminations based on only wavelength information were examined in considerable detail in several animals. Figure 16.2 shows data obtained from two monkeys using the oddity task. Eight stimuli were presented equidistant from the fixation spot, one of which varied either in color angle (left graph) or in color saturation (right graph). The results show a distinct but rather mild deficit in color discrimination following V4 lesions. On the color saturation task the normal 50% difference threshold is 1%; after V4 lesions it is about 3%. This is a rather mild deficit suggesting that other cortical areas can make an important contribution toward wavelength discrimination. The data also show that there was no discernible deficit following MT lesions. The small magnitude of the deficits obtained with V4 lesions stands out when compared with the deficits that are incurred following lesions of the parvocellular lateral geniculate nucleus after which the performance of monkeys on any color discrimination task is devastated (Schiller et al., 1990).

The Perception of Form

Several different tests were administered to assess deficits in form vision. These included the discrimination of various shapes and sizes of stimuli, textures, and checkerboard patterns. The magnitude of the deficits with V4 lesions varied to some degree among the tasks as well as among the animals. The results using texture arrays consisting of oriented line segments in which monkeys had to detect a small area of differently oriented lines showed only minor deficits. The discrimination of various geometric shapes yielded mild deficits provided the overall size of the target and comparison stimuli was similar (see "The Selection of 'Greater' and 'Lesser' Stimuli" below). The discrimination of checkerboard patterns of different spatial frequencies provided mild to moderate deficits. One of the more pronounced deficits obtained in one of our animals is shown in figure 16.3. This animal had a V4 lesion in one hemisphere and MT lesion in the other. The lesions were made serially. The deficit is quite pronounced at the site where the V4 visual field representation was lesioned. This can be seen both in the percent correct and response latency data. At the MT lesion site the deficit is not significant in percent correct performance, but there is a significant latency increase on the task. It appears, therefore, that both areas make some sort of contribution to pattern discrimination, but that V4 plays a more significant role. Other studies have also shown that area V4 contributes to form perception. Since the deficits on the various form perception tasks range from mild to moderate, it is likely that other extrastriate areas are also involved in the processing of form information. The results obtained with the V4 lesions stand in strong contrast with the deficits we had obtained in an earlier study following lesions of the parvocellular lateral

geniculate nucleus (Schiller et al., 1990) after which form discrimination of high spatial-frequency stimuli is virtually eliminated.

The Perception of Stereoscopic Depth

As described earlier, monkeys were tested on three kinds of stereoscopic displays: static random-dot stereograms, dynamic random-dot stereograms, and static Gaussian stimuli, using both detection and discrimination paradigms in which the degree of disparity was systematically varied. Neither V4 nor MT lesions produced any deficits in percent correct performance on these tasks. Examples of this appear in figure 16.4. The monkeys did, however, show significant increases in saccadic response latencies. Increased reaction times, as already noted, were obtained on many of the tasks studied. In earlier work we have shown that, following parvocellular but not magnocellular lesions, monkeys show a dramatic loss in stereoscopic depth perception, especially with small disparity differences and high spatial frequency displays (Schiller et al., 1990).

The Perception of Motion

Figure 16.5 shows performance on two kinds of motion perception tasks. In the first, on the left, a discrimination task was used in which the velocity of the target was kept constant and the velocity of the comparison stimuli was

Pattern Discrimination

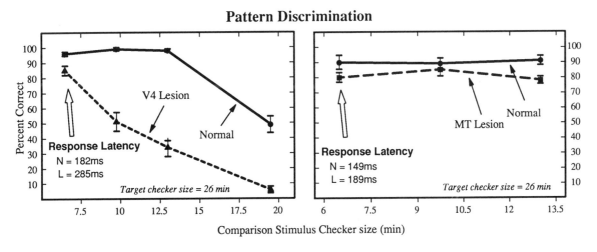

Figure 16.3
The effects of V4 and MT lesions on pattern discrimination. Data are shown from two animals. High contrast (84%) checkerboard patterns were used. The size of the comparison stimuli was varied as indicated on the abscissa. Latency data are shown for the easiest discrimination point in each of the panels.

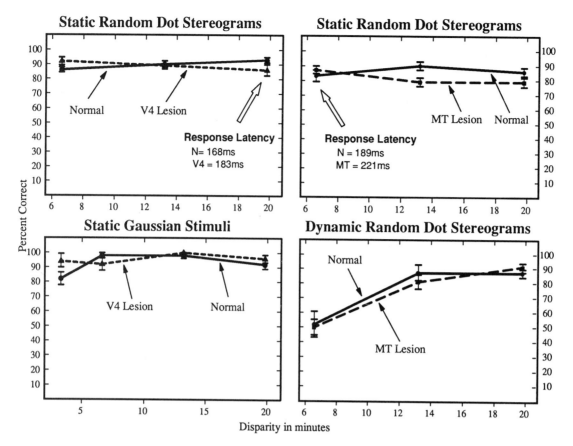

Figure 16.4

The effects of V4 and MT lesions on stereoscopic depth perception. Data are shown from four monkeys using three kinds of tasks: *static random-dot stereograms, dynamic random-dot stereograms, and static Gaussian stimuli.* Summary latency data are shown for two sets of conditions with static random-dot stereograms obtained at normal, V4, and MT lesion sites. In all cases disparity, as shown on the abscissa, was varied randomly by trial.

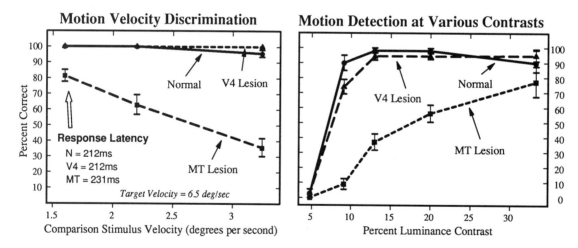

Figure 16.5

The effects of V4 and MT lesions on motion perception. *Motion velocity discrimination*: Target velocity was constant at 6.5° sec. The velocity of the comparison stimuli was varied as shown on the abscissa. Latency data are shown for the easiest discrimination point.

Motion detection at various stimulus contrasts: The target was a small array of dots moving within a large array of stationary dots. Percent correct data are shown.

varied. In the second task, on the right, a detection task was used in which velocity of the moving dots was kept constant and the contrast of the display was varied. Both tasks show a deficit after MT but not after V4 lesions. The deficits seem moderate suggesting that other cortical areas besides area MT can contribute to the perception of motion.

The Selection of "Greater" and "Lesser" Stimuli in the Oddity Task

Using the oddity task, as described earlier, we tested animals on a variety of tasks in which the target stimulus was either "greater" or "lesser" than the comparison stimuli. The tasks included varying the relative luminance of the target and comparison stimuli, their rate of motion and

their relative size. Figure 16.6 shows normal, V4, and MT lesion data for conditions when the target was either larger (left side) or smaller (right side) by various amounts than the comparison stimuli. The MT lesions produced little or no deficit on these tasks. On the other hand, performance for the task where the target was smaller than the comparison stimuli was devastated after the V4 lesion. These dramatic findings suggest that area V4 plays a significant role in a hitherto not noted visual function: to select physically less prominent stimuli from the visual scene, stimuli that presumably elicit less neural activity in early portions of the visual system than do other stimuli in the visual scene. Recent work by Braun (1992) has shown that attentional manipulation in human subjects can yield an effect similar to those found in monkeys with V4 lesions when stimulus prominence is varied in an oddity task.

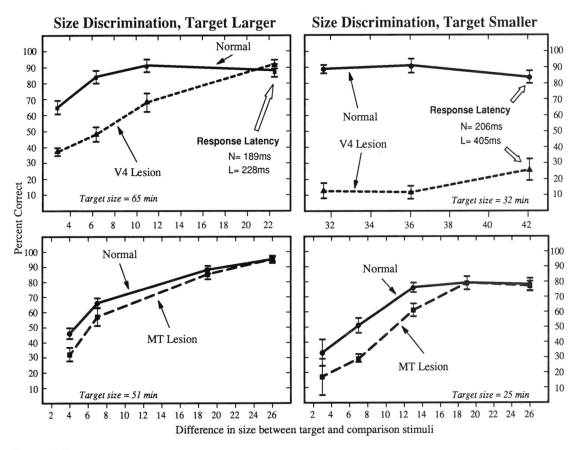

Figure 16.6
The effects of V4 and MT lesions on the discrimination of size with targets that were either larger (*left panels*) or smaller (*right panels*) than the comparison stimuli whose sizes were varied as indicated on the abscissa. The abscissa shows the difference in the diameter of the

targets and the comparison stimuli in minutes of visual angle. Target size diameter is indicated separately in each panel in minutes of visual angle. In addition to the percent correct data, summary latency results are shown in the upper two panels.

The Effects of Paired V4 and MT Lesions

In two animals the visual capacities already described were examined after paired lesions of V4 and MT. Surprisingly, the deficits were for the most part not greater than the sum of the deficits incurred with individual lesions. Figure 16.7 shows latency and percent correct data collected for stereopsis. Although there is a notable increase in saccadic latencies, as already obtained with individual lesions, there was very little deficit on percent correct performance. These findings suggest first that stereopsis can be quite efficiently processed by areas other than V4 and MT and second that there must be more than just two major streams reaching higher cortical centers, with one coursing through V4 and the other through MT.

The Learning of New Tasks after the Lesions

Prior to the making of lesions each animal was trained for a long time and was exposed to many of the tasks we studied. Some tasks, however, were introduced only after the lesions. Doing so uncovered another significant effect. Performance on new tasks was much worse at V4 lesion sites and the rate of learning was much slower than at normal sites. Furthermore, once a task was learned at a

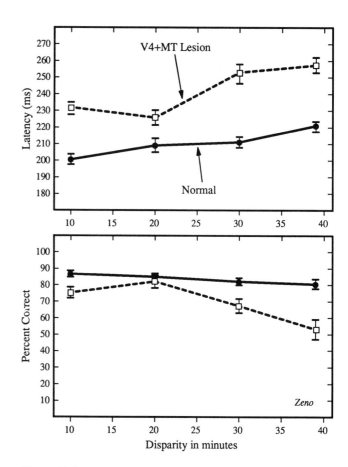

Figure 16.7
The effect of paired V4 and MT lesion on stereopsis using static random-dot stereograms.

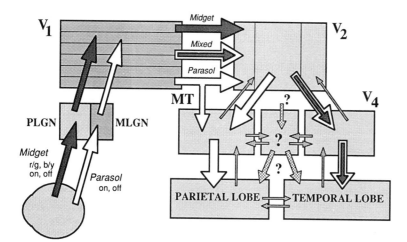

Figure 16.8
Diagram of the major connections derived from the work described. Originating in the retina are the midget and parasol systems that project to the parvocellular (PLGN) and magnocellular (MLGN) portions of the lateral geniculate nucleus. The midget system comprises red/green (r/g) and blue/yellow (b/y) ON and OFF cells. The parasol system has ON and OFF cells. In the striate cortex (V1) some cells are driven selectively by the midget and parasol systems whereas others receive a convergent input from both of these systems. The input to area MT, either directly from the striate cortex or from area V2, is dominated by the parasol system as is the output from MT to the parietal lobe. Area V4 and the temporal lobe on the other hand receive a mixed input from these two systems. In addition to these two major pathways other regions with inputs and outputs not yet characterized (indicated by question marks) must contribute to perception since paired lesions of areas MT and V4 leave some functions intact (stereopsis) and affect others only to a moderate degree. All areas shown are extensively interconnected.

particular location in the visual field it showed very poor transfer to new locations within the lesioned area. Transfer was typically quite rapid at intact sites. These observations, reported in more detail elsewhere (Schiller, 1993), suggest that area V4 and the areas with which it connects make an important contribution to visual learning and to the generalization of the learned task to other locations in the visual field.

The conclusions we derive from these lesion studies are the following:

1. Area V4 is part of neural circuitry that makes an important contribution to the selection of crucial, physically less prominent stimuli in the environment, which in the early parts of the visual system elicit less neural activity than do other stimuli that appear in the visual scene.

2. Lesions of area V4 and MT produce both specific and general deficits; impairment on basic visual functions ranges from mild to moderate. While these findings do not negate the notion that some areas are specialized in the visual processing they perform, they also suggest redundancy and interactive processing in extrastriate cortex.

3. Since paired V4 and MT lesions also produce only relatively mild deficits on many visual functions and virtually none in stereopsis, there must be more than just two major streams that project from area V1 to higher cortical areas.

4. Area V4 may be part of neural circuitry involved in perceptual learning and the generalization of such learned material to other locations of the visual field.

The results of this work suggest that the extrastriate visual areas may have evolved for reasons other than separately analyzing various basic visual capacities such as color, form, motion, or depth. Instead, some of these areas may be involved in more complex aspects of perception, one of which involves the rapid and efficient identification and selection of visual stimuli based on a variety of criteria possibly dictated by feedback from higher cortical areas. The findings furthermore suggest that more than just two major cortical streams must be involved in visual information processing. The basic connections inferred from the recent anatomical, physiological, and lesion studies that have been discussed in this chapter are shown in figure 16.8.

References

Braun, J. (1992). Absence of visual attention mimics a lesion of V4. *Invest. Ophthalmol. Visual Sci. 33*, 1354.

Brodmann, K. (1909). *Vergleichende Lokalisationslehre der Grosshirnrinde.* Leipzig: Barth.

Dean, P. (1979). Visual cortex ablation and thresholds for successively presented stimuli in rhesus monkeys: II. Hue. *Exp. Brain Res. 35*, 69–83.

Derrington, A. M., Krauskopf, J., and Lennie, P. (1984). Chromatic mechanisms in lateral geniculate nucleus of macaque. *J. Physiol. (London) 357*, 241–265.

Desimone, R., and Schein, J. (1987). Visual properties of neurons in area V4 of the macaque: Sensitivity to stimulus form. *J. Neurophysiol. 57*, 835–868.

Desimone, R., Schein, S. J., Moran, J., and Ungerleider, L. G. (1985). Contour, color, and shape analysis beyond the striate cortex. *Vision Res. 25*, 441–452.

Felleman, D. J., and Van Essen, D. C. (1991). Distributed hierarchical processing in the primate cerebral cortex. *Cerebral Cortex 1*, 1–47.

Ferrera, V. P., Nealy, T. A., and Maunsell, J. H. R. (1992). Mixed parvocellular and magnocellular geniculate signals in visual area V4. *Nature (London) 358*, 756–758.

Haenny, P. E., and Schiller, P. H. (1988). State dependent activity in monkey visual cortex. I. Single cell activity in V1 and V4 on visual tasks. *Exp. Brain Res. 69*, 225–244.

Haenny, P. E., Maunsell, J. H. R., and Schiller, P. H. (1988). State dependent activity in monkey visual cortex. II. Retinal and extraretinal factors in V4. *Exp. Brain Res. 69*, 245–259.

Heywood, C. A., and Cowey, A. (1987). On the role of cortical area V4 in the discrimination of hue and pattern in macaque monkeys. *J. Neurosci. 7*, 2601–2617.

Hubel, D. H., and Wiesel, T. N. (1962) Receptive fields, binocular interaction and functional architecture in the cat's visual cortex. *J. Physiol. (London) 160*, 106–154.

Hubel, D. H., and Wiesel, T. N. (1965). Receptive fields and functional architecture in two nonstriate visual areas (18 and 19) of the cat. *J. Neurophysiol. 28*, 229–289.

Hubel, D. H., and Wiesel, T. N. (1970). Cells sensitive to binocular depth in area 18 of the macaque cortex. *Nature (London) 225*, 41–42.

Livingstone, M. S., and Hubel, D. H. (1987). Psychophysical evidence for separate channels for the perception of form, color, movement, and stereopsis. *J. Neurosci. 7*, 3416–3468.

Livingstone, M. S., and Hubel, D. H. (1988). Segregation of form, color, movement, and depth: Anatomy, physiology, and perception. *Science 240*, 740–749.

Malpeli, J., Schiller, P. H., and Colby, C. L. (1981). Response properties of single cells in monkey striate cortex during reversible inactivation of individual lateral geniculate laminae. *J. Neurophysiol. 46*, 1102–1119.

Maunsell, J. H. R., Nealey, T. A., and Depriest, D. D. (1990). Magnocellular and parvocellular contributions to responses in the middle temporal visual area (MT) of the macaque monkey. *J. Neurosci. 10*, 3323–3334.

Moran, J., and Desimone, R. (1985). Selective attention gates visual processing in the extrastriate cortex. *Science 229*, 782–784.

Newsome, W. T., and Wurtz, R. H. (1988). Probing visual cortical function with discrete chemical lesions. *Trends Neurosci. 11*, 394–400.

Poggio, G. F., and Poggio, T. (1984). The analysis of stereopsis. *Annu. Rev. Neurosci. 7*, 379–412.

Schein, S. J., and Desimone, R. (1990). Spectral properties of V4 neurons on the macaque. *J. Neurosci. 10*, 3369–3389.

Schiller, P. H. (1993). The effects of V4 and middle temporal (MT) area lesions on visual performance in the rhesus monkey. *Visual Neurosci. 10*, 717–746.

Schiller, P. H., Logothetis, N. K., and Charles, E. R. (1990). Role of color-opponent and broad-band channels in vision. *Visual Neurosci. 5*, 321–346.

Ungerleider, L. G., and Mishkin, M. (1982). Two cortical visual systems. In D. J. Ingle, M. A. Goodale, and R. J. W. Mansfield (Eds.), *Analysis of Visual Behavior* (pp. 549–586). Cambridge, Ma: MIT Press.

Zeki, S. M. (1973). Colour coding in rhesus monkey prestriate cortex. *Brain Res. 53*, 422–427.

Zeki, S. M. (1974). Functional organization of a visual area in the posterior bank of the superior temporal sulcus of the rhesus monkey. *J. Physiol. (London) 236*, 549–573.

Zeki, S. M. (1980). The representation of colours in the cerebral cortex. *Nature (London) 284*, 412–418.

Part IV

Attention

Eileen Kowler

When I talk about attention in my undergraduate perception classes, I start out with the ideas of William James. Not just his famous definition of attention: "Everyone knows what attention is. It is the taking possession by the mind, in clear and vivid form, of one out of what seem several simultaneously possible objects or trains of thought." Nor do I limit discussion to his colorful anecdote about the group of dogs raised in a sculpture garden, who never learn anything about art, but who become expert in organizing the smells at the bases of the statues. Experience—for dogs or for humans—is what we "agree to attend to."

James's writings on attention anticipated so closely, and described so clearly, the dilemmas that occupy contemporary researchers in attention that I will organize this introduction around the problems he raised. Consider, for example, the very broad question of precisely how attention affects human conscious experience. Undoubtedly, says James, attention enhances memory (see Reeves and Sperling, 1986, for a model of the attention-memory link). But the relationship between attention and perception is far less clear:

Most people would say that a sensation attended to becomes stronger than it otherwise would be. This point, is however, not quite plain, and has occasioned some discussion. From the strength of intensity of a sensation must be distinguished its clearness; and to increase this is, for some psychologists, the utmost that attention can do. When the facts are surveyed, however, it must be admitted that to some extent the relative intensities of two sensations may be changed when one of them is attended to and the other not. . . . Confident expectation of a certain intensity or quality of impression will often make us sensibly see or hear it in an object which really falls far short of it. In face of such facts it is rash to say that attention cannot make a sense-impression more intense.

Thus, as James' intellectual descendents might say today, attention may exert its influence by enhancing the activity in early levels of visual processing. Indeed, physiological evidence for enhancement of neural activity as early as the primary visual cortex (V1) is cited in the chapter (21) by Desimone et al. and is predicted as well by the model described by Tsotsos (chapter 20). There is also the work of Posner and his colleagues, whose studies of the effect of expectations on the reaction time for detection of targets implies possible low-level attentional contributions to perception (see Posner and Petersen, 1990, for a review).

However, not all agree that attention can influence early vision. For alternative views of the reaction time work, see, for example, Sperling and Dosher (1986), Shaw (1984), and Kinchla (1992). James anticipated such controversies:

But on the other hand, the intensification which may be brought about seems never to lead the judgment astray. As we rightly perceive and name the same color under various lights, the same sound at various distances; so we seem to make an analogous sort of allowance for the varying amounts of attention with which objects are viewed; and whatever changes of feeling the attention may bring we charge, as it were, to the attention's account, and still perceive and conceive the object as the same.

And then, James quotes Fechner:

A gray paper appears to us no lighter, the pendulum-beat of a clock no louder, no matter how much we increase the strain of our attention upon them. No one, by doing this, can make the gray paper look white, or the stroke of the pendulum sound like the blow of a strong hammer.

James's focus on what attention *cannot* do anticipates much of the modern thinking about the role of attention in perception. Bela Julesz's work on texture segmentation, for example, demonstrated the existence of visual processes that, if not completely immune to effects of attention, certainly do not depend much on attention in order to succeed. Julesz drew a distinction between "preattentive" processing, which allowed boundaries between different texture patterns to appear quickly and effortlessly, regardless of where in the visual field the boundary was located, and the slower, serial, attentionally driven search for boundaries, which would need to be invoked whenever preattentive, effortless segmentation failed. Anne Treisman took a similar tack, distinguishing between preattentive and attentive visual search. For a comprehensive review, see Julesz (1991), as well as part II, "Visual Texture," in this volume. See also He and Kowler (1992) for a comparison of attentional vs. saccadically mediated inspection of textures. Julesz collaborated with Dov Sagi on a number of studies that explored the issue of what and how attention contributes to visual processing (Sagi and Julesz, 1985a,b; 1986; also Kröse and Julesz, 1989).

The chapters in this section reflect various aspects of the attention–perception dilemma introduced by James

just over a century ago. Nakayama and He (chapter 17) provide convincing evidence that the appearance of attention in the processing stream should be delayed to a level beyond feature extraction—a level at which the visual system begins to construct representations of surfaces. Wolfe, Chun, and Friedman-Hill (chapter 18), on the other hand, who study segmentation and search, concentrate on feature-based approaches. Ahissar and Hochstein (chapter 19) also focus on features, and show that attention is a requirement of some intriguing phenomena in perceptual learning. Tsotsos (chapter 20) represents a point of view originating from computer science and AI. He summarizes various computational models of attention (including his own recent work) that attempt to show, in neurophysiologically plausible ways, how a selective mechanism might operate to avoid overload of higher order processing centers. Desimone, Chelazzi, Miller, and Duncan (chapter 21) review the way in which various neurons in IT adjust their firing, depending on both past history and the significance of the stimulus, and summarize new studies on neural and attentional dynamics during active visual search. Ramachandran (chapter 22) picks up the theme of the modulation of neural activity due to learning, and, departing somewhat from the section's focus on attention, describes some new and surprising demonstrations of cortical plasticity in patients with scotomas.

When one steps back from these chapters, it is not the diversity of points of view that stands out, but rather the surprising degree of overlap among the psychophysicists, electrophysiologists, and computer-modelers, despite the different tools and goals that each has brought to the work. While there is still disagreement about the level at which attention influences perception, there is now obvious consensus that we will not get very far in understanding perception itself without understanding this remarkable capacity to alter perceptual processing on the basis of the salience of items, the novelty of items, or even whimsical choice.

References

He, P., and Kowler, E. (1992). The role of saccades in the perception of texture patterns. *Vision Res. 32,* 2151–2163.

James, W. (1890). *Principles of Psychology.* New York: Dover.

Julesz, B. (1991). Early vision and focal attention. *Rev. Modern Phys. 63,* 735–772.

Kinchla, R. A. (1992). Attention. *Annu. Rev. Psychol. 43,* 711–742.

Kröse, B. J. A., and Julesz, B. (1989). The control and speed of shifts of attention. *Vision Res. 29,* 1607–1619.

Posner, M. I., and Petersen, S. E. (1990). The attention system of the human brain. *Annu. Rev. Neurosci. 13*, 25–42.

Reeves, A., and Sperling, G. (1986). Attention gating in short-term memory. *Psychol. Rev. 93*, 180–206.

Sagi, D., and Julesz, B. (1985a). Fast noninertial shifts of attention. *Spatial Vision 1*, 141–149.

Sagi, D., and Julesz, B. (1985b). "Where" and "What" in vision. *Science 228*, 1217–1219.

Sagi, D., and Julesz, B. (1986). Enhanced detection in the aperture of focal attention during simple discrimination tasks. *Nature (London) 321*, 693–695.

Shaw, M. L. (1984). Division of attention among spatial location: a fundamental difference between detection of letters and detection of luminance increments. In H. Bouma and D. G. Bouwhuis (Eds.), *Attention and Performance, 10*. Hillsdale, NJ: Erlbaum.

Sperling, G., and Dosher, B. (1986). Strategy and optimization in human information processing. In K. Boff, L. Kaufman, and J. Thomas (Eds.). *Handbook of Perception and Performance*. New York: Wiley.

17

Attention to Surfaces: Beyond a Cartesian Understanding of Focal Attention

Ken Nakayama and Zijiang J. He

In the early 1980s, the study of visual attention gained increased prominence thanks largely to the foundation laid earlier by Bela Julesz and followed by studies by Anne Treisman. Both took approaches generating more widespread interest than prior investigations in part because they attempted to link their work to emerging ideas about early visual coding.

In this chapter, we would like to outline the theoretical conclusions that were implicitly drawn from these and related studies. In particular, we wish to make explicit the underlying supposition that attention can be deployed in a "content-free" coordinate geometric framework, a hypothetical function that could be plausibly mediated by the activity in units that are analogous to cells in the early visual pathway with relatively uncomplicated receptive fields. Then, we shall discuss some recent work that we hope will cast doubt on this general conception and to open the door to different understanding of how attention might be deployed to surfaces and objects in the world.

Let us start with Anne Treisman's early work on visual search (Treisman and Gelade, 1980; Treisman, 1985). She made the strong assertion that all else being equal, visual search for items differing on just a single feature will proceed equally efficiently independent of the number of distractors. The assumption here is that there exist a number of parallel processes, composed of independent detecting entities that would function equally well no matter how many distractors were present in a search array. In contrast to this, she proposed that in a conjunctive search array, where the observer had to find an odd target defined by two attributes, there is in general no set of more complex detectors that can passively decode an arbitrary combination of features across the visual field. In this case, search must be item-by-item using the full operation of focal attention to examine whether such a conjunction is present or not.

Bela Julesz also assumed attention could be drawn to textons, elemental primitives of vision (Julesz, 1975, 1981, 1986). Textons were more complex than Treisman's features in that there could be lateral interactions between them. In particular, the attention-directing system was sensitive to texton gradients, providing an opportunity for a bottom-up early selection mechanism to determine the deployment of focal attention.

Nakayama and Silverman's (1986) visual search study was motivated by the desire to critically examine Treisman's assertion that conjunctive search required an item-by-item serial search. In particular, and following Bela Julesz's lead, we wanted to use stimuli more likely to be understood in terms of visual cortical mechanisms. As a start, we hypothesized that perhaps a conjunctive search where binocular disparity was one of the dimensions might prove to be an exception to the rule proposed by Treisman. So we examined whether the coupling of disparity with other dimensions (namely color and motion) would not be subject to the distractor number dependence common to all other conjunctive search tasks (figure 17.1A). Indeed, in our study we were able to demonstrate that conjunctions of stereoscopic disparity and color, as well as stereoscopic disparity and motion, were altogether different (Nakayama and Silverman, 1986). Instead of increasing reaction times for increasing number of distractors, flat search functions were observed (see figure 17.1B).

At first glance, the findings originally served to cast doubt on Treisman's notion, providing a counterexample in which search for conjunctions did not depend on distractor number. Yet, in thinking about the underlying neural mechanisms, the apparently contradictory results still seemed to fit into a broader synthetic view of how cortical receptive fields might be linked to the deployment of attention. Because binocular disparity has an early representation in cortical processing (Barlow et al., 1967) and because many cells sensitive to binocular disparity are also selective to stimulus dimensions such as motion and color (Maunsell and Van Essen, 1983; Burkhalter and Van Essen, 1986), it actually reinforced the view that attention could be drawn to isolated activity in certain classes of stimuli coded by binocular receptive fields. That binocular disparity was co-coded with other dimensions such as color and motion provided an exception to the notion that combinations of features could not be arbitrarily coded without visual attention. Binocular disparity, according to this view, is more like retinal location, both providing a fundamental way to tag visual information in terms of position and depth in the visual field. The addition of disparity thus allows for the possibility that attention can be drawn to particular depths in addition to particular features and locations in $X-Y$ space (figure 17.1C).

These general ideas can be incorporated into a fairly simple model of cortical facilitation to explain focal attention (see figure 17.2). In this model, closely related to a searchlight (Crick, 1984), or zoom lens model (Ericksen and James, 1986), one can conceive of increasing the responsiveness of a subset of cortical neurons, sharing the same general region of the visual field and also sharing the same binocular disparity and the same receptive field types. As such, one can conceive of attention as a simple facilitation of certain set of neurons, thus highlighting particular features at a particular XYZ position in the visual field. We call this a Cartesian view of attention because it is specified simply in terms of coordinates in a viewer-centered geometric feature space, all plausibly mediated by activities in fairly low-level receptive fields similar to those characterized in primate striate cortex.

Nakayama and Silverman's (1986) experiment seemed to fall well within this general conception insofar as one could easily see how various frontoparallel slabs of space might get potentiated because they shared a common binocular disparity (as in figure 17.1C).

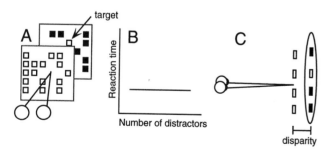

Figure 17.1
(A) Conjunctive search experiment where an observer must find the odd color in a particular disparity plane (redrawn from Nakayama and Silverman, 1986). (B) Schematic of the results, no increase in manual reaction time with increasing numbers of distractors. (C) Hypothetical mechanism that might account for the results, an ability of the visual system to selectively attend to a particular binocular disparity value.

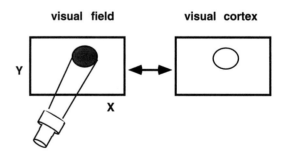

Figure 17.2
Theoretical deployment of attention to a portion of the visual field (searchlight model) that might be conceived as selective activation of a class of visual cortical cells that could have particular values of binocular disparity, thus enabling attention to be directed to particular frontoparallel slabs in a Cartesian coordinate representation (as shown in figure 17.1C).

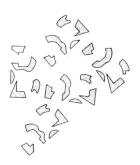
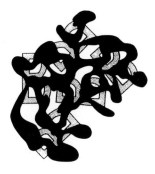

Figure 17.3
Bregman Bs. Fragments (denoted by stipled regions) are seen as separate entities on the left but group to form capital letter Bs on the right. (From Bregman, 1981.)

Associated with and supporting this general point of view are two key empirical propositions:

1. Attention can be directed to features in the visual field.
2. Attention can be deployed to loci in the visual field, determined by local retinal position (plus disparity).

In the next two sections, we would like to describe results that are at odds with these assertions and, in so doing, lay the groundwork for an alternate view of attentional deployment. First, however, we need to review some recent experimental work that indicates that visual perception is strongly determined not by what happens at a feature or receptive field level, but by how the visual system parses the scene into distinct surfaces. In particular, we review evidence that perceived depth can determine whether image fragments can be seen in isolation or join together to complete "amodally" behind occluders.

Well known is the figure from Bregman (1981), showing that when the fragmented Bs are adjacent to a visible occluder, they are readily visible as identifiable grouped fragments (figure 17.3). This is in stark contrast to the case where the occluder is invisible. We have hypothesized that the Bs amodally complete behind the occluder and thus form entities available for pattern recognition (Nakayama, Shimojo, and Silverman, 1989).

Previous work manipulating binocular disparity indicated that amodal completion requires that the image fragments be seen in back and that they must be contiguous with an occluding edge. Thus, the separate U-shaped black pieces in figure 17.4 become joined as a C when an occluder is perceived to be in front of the Us (Nakayama and Shimojo, 1990b). Yet, when the occluder is perceived to be in back via stereopsis, the C disappears and the observer sees two U-shaped disconnected fragments. A similar result can also be seen for face recognition (Nakayama et al., 1989).

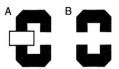

Figure 17.4
(A) Observers normally see pattern of two U-shaped black figures as part of an occluded letter C. However, if the "occluder" is placed behind the U-shaped figures using binocular stereopsis, the C breaks up into the two U-shaped figures (as in B). (From Nakayama et al., 1989.)

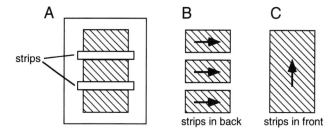

Figure 17.5
Barber pole stimulus. Diagonal bars moving in three separate barber poles appear to move with horizontal motion (shown in B). If, however, the horizontal strips are seen as in front of the diagonal moving stripes, then the whole pattern of moving stripes appears as a large vertical pattern (as in C) and vertical motion is seen. (From Shimojo et al., 1989.)

In addition to showing that image fragments can complete behind under a restricted yet well-defined set of conditions, we have also shown that this has dramatic consequences on other aspects of vision, including those that have been thought to be mediated by early mechanisms, namely, motion. For example, in a column of three separate barber pole stimuli (see Figure 17.5A) one would ordinarily see horizontal motion in each panel because the elongated axis of each barber pole is horizontal (Wallach, 1935). Yet, the horizontal motion changes to vertical motion if by manipulating binocular disparity the strips separating the three sections are seen as in front of the moving diagonal lines (Shimojo, Silverman, and Nakayama, 1989). Here the three separate patches can be seen as a single vertical barber pole (as in figure 17.5C) "completing" behind the strips and the motion now conforms to the perceived major axis, i.e., vertical.

These examples, taken together with others (see Shimojo and Nakayama, 1990), strongly indicate a surface level of visual representation that determines whether image patches are seen to extend beyond their physically present borders. The rules governing surface formation and completion are outlined in previous papers (Nakayama et al., 1989; Nakayama and Shimojo, 1990a,b,

1992). What is important to note, however, is that not only does surface formation determine what is seen to complete, surface formation can also have decisive effects in terms of visual performance. It can, for example, determine what direction of motion will be perceived.

Attention Drawn to Completed Surfaces Not Features

At this point, we wondered whether such completion phenomena might also be relevant to understanding visual search and texture segregation, topics usually thought to be closely associated with the directing and deploying of visual attention. Would it be possible that instead of features, the visual system was responsive to surfaces in performing visual search and texture segregation tasks?

To conduct such a study we first used visual stimuli that were easily discriminable and that supported visual search with no increase in reaction times with increasing distractor numbers (He and Nakayama, 1992). In this case, we examined visual search for seeing an L among reversed Ls or vice versa. Using a stereoscope we added a square adjacent to the Ls and reversed Ls, so that when the squares were in front, the Ls tended to amodally complete behind as larger less L-like surfaces (figure 17.6). This was contrasted to the case where the Ls were located in front so that they maintained their distinct L shape. The results of such an experiment were clear. Visual search for finding the odd L (reversed or not) became much more difficult if the L was behind (figure 17.7a). Furthermore, this effect could not be due to the disparity manipulation alone because we also conducted a control experiment where there was a small separation between the L shape and the occluder (see figure 17.6), thus preventing amodal surface completion (figure 17.7b). In this case, there was no difference in performance between the in front and back case.

Rapid texture segregation is often studied alongside of visual search, because there has been the underlying assumption that it too is mediated at a similar level, by operating on a feature representation. Here again, however, it is possible to ask more or less the same question posed in our studies of visual search. In this case we measured the ability of an observer to discern the orientation of a rectangular region made up of different texture elements, defined by Is and Ls (He and Nakayama, 1994). The Is could comprise the texture and the Ls the background or vice versa. Again we placed these texture ele-

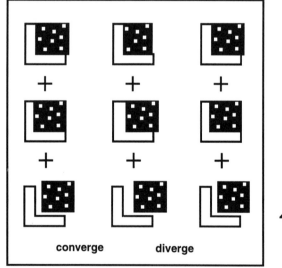
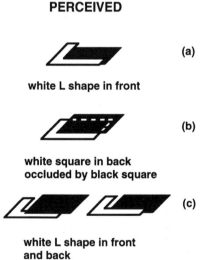

PERCEIVED

(a)
white L shape in front

(b)
white square in back occluded by black square

(c)
white L shape in front and back

converge   diverge

Figure 17.6
Stimulus elements used for visual search experiments. Three paneled stereograms (in box) designed for convergent or divergent fusion. For convergent fusion, left and center images should be used, ignoring the right image. For divergent fusion, center and right images should be used, ignoring the left image. Perceived shapes are illustrated at right of the frame where an L shape is seen in front for row (a), and seen in back for row (b). Note that in row (b), the L becomes extended to form a larger surface, "amodally" completing behind the square occluder. Row (c) illustrates stimuli used in the second experiment, which have the same disparity differences but with a 9.2 arc min separation between Ls and square. In both experiments, target and distractors were distributed randomly within a rectangular area (13.4 deg × 9.6 deg). The size of the L is 1 deg × 1 deg with the horizontal limb subtending 11.5 min. (From He and Nakayama, 1992.)

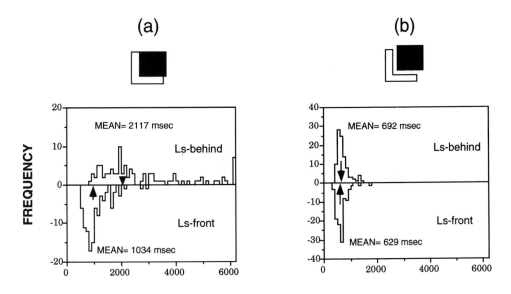

REACTION TIME (msec)

Figure 17.7
Reaction time histograms for the visual search of an L among reversed Ls (or vice versa), showing the role of relative binocular disparity between the local occluding square and the L. On the left are cases where the L is adjacent to the occluding square and where depth can determine amodal completion. As expected, reaction times are longer for the Ls in back vs. Ls in front case. Note, however, that this difference disappears when binocular disparity has no influence on amodal occlusion because there is a gap between the Ls and the square (as in the histograms on the right). (From He and Nakayama, 1992.)

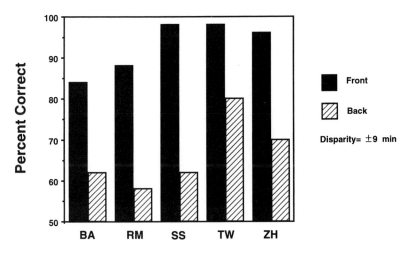

Figure 17.8
Results of texture discrimination experiment. Observer's task is to identify the orientation of a differently textured region, comprised of Is vs. Ls (or the reverse). To vary the element's surface representation, we placed these texture elements adjacent to black squares. The texture elements could either be in front of (leading to no surface completion) or in back of (leading to completion). Solid and hatched bars show performance for the front and back case, respectively. Note that for each of the five observers, texture segregation is far superior when the texture elements are in front of their adjacent occluders, i.e., for the case where no surface completion occurs (From He and Nakayama, 1994.)

ments adjacent to local occluders and noted the effect of their relative stereoscopic depth. In this case, it was also clear that performance in this texture segregation task was clearly influenced by whether the texture elements were in front or behind of neighboring "occluders." When they were in front, texture segregation was quite reliable at very short durations. This should be compared (figure 17.8) to the case where the Is and Ls were in the back where performance was much worse.

In both our visual search and visual texture segregation experiments, perceptual completion rendered the target and the background less distinctive. If we think of visual search and visual texture segregation occurring only at an early feature level, the experimental results would have no coherent explanation. Only if we assume that the inputs to visual search and visual texture segregation are at a surface representation level, do the results become comprehensible. Thus we attach special significance to the fact that visual search is impaired by changing a surface representation yet leaving a presumed feature level of representation intact. It indicates that a feature level of representation cannot be directly accessed by visual search or texture segregation mechanisms, that in order to perform these operations, the system must operate at a level beyond that of feature registration.

Attention Can Spread to Well-Formed Surfaces in Space, Not to Elements Having a Common Disparity

Recall that in the Nakayama and Silverman (1986) experiment the observer was able to find the odd target defined by both binocular disparity and one other stimulus dimension, color or motion. Our original interpretation to explain the ease of such a search was that one can attend to a given surface plane defined by a common binocular disparity, an explanation in keeping with the Cartesian framework mentioned above. Yet one must also be open to an alternative explanation. Perhaps the task is easy because the observer can simply focus on any surface, not one just defined by a single disparity.

To examine this issue, we constructed a set of stereograms (He and Nakayama, 1993) where the local 3D

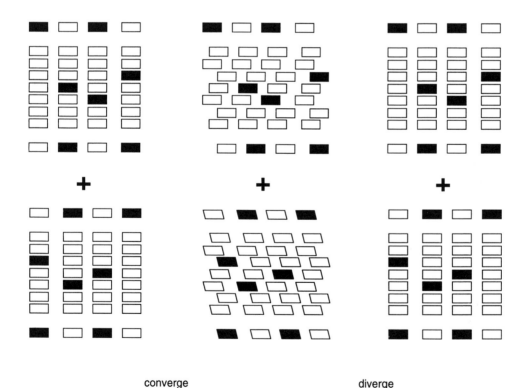

converge   diverge

Figure 17.9
Stereograms used to search for an odd target in a planar array of elements. Each stereogram consists of a 3D matrix, four elements wide, three elements high, and three elements deep. As such, we can conceive of this matrix as a set of arbitrary slices, for example, a set of three frontoparallel arrays (with 4 × 3 elements) or a set of three horizontal arrays (also with 4 × 3 elements). In each case, the observer's task is to find the odd colored target in the middle fronto-parallel array or the middle horizontal array. Note that the search is relatively effortless when individual elements are coplanar with the array to be searched.

spatial orientation of individual elements could vary in relation to the global plane in which the observer was instructed to search for an odd color (figure 17.9). These stereograms depict a three-dimensional matrix of colored stimuli, four elements wide, three elements deep, and three elements high. For our purposes, we asked the observer to conceptualize the matrix as either three vertical frontoparallel (4 × 3 element) arrays or three horizontal (4 × 3 element) arrays. In the first task, the observer is to find an odd color in the middle frontoparallel array where the individual tokens could either lie in this plane (upper stereogram) or where they instead were arranged to lie in a "horizontal" plane receding back from the observer (lower stereogram). Note in the upper case the observer's task was very similar to that confronting observers in Nakayama and Silverman's (1986) original experiment. Furthermore, if disparity was decisive, then the orientation of the individual tokens should have little effect on the search process, that is, the search effort to find the odd colored target in the lower stereogram should be approximately the same. It should be clear that this is not the case. This mid-frontoparallel plane in the lower stereogram is very hard to discern because the individual elements are not in this plane and visual search is much more effortful. This result by itself indicates that there is likely to be something much more powerful than a common disparity because despite the equivalency of disparity in both cases, there was a large difference in search effort.

In a second demonstration, we use exactly the same stimulus arrangement, except that now the observer is asked to search for the odd color in the middle of the three horizontal arrays. Now the results are reversed. The observer finds it very hard to find the odd target in the upper stereogram of figure 17.9 where the local elements are not coplanar with the horizontal array to be searched. The horizontal array is difficult to discern without effort. It becomes very easy to search for the odd colored target in the lower stereogram, however, where the local orientation of the individual elements is coplanar with the horizontal arrays. This occurs despite the fact that within this plane many different binocular disparities are represented. This result by itself indicates that the visual system is perfectly adept at attending to groups of stimuli having a very wide range of binocular disparities. What is important is that the elements form a well-defined perceptual surface via local coplanarity. That there are large differences in binocular disparity is irrelevant. These results taken together indicate that any arbitrary well-formed plane not confined to a single disparity can be attended to and searched with ease.

Conclusion

In examining the two assertions critical for a Cartesian understanding of attentional deployment, we have presented two sets of experiments. First, we have shown that visual attention is not directed to features but to surface shape. Employing visual search and texture segregation paradigms, we show that simply changing the surface representation of individual elements while leaving their featural representation intact leads to dramatic deficits in performance. This indicates that the visual system is not responding to differences that could be plausibly coded by the known properties of early receptive fields. In our second set of demonstrations, we show that attention is not, as previously thought, directed most easily to specific amounts of binocular disparity but to well-formed surfaces. This can occur independently of the orientation of the surface and despite the fact that elements within a surface may span many different binocular disparities.

Taken together, these results also indicate that one cannot sustain the view that visual attention is directed via the modulation of known cortical receptive fields such as those that have been found in striate cortex. What seems to be needed is the neural machinery that is involved in the representation of surfaces. This is consistent at least so far with the fact that there appears to be little in the way of attentional modulation in V1 (Moran and Desimone, 1985). One can speculate that visual attention will be evident only at a neurophysiological level where surface or object representation is made explicit.

Acknowledgment

This research has been supported from a grant from the Life Sciences Directorate, AFOSR.

References

Barlow, H. B., Blakemore, C., and Pettigrew, J. D. (1967). The neural mechanism of binocular depth discrimination. *J. Physiol. (London) 193*, 327–342.

Bregman, A. L. (1981). Asking the "what for" question in auditory perception. In *M. Kubovy and J. R. Pomerantz (Eds.), Perceptual Organization* (pp. 99–118). Hillsdale, NJ: Lawrence Erlbaum.

Burkhalter, A., and Van Essen, D. (1986). Processing of color, form and disparity information in visual area VP and V2 of the ventral extrastriate cortex in the macaque monkey. *J. Neurosci. 6*, 2327.

Crick, F. (1984). The function of the thalamic reticular complex: The searchlight hypothesis. *Proc. Natl. Acad. Sci. U.S.A. 81*, 4586–4590.

Eriksen, C. W., and St. James, J. D. (1986). Visual attention within and around the field of focal attention: A zoom lense model. *Percept. Psychophys. 40*, 225–240.

He, Z. J., and Nakayama, K. (1992). Surfaces vs. features in visual search. *Nature (London) 359*, 231–233.

He, Z. J., and Nakayama, K. (1994). Perceiving textures: Beyond filtering. *Vision Res. 34*, 151–162.

He, Z. J., and Nakayama, K. (1993). Common surface rather than common depth determines attention in 3-D search. *Neurosci. Abstr.*

Julesz, B. (1975). Experiments in the visual perception of texture. *Sci. Am. 232*, 34–43.

Julesz, B. (1981). Textons, the elements of texture perception and their interactions. *Nature (London) 290*, 91–97.

Julesz, B. (1986). Texton gradients: The texton theory revisited. *Biol. Cybern. 54*, 245–251.

Maunsell, J. H. R., and Van Essen, D. C. (1983). Functional properties of neurons in middle temporal visual area of the macaque monkey. II. Binocular interactions and sensitivity to binocular disparity. *J. Neurophysiol. 49*, 1148–1166.

Moran, J., and Desimone, R. (1985). Selective attention gates visual processing in the extrastriate cortex. *Science 229*, 782–784.

Nakayama, K., and Shimojo, S. (1990a). DaVinci stereopsis: Depth and subjective occluding contours from unpaired image points. *Vision Res. 30*, 1811–1830.

Nakayama, K., and Shimojo, S. (1990b). Towards a neural understanding of visual surface representation. In T. Sejnowski, E. R. Kandel, C. F. Stevens, and J. D. Watson (Eds.), *The Brain* (Vol. 55, pp. 911–924). Cold Spring Harbor Laboratory, NY: Cold Spring Harbor Symposium on Quantitative Biology.

Nakayama, K., and Shimojo, S. (1992). Experiencing and perceiving visual surfaces. *Science 257*, 1357–1363.

Nakayama, K., and Silverman, G. H. (1986). Serial and parallel processing of visual feature conjunctions. *Nature (London) 320*, 264–265.

Nakayama, K., Shimojo, S., and Silverman, G. H. (1989). Stereoscopic depth: Its relation to image segmentation, grouping and the recognition of occluded objects. *Perception 18*, 55–68.

Shimojo, S., and Nakayama, K. (1990). Amodal presence of partially occluded surfaces determines apparent motion. *Perception 19*, 285–299.

Shimojo, S., Silverman, G. H., and Nakayama, K. (1989). Occlusion and the solution to the aperture problem for motion. *Vision Res. 29*, 619–626.

Treisman, A. (1985). Preattentive processing. *Comput. Vision Graphics Image Process. 31*, 156–177.

Treisman, A. and Gelade, G. (1980). A feature integration theory of attention. *Cog. Psychol. 12*, 97–136.

Wallach, H. (1935). Ueber visuell wahrgenommene Bewegungrichtung. *Psychol. Forsch. 20*, 325–380.

18

Making Use of Texton Gradients: Visual Search and Perceptual Grouping Exploit the Same Parallel Processes in Different Ways

Jeremy M. Wolfe,
Marvin M. Chun, and
Stacia R. Friedman-Hill

When I was a high school senior, I had a summer job at Bell Laboratories biting a bite bar and looking for impossibly dim spots of light somewhere in the depths of John Krauskopf's optical bench. One can do that only for a limited number of hours per day and so I, a would-be English major, roamed the halls talking to everyone and was converted to a career in vision research. I met Bela Julesz in this way. At that time, in the early 1970s, one of the hot topics in Julesz's lab was texture perception. Specifically, Julesz had proposed that humans could not effortlessly perceive a border between regions that did not differ in their second-order statistics (Julesz, 1962; Julesz et al., 1973). Frankly, as an introduction to vision research, this was pretty confusing to an 18-year-old, but the pictures were compelling. Using two micropatterns that were clearly different from each other, textures could be created where borders of a region composed of one pattern were completely invisible when embedded in a region composed of the other pattern. (See Julesz et al., 1973 for a number of good illustrations.)

Like most good theories, the second-order conjecture was wrong. By the end of the decade, it was clear that there was a small set of basic features that would support texture segmentation and other forms of preattentive processing even if the second-order statistics remained unchanged across the figure. Julesz named these "atoms" of texture perception "textons" (Julesz, 1981; Julesz and Bergen, 1983). These were "elongated blobs ... with specific colors, angular orientations, widths, and lengths ... terminators of line segments ... crossings of line segments" (Julesz, 1984). Thus Julesz came to a conclusion that others were working toward at the same time: A set of basic features is processed in parallel across large portions of the visual field (see Treisman, 1986b for a review).

There are two aspects to this parallel processing of basic features. There is "bottom-up," stimulus-driven processing based on local differences in a specific feature, what Julesz called "texton gradients" (Julesz, 1986), and there is top-down, user-driven use of parallel processing to find elements having a specific color, size, orientation, etc. (e.g., Egeth, Virzi, and Garbart, 1984; Wolfe et al., 1992). It is the bottom-up texton gradients and not the top-down identity of the items that seems to make texture segmentation possible (Nothdurft, 1990; Wolfe, 1992a). The processing of these texton gradients is the subject of this chapter.

In this chapter, we consider the ability of isolated texton gradients to define forms. An example, based on the work of (Nothdurft, 1992), is shown in figure 18.1a. In these tasks, subjects were asked to indicate the orientation of a virtual triangle that was defined by three texton gradients. Nothdurft found that it did not matter if all of the vertices of the triangle were defined by the same orientation or if they were all different. Nor did it matter if there was a slow variation in the orientations of the background elements. What mattered was the salience of the local contrast, texton gradient created by each vertex. Three salient orientation texton gradients could produce a triangle no matter how the gradients were produced

**Find the triangle
defined by three orientation texton gradients.**

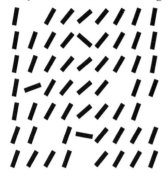

**Find the triangle
defined by three lines of the same orientation.**

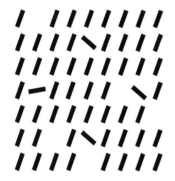

Figure 18.1
Nothdurft's paradigm for studying grouping of texton gradients. Subjects identify the orientation of a triangle created by three texton gradients. (*Top*) A triangle is easily found even though each vertex is a different orientation and background orientation is not homogeneous. (*Bottom*) A triangle created by three lines of one orientation is masked by the presence of a fourth item of a different but salient orientation.

(see Moraglia, 1989 for a related point). In a complementary finding, Nothdurft (1992) showed that the triangle created by three identically oriented lines could be masked by the addition of a fourth line of different orientation as long as that fourth line created a texton gradient (figure 18.1b). The four vertices created a virtual square and made it hard to determine the orientation of the triangle formed by the three identical vertices. The conclusion was that the ability of a texton gradient to support perception of a form was based only on the salience of the gradient and not on the identity of item producing the gradient. Ignoring variations in salience, all texton gradients were created equal.

Where are these virtual triangles produced? There are, at least, two possibilities. (1) The orientation texton gradients in figure 18.1 might produce bumps of activation in an orientation "feature map," a parallel process specific for orientation (e.g., Treisman, 1988; Treisman and Sato, 1990) and the perception of virtual triangle might be based on form extracting operations within that feature process. Alternatively, (2) texton gradients might produce bumps of activation in some general, feature-blind map where all gradients would, indeed, be treated as equal regardless of their featural origins. The perception of the triangle might be based on operations in this feature-blind representation. In the experiments described below, we provide data against hypothesis 2. Triangles with vertices defined by gradients in three different features are harder to see than triangles with vertices defined by variation within a single feature (experiment 1). This argues against a feature-blind locus for the generation of these virtual triangles. In experiments 1 and 2, we show that color behaves differently from orientation in tasks of this sort. Triangles defined by three colors are harder to see than triangles defined by a single color, while, as Nothdurft has shown, triangles defined by three orientations are no harder to see than triangles defined by a single orientation. Finally, in experiment 3, we find that triangles defined by conjunctions of color and orientation fail to "pop-out," providing further evidence that the emergence of form from texton gradients is accomplished in feature-specific maps.

General Methods

The basic design of all experiments was similar and is schematized in figure 18.2. On each trial, a test stimulus was presented for 50 msec followed by a blank ISI (interstimulus interval) of variable duration followed by a mask that remained visible until the subject responded. The test

THE PARADIGM

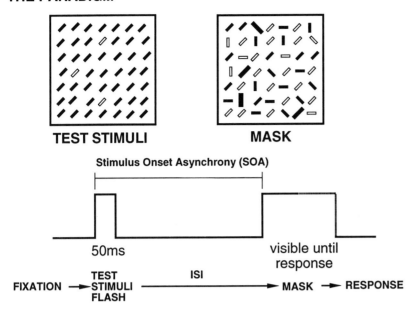

TEST STIMULI **MASK**

Stimulus Onset Asynchrony (SOA)

50ms   visible until response

FIXATION → TEST STIMULI FLASH ——— ISI ——→ MASK → RESPONSE

Figure 18.2
The basic paradigm for experiments reported in this chapter. A test stimulus is briefly presented. Following a variable interstimulus interval (ISI) a mask appears. The mask remains until the subject gives a response. The response is a 4-alternative, forced-choice specifying the orientation of the triangle (pointing left in the illustration).

stimulus contained a virtual triangle defined by distinctive stimuli marking its vertices. The vertices were chosen from a set of eight possible locations in a 7 × 7 array. Eight loci were used in order to minimize the utility of guessing strategies. One could use just four vertices but with triangles defined by the choice of three out of four vertices, detection of any one vertex increases the probability of successful guessing to 33%. Detection of two increases guessing success to 50%. Worse, a more sophisticated observer might note that the absence of a vertex at one location predicts triangle orientation with 100% accuracy. It is easy to show that a strategy of attending to just two of four possible locations yields 75% correct performance. These problems are much reduced if eight vertices are used. These eight vertex locations are shown in figure 18.3.

In some conditions, an additional vertex was added. Nothdurft (1992) found that a perception of a triangle defined by three vertices of the same orientation could be impaired by the addition of a fourth vertex, even if that vertex was of a different orientation. This bolstered the conclusion that texton gradients, rather than the specific orientations of the vertices, were important in the perception of the virtual triangles.

Masks were composed of randomly chosen elements from the display set. Set sizes of 37, 43, and 49 were used for displays and masks. In a 7 × 7 texture, 37- and 43-

Possible vertex locations

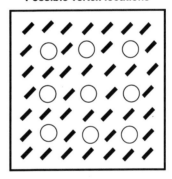

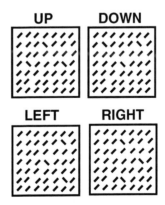

UP **DOWN**

LEFT **RIGHT**

Figure 18.3
Vertices were drawn from eight possible locations. Previous work has used four locations. Eight locations reduces the probability of successful guessing.

element arrays had "holes" where texture elements were missing. The presence of these "holes" meant that a subject could not find the triangles by looking for the position of "holes" in some internal representation. Thus, suppose that there existed an orientation map that registered the presence of "steep" lines (-45 to $+45$ around a $0°$ vertical) and suppose that the triangle was defined by three $90°$, horizontal lines. Since these vertex lines would not be seen, the triangle could be inferred from holes in the "steep" map unless other holes are introduced.

Stimuli were presented on the monitors of PC or Macintosh computers. Subjects ranged in expertise from naive paid volunteers to the authors. All volunteer subjects gave informed consent. Data consisted of measures of accuracy (percentage correct) as a function of ISI.

Experiment 1: Grouping within and across Features

Experiment 1 had three purposes and eight types of triangles:

1. To replicate Nothdurft's (1992) finding that texton gradients and not specific orientations determined the perception of virtual triangles. The relevant conditions here were

   a. SAME-ORIENT: triangles where all three vertices were of the same orientation;

   b. MIX-ORIENT: triangles where each vertex was a different orientation;

   c. ORIENT + 1: three vertices of the same orientation and a fourth of different orientation.

The expected results would be that the SAME-ORIENT and MIX-ORIENT conditions should be equally easy. The ORIENT + 1 condition should be more difficult as the extra texton gradient groups with the other three and disrupts perception of the triangle.

2. To determine if the results for orientation generalize to another feature, e.g., color. The relevant conditions were

   d. SAME-COLOR: triangles where all three vertices were of the same color;

   e. MIX-COLOR: triangles where each vertex was a different color;

   f. COLOR + 1: 3 vertices of the same color and a fourth of different color.

If color were like orientation, SAME-COLOR and MIX-COLOR conditions should be equally easy. The COLOR + 1 condition should be more difficult as the extra texton gradient disrupts perception of the triangle.

3. To determine if texton gradients group across features. In addition to the SAME-COLOR and SAME-ORIENTA-

TION conditions, the relevant conditions were

   g. SAME-SIZE: triangles where all three vertices were of the same size;

   h. MIX: triangles where each vertex is a different feature (color, orientation, and size).

If each texton gradient could be grouped with any other gradient, then the MIX condition should be no harder than the least salient of the SAME-(FEATURE) conditions.

Each of nine subjects ran 100 trials of each of the eight conditions. These were run in three blocks. In two blocks, the six conditions with three vertices were intermixed. Each block consisted of 30 practice and 300 data trials. In the third block, the two conditions with four vertices were intermixed. That block consisted of 20 practice and 200 data trials.

ISIs in experiment 1 were 50, 100, 150, 250, and 350 msec.

Results

Replication of Nothdurft (1992)

Results for the replication of the orientation results are shown in figure 18.4. Here and elsewhere results are given as proportion correct as a function of SOA (stimulus onset asynchrony), here equal to ISI + the 50 msec flash duration. As Nothdurft found, the SAME-ORIENT and MIX-ORIENT conditions are not significantly different [$F(1,8) = 1.40, p > 0.25$] while the ORIENT + 1 condition is worse than either of the conditions with only three vertices [$F(1,8) > 14, p < 0.01$, for both comparisons].

Color Texton Gradients

Results for the color results are shown in figure 18.5. Color is different from orientation. The MIX-COLOR condition is significantly worse than the SAME-COLOR condition ($F(1,8) = 27.17, p < 0.001$) while the addition of an extra color vertex in the COLOR + 1 condition does not impair performance relative to the SAME-COLOR condition ($F(1, 8) = 0.04, p > 0.8$). The decrease in performance with heterogeneously colored vertices suggests that the identity of the colored vertices is important in a way the identity of the oriented vertices is not. Nothdurft (1993) has recently reported similar results.

Combining Different Features

Can texton gradients from three different features support the perception of a virtual triangle as readily as texton gradients drawn from a single feature? Apparently not.

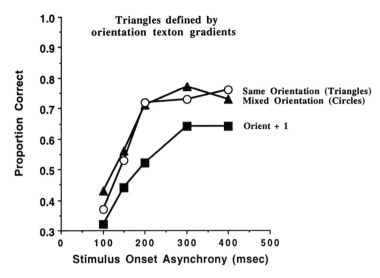

Figure 18.4

Performance as a function of stimulus onset asynchrony for triangles defined by orientation gradients. As Nothdurft found, there is no difference between triangles defined by three identical or three different orientations. When a fourth differently oriented vertex is added to a triangle defined by three identical orientations, performance is impaired (Orient +1 condition).

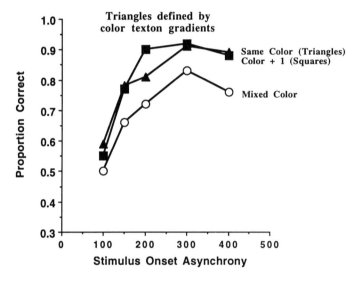

Figure 18.5

Performance as a function of stimulus onset asynchrony for triangles defined by color gradients. Triangles defined by three identical colors are easier to identify than triangles defined by three different colors (Same vs. Mixed conditions). When a fourth differently colored vertex is added to a triangle defined by three identical colored vertices, performance is not impaired (Color +1 condition). These results are different from those for orientation (figure 18.4).

The MIX condition is worse than any of the single feature conditions as shown in figure 18.6. The MIX condition is significantly worse than any of the single feature conditions $(F(1,9) > 14, p < 0.01$ for all comparisons). In a control condition, we found that intermixing all types of triangles was not a critical factor. When COLOR, SIZE, ORIENTATION, and MIX conditions were presented in separate blocks, MIX was still significantly worse than

any of the single feature cases $(F(1,9) > 7.6, p < 0.05$ for all comparisons).

Discussion

The results of experiment 1 show that the identity of an item producing a texton gradient may be important after all. We replicate Nothdurft's (1992) finding that identity is not critical in grouping of orientation texton gradients.

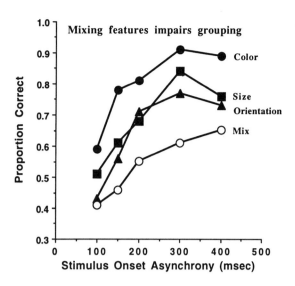

Figure 18.6
Performance as a function of stimulus onset asynchrony for triangles defined by texton gradients. Triangles defined by three identical colors, sizes, or orientations are easier to identify than triangles having each vertex defined by a different feature (Mix condition).

However, gradients do not group so readily across different features. Three highly salient items form a better virtual triangle if they are "vertical," "horizontal," and "left oblique" than if they are vertical," "red," and "big." This finding suggests that the grouping processes that produce the percept of the triangle operate more effectively within the representation of a specific feature.

The results from color suggest there may be a further restriction on grouping in that dimension. Three vertices of different colors produced a weaker triangle than did three vertices of the same color. This suggests that, unlike orientation, grouping in the color domain is better when colors are similar. However, in this case, the data allow alternative explanations. First, the colors were not equiluminant so that some single-color triangles were composed of three vertices brighter (or dimmer) than all other items. Second, different colors differed in their ability to support perception of the triangle. The difficulty with the MIX-COLOR triangle could have been due to reduced visibility of a single vertex rather than difficulty in combining the three vertices. Accordingly, the color conditions of the experiment were rerun to eliminate these hypotheses.

Experiment 2: Grouping by Color—Revisited

Methods

Methods were similar to those in experiment 1 with the following changes. Three vertex colors were picked: red,

green, and blue. The background items were gray. Approximate equiluminant values were found for each color by flicker photometry. The luminance values for each color that were used in the experiment were chosen from a range of luminances around the nominal equiluminant point for that color. As a result, luminance information would not have been a useful cue. The colored triangles were defined by three red, three green, or three blue vertices or by one vertex of each color in the MIX condition. Set sizes were 40, 43, and 46 items. Flash duration was 45 msec. ISIs were 45, 90, 135, 240, and 330 msec. Ten subjects were tested on 40 trials at each ISI for each condition.

Results and Discussion

Results are shown in figure 18.7. The MIX COLOR condition is significantly worse than any of the SAME COLOR conditions ($F(1,9) > 5.3, p < 0.05$ for all comparisons). Having eliminated two less interesting accounts of the MIX COLOR results, the results of experiment 2 confirm an interesting difference between grouping of orientation texton gradients and grouping of color. In orientation, the identity of the vertex does not matter. In color it does. The finding in the color dimension further strengthens the conclusion that grouping is not based entirely on a feature-independent analysis of local texton gradients.

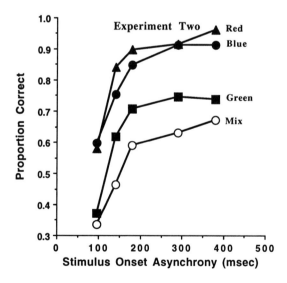

Figure 18.7
Experiment 2: performance as a function of stimulus onset asynchrony for triangles defined by color texton gradients. Even with luminance cues removed, triangles defined by three identical colors (red, green, or blue) are easier to identify than triangles having each vertex defined by a different color (Mix condition).

Experiment 3: Failure to Group Conjunctively Defined Items

We have argued that tasks like texture segmentation make different use of parallel processing than do visual search tasks (Wolfe, 1992a). Specifically, we suggested that texture processes work within feature maps while search tasks can combine information from two or more feature maps (Cohen, 1993; Driver, McLeod, and Dienes, 1992; Muller, Humphreys, and Donnelly, 1994; Poisson and Wilkinson, 1992; Treisman et al., 1990; Wolfe, 1992b). Thus, in a search for a red vertical item among red horizontals and green verticals, color information about the location of red items can be combined with orientation information about the locations of vertical items to guide attention to the likely locations of red vertical items. The results from the MIX conditions in figures 18.6 and 18.7 support this dissociation by showing that grouping of texture elements is weaker when the elements to be grouped differ in type or even just in color. However, the task is still possible in these MIXED conditions. To bolster the argument that information from multiple features is *not* combined in the grouping of texture elements, triangles with conjunctively defined vertices were used in experiment 3.

Methods

In experiment 3, the vertices of the triangle were red vertical items. The other items in the field were red horizontal and green vertical. Stimulus duration was 100 msec (rather than 50 msec in previous experiments). ISIs were 100, 200, 300, 400, 600, and 800 msec (much longer than for the other experiments). Set sizes were 24, 36, and 48 items out of a 7 × 7 array. There were 30 practice and 300 data trials. Ten subjects were tested. These subjects were also tested on a standard visual search paradigm with the same stimuli (see Wolfe et al., 1989 for methodological details). In the search task, one red vertical element was present on 50% of the trials. Set sizes were 24, 36, and 48 items. RTs were the dependent measure.

Results and Discussion

The standard visual search was very efficient, yielding slopes of 2.3 msec/item for target trials and 7.6 msec/item for blank trials. These slopes are comparable to "parallel" searches for items defined by a single, salient target feature (though we would consider them to be "guided" searches (Cave and Wolfe, 1990; Wolfe, 1992b). Nevertheless, grouping of three of these easily found items fails

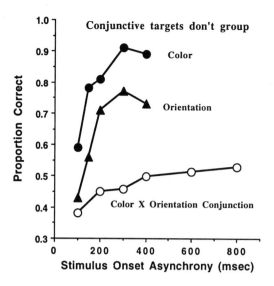

Figure 18.8
Performance as a function of stimulus onset asynchrony for triangles defined by conjunctions. Triangles with vertices defined by a conjunction of color and orientation are very hard to identify: much harder than triangles defined by color or orientation alone. Visual search for this particular conjunction of color and orientation is very efficient (target trial slope = 2.3 msec/item).

miserably. Figure 18.8 shows results from experiment 3 compared to the results for the SAME-COLOR and SAME-ORIENTATION conditions of experiment 1. It is obvious that the conjunctive targets simply fail to group in any compelling manner. Performance is only about 50% even after 800 msec (chance is 25%). Introspection suggests that the triangle can be found only by successively locating each vertex and combining them by some act of will. This is very different from what seems to be the automatic, preattentive perception of a triangle in the single feature cases. Conjunctive targets do not participate in grouping. This should be taken as further evidence that visual search and grouping make different use of the same preattentive information (Wolfe, 1992a). Specifically, search mechanisms can combine information from two or more feature processors. Texture grouping mechanisms appear to lack this ability.

General Discussion

Based on the results of these experiments, an architecture for the preattentive grouping of texture elements can be proposed. The work on visual search has led to several candidate architectures for the preattentive processing of basic feature information. There could be functionally separate representations for each instance of a basic feature (e.g., Treisman, 1985). In this model, there might

Wolfe et al.: Making Use of Texton Gradients

be separate maps for red, green, steep, big, and so forth. Alternatively, there could be one representation for each type of feature (e.g., Treisman, 1986a; Wolfe et al., 1990). In this model, there would be maps for orientation, color, size, etc, but no division of those into specific features. One could even propose that all the features are processed together in a single, multidimensional space (Duncan and Humphreys, 1989, but see Duncan and Humphreys, 1992 for later modifications).

For the grouping of texture elements, the results of these experiments argue against a representation where all features are treated as equal. Were this the case, texton gradients drawn from three different features should be just as effective as texton gradients drawn from within a single feature. Experiment 1 (figure 18.6) shows that this is not the case. The substantial loss of performance with conjunctively defined vertices is further evidence that grouping is not performed in a multidimensional representation. The results for orientation-defined triangles (figure 18.4) support the idea of grouping based solely on local differences in a single feature. However, the results for color (figure 18.5) show that stimulus identity has a role to play in some cases. Vertices of three different colors do not produce as good a triangle as do three vertices of the same color. This finding suggests that the representation of color may be further divided into subrepresentations for specific colors, an architecture different from that for orientation.

It is interesting that the preattentive architecture of color is different from that for orientation. In an earlier paper (Wolfe et al., 1990), we argued against the existence of subfeature representations because of our failure to find evidence for guided search for color × color or orientation × orientation conjunctions. That is, attention could be guided to the item that is red and vertical but not to an item that is red and green or vertical and oblique. We took this to show that one could not combine information about the location of "redness" with information about the location of "greenness." More recently, we have found an exception to this failure of guidance for same-feature conjunctions. Search for a *whole* red item with a green *part* is quite efficient even if search for an item with red and green *parts* is not (Wolfe and Friedman-Hill, 1992; Wolfe, Friedman-Hill, and Bilsky, 1994). Curiously, in spite of many efforts, we have been unable to show the same *part-whole* effect with conjunctions of two orientations. This may be taken as converging evidence for a difference in the preattentive processing of color and orientation.

In summary, the preattentive grouping of texture elements into forms appears to occur in feature-specific representations rather than in a general representation where all texton gradients are treated as equal. The combination of information from multiple features that allows for efficient visual search for conjunctions does not occur for texture grouping. Even vertices defined by single-feature texton gradients do not group well if those textons are created by variation in different features. Indeed, evidence suggests that for some features (here, color but not orientation) texton gradients group better within subfeature maps, making it easier to find a triangle with three red vertices than to find a triangle with three equally salient but heterogeneously colored vertices. These results underline the modular nature of visual processing and show that information available to one process (e.g., visual search) may not be available to another (e.g., texture grouping).

Acknowledgments

We thank Patricia O'Neill for comments on the manuscript and Alex Bilsky and Yurah Kim for help with the project. Our thinking was aided by conversations with Hans-Christoph Nothdurft. Research was supported by NEI EYO5087.

References

Cave, K. R, and Wolfe, J. M. (1990). Modeling the role of parallel processing in visual search. *Cog. Psychol.* 22, 225–271.

Cohen, A. (1993). Asymmetries in visual search for conjunctive targets. *J. Exp. Psychol. Human Percept. Perform.* 19, 775–797.

Driver, J., McLeod, P., and Dienes, Z. (1992). Motion coherence and conjunction search: Implications for guided search theory. *Percept. Psychophys.* 51(1). 79–85.

Duncan, J., and Humphreys, G. W. (1989). Visual search and stimulus similarity. *Psychol. Rev. 96*, 433–458.

Duncan, J., and Humphreys, G. W. (1992). Beyond the search surface: Visual search and attentional engagement. *J. Exp. Psychol. Human Percept. Perform.* 18(2), 578–588.

Egeth, H. E., Virzi, R. A., and Garbart. H. (1984). Searching for conjunctively defined targets. *J. Exp. Psychol. Human Percept. Perform. 10*, 32–39.

Julesz, B. (1962). Visual pattern discrimination. *IRE Trans. Inf. Theory IT-8*, 84–92.

Julesz, B. (1981). A theory of preattentive texture discrimination based on first order statistics of textons. *Biol. Cybern. 41*, 131–138.

Julesz, B. (1984). A brief outline of the texton theory of human vision. *Trends Neurosci. Feb*, 41–45.

Julesz, B. (1986). Texton gradients: The texton theory revisited. *Biol. Cybern. 54*, 245–251.

Julesz, B., and Bergen, J. R. (1983). Textons, the fundamental elements in preattentive vision and perceptions of textures. *Bell Syst. Tech. J. 62*, 1619–1646.

Julesz, B., Gilbert, E. N., Shepp, L. A., and Frisch, H. L. (1973). Inability of humans to discriminate between visual textures that agree in second-order statistics—revisited. *Perception 2*, 391–405.

Moraglia, G. (1989). Display organization and the detection of horizontal line segments. *Percept. Psychophys. 45*, 265–272.

Muller, H. M., Humphreys, G. W., and Donnelly, N. (1994). SEarch via Recursive Rejection (SERR): Visual search for single and dual form conjunction targets. *J. Exp. Psychol. Hum. Percept. Perf. 20*, 235–258.

Nothdurft, H. C. (1990). Texture segmentation by associated differences in global and local luminance distribution. *Proc. R. Soc. London B 239*, 295–320.

Nothdurft, H. C. (1992). Feature analysis and the role of similarity in pre-attentive vision. *Percept. Psychophys. 52*(4), 355–375.

Nothdurft, H.-C. (1993). The role of features in preattentive vision: Comparison of orientation, motion and color cues. *Vision Res. 33*, 1937–1958.

Poisson, M. E., and Wilkinson, F. (1992). Distractor ratio and grouping processes in visual conjunction search. *Perception 21*, 21–38.

Treisman, A. (1985). Preattentive processing in vision. *Comput. Vision Graphics Image Process. 31*, 156–177.

Treisman, A. (1986a). Features and objects in visual processing. *Sci. Am. 255*(Nov), 114B–125.

Treisman, A. (1986b). Properties, parts, and objects. In K. R. Boff, L. Kaufmann, and J. P. Thomas (Eds.), *Handbook of Human Perception and Performance* (pp. 37.1–35.70). New York: John Wiley.

Treisman, A. (1988). Features and objects: the fourteenth Bartlett memorial lecture. *Quart. J. Exp. Psychol. 40A*(2), 201–237.

Treisman, A., and Sato, S. (1990). Conjunction search revisited. *J. Exp. Psychol. Human Percept. Perform. 16*(3), 459–478.

Wolfe, J. M. (1992a). "Effortless" texture segmentation and "parallel" visual search are *not* the same thing. *Vision Res. 32*(4), 757–763.

Wolfe, J. M. (1992b). The parallel guidance of visual attention. *Curr. Direct. Psychol. Sci. 1*(4), 125–128.

Wolfe, J. M., and Friedman-Hill, S. R. (1992). Part-whole relationships in visual search. *Invest. Ophthalmol. Visual Sci. 33*, 1355.

Wolfe, J. M., Cave, K. R., and Franzel, S. L. (1989). Guided Search: An alternative to the Feature Integration model for visual search. *J. Exp. Psychol. Hum. Percept. Perf. 15*, 419–433.

Wolfe, J. M., Yu, K. P., Stewart, M. I., Shorter, A. D., Friedman-Hill, S. R., and Cave, K. R. (1990). Limitations on the parallel guidance of visual search: Color × color and orientation × orientation conjunctions. *J. Exp. Psychol. Human Percept. Perform. 16*(4), 879–892.

Wolfe, J. M., Friedman-Hill, S. R., Stewart, M. I., and O'Connell, K. M. (1992). The role of categorization in visual search for orientation. *J. Exp. Psychol. Human Percept. Perform. 18*(1), 34–49.

Wolfe, J. M., Friedman-Hill, S. R., and Bilsky, A. B. (1994). Parallel processing of part/whole information in visual search tasks. *Percept. Psychophys. 55*, 537–550.

19

How Early Is Early Vision? Evidence from Perceptual Learning

Merav Ahissar and
Shaul Hochstein

Early vision is said to be *bottom-up*, affected only by retinal images and fixed neuronal characteristics. Higher vision uses the results of integrative computations, expectation, attention, etc. to further process salient and behaviorally important features in a scene and interpret its meaning. A classic preattentive visual task is detection of an odd element among distractors (Julesz, 1981, 1984). Using arrays of short line elements with a differently oriented target, we found that practicing target detection improves performance by shortening the threshold stimulus-mask onset asynchrony by a factor of 2−4. Thus, even performance of early visual tasks may be improved. Studying the transfer of training effects to novel situations, we find that training is indeed specific to basic stimulus attributes including position, size, and orientation, in accordance with the expected specificity of early mechanisms and previous results. However, other characteristics of learning specificity are commensurate with higher order processing. First, substantial learning requires selective attention: Viewing the stimuli thousands of times hardly improves pop-out detection if the odd element is not searched for intentionally. Moreover, stimulus specificity is rather complex: Transfer is greater across mirror-image orientation shifts than for simple rotations; and size specificity is asymmetric (transfer is greater for changes to larger than to smaller images). We conclude that this perceptual learning occurs at an early processing level where fine retinotopic locations, and different orientations and sizes are separately handled. Yet, processing and learning here involve complex interneuron computations and are *top-down* controlled.

Among a large variety of visual search tasks, one that has been specifically noted and studied, especially by Bela Julesz and his colleagues, is the search for a target that is saliently different from the surrounding distractor elements (Bergen and Julesz, 1983a,b; Julesz, 1984, 1986). When it is salient to the extent that its presence "pops out" to the observer even without intended attentional search, this task is considered to be performed by the visual system at an early "preattentive" processing stage (Bergen and Julesz, 1983a,b; Treisman and Gelade, 1980). Under these conditions, search time is independent of the number of distractors, and is, therefore, assumed to be performed in parallel for the various elements in the display. The saliency that produces these search characteristics may derive from basic primitives that the visual system detects directly ("textons"; Julesz, 1984), or from basic features for which the system dedicates specific representations (Treisman and Gelade, 1980). The range of basic primitives or features that "pop out" has not yet been characterized fully (Fahle, 1991; Wolfe et al., 1992b).

One of the best studied, and perhaps the most typical example of effortless detection is the search for a line bar at an orientation that differs greatly from the common orientation of the surrounding distractor line bars. This task also has the virtue of possessing a known potential physiological correlate for its performance: A large proportion of the neurons in the primary visual area are selective in their responses to the orientation of a bar presented within a specific area of the visual field (Hubel and Wiesel, 1968). At this processing stage computations are considered to be mainly local as the majority of connecting fibers run perpendicular to the cortical surface (Gilbert and Wiesel, 1989). Indeed it has been shown that this pop-out task depends on local interactions (Julesz, 1986; Sagi and Julesz, 1987; Nothdurft, 1992). In addition, neuronal responses in this area are largely determined by retinal stimulation and are hardly affected by extraretinal attentional task-related influences (Wurtz et al., 1982; Haenny and Schiller, 1988). Since pop-out detection also needs no intended attentional resources, its characteristics match those of this primary visual cortical area. This match is significant since responses in higher visual areas are indeed more affected by extraretinal influences (Moran and Desimone, 1985; Haenny et al., 1988; Maunsell and Newsome, 1987; Maunsell and Hochstein, 1991). Based on these correlations, processing suitable for preattentive pop-out tasks has been sought and attributed to the primary-visual cortex (Nothdurft and Li, 1985; Knierim and Van Essen, 1992; see also Gallant et al., this volume). This behavior-to-anatomy mapping (called psychoanatomy by Julesz) has received support recently by results from lesion experiments: Monkeys trained to perform a pop-out task retained this skill even when their secondary visual area (V2) was lesioned, though other trained tasks did depend on the presence of area V2 (Merigan et al., 1992).

In this chapter we present evidence from studies of the improvement characteristics of pop-out task training that question the apparent simplicity of the underlying processes. These findings indicate that if improvement does involve an early visual cortical area (e.g., area V1 or V2) as indicated by its fine retinotopic specificity, then we must conclude that processing already in this area is strongly affected by specific attentional mechanisms. In addition this area must include processing of basic two-dimensional transformations, such as left–right mirror reversal.

Methods

We have been studying the characteristics of learning and the improvement of performance in a pop-out task. As described above, initial performance in detecting an odd element is very impressive. On the average, it was sufficient that the display be available for about 130 msec, so that a target whose orientation deviated by 30° from that of the distractors would be detected with more than 80% of the decisions correct. This time interval depends on the parameters used. The paradigm we designed is described in figure 19.1 (further details about the experimental procedure have been described elsewhere; see Ahissar and Hochstein, 1993). During the first session subjects substantially improved, and through the next 2–10 following sessions subjects continued to improve. On the whole, the time interval (stimulus onset asynchrony) needed to achieve 82% correct (threshold) was reduced to about a third, from that averaged over the first session to that of the last session (when improvement ceased). Examples of the shift in the psychometric curve for two subjects are illustrated in figure 19.2. The strong learning effect indicates that even for this preattentive task, processing is not hard-wired even in adults.

Results

If processing of the pop-out task is indeed accomplished by the primary visual area then the most straightforward assumption is that improvement in its performance involves neuronal changes in this area. Neuronal plasticity in primary sensory areas of adult behaving animals has been demonstrated recently (Recanzone et al., 1992; Ahissar et al., 1992). Since V1 receptive fields are specific to a small retinal location, as well as to a limited range of sizes and orientations, this assumption implies that learning will be similarly specific. If the target is consistently presented in a given retinal area, and learning is dependent on the activation of the neurons that respond to the target element, then learning will mainly occur for those neurons whose excitatory receptive field contains this retinal area. If the target is then moved to a retinal location that excites a nonoverlapping neuronal population, performance is expected to be degraded. This approach of using learning specificity as a probe to the underlying

A stimuli for two tasks

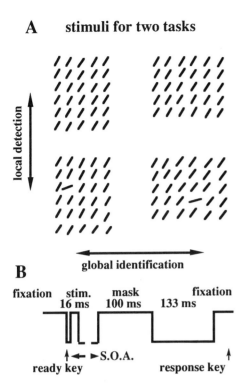

B

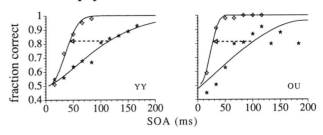

Figure 19.1

(*A*) The stimulus set: arrays that contain an odd element (*bottom*) versus arrays that do not (*top*) for the odd-element pop-out task. In addition, vertical arrays (6 × 5 elements, *left*) versus horizontal arrays (5 × 6 elements, *right*) denote a global orientation difference (see text for details). To ensure viewing of the entire stimulus, the position of the array relative to a preceding fixation point was randomly varied (within a 7 × 7 stimulus lattice that subtended 4.5° × 4.5°). Similarly, the odd element (present in half of the trials) was randomly positioned at any location within the array (except at the fixation point). Element position was jittered within the grid by ± 8 min. A mask followed each stimulus. The mask was composed of a 7 × 7 array of asterisk-like elements located at the grid points (± jitter) of the stimulus lattice. The mask elements were superpositions of four lines (two of which were the trained target and distractor orientations, e.g., 30, 60, 120, and 150°). Each stimulus element subtended 22 × 1 min. The distance between element centers was 42.6 min. (*B*) Trial temporal sequence. Each trial started with a fixation cross. When the observer pressed the ready key, the stimulus appeared for 16 msec. Following a variable delay between presentation of the stimulus and a subsequent mask (the stimulus onset asynchrony, SOA), the mask was displayed for 100 msec. Finally, following a 133-msec dark period, the fixation point reappeared while the subject pressed a response key. A computer tone confirmed correct responses. Stimuli were presented in blocks of 20 trials with the same SOA. Each session comprised 70 blocks of 20 trials each. The SOAs were chosen so that average performance was kept around 75% correct, within and throughout sessions.

psychometric curve shift

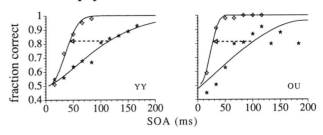

Figure 19.2

Performance improvement from the initial sessions (filled symbols) to the posttraining final sessions (open symbols). The data for two subjects (YY and OU) are fit to Quick psychometric functions (Quick, 1974). Training induces a leftward shift and a steepening of the psychometric curves, substantially decreasing the threshold SOA (arrows). In the following figures the threshold decrease is used as a measure of the learning.

anatomical site has been used recently to show that mechanisms involved in a variety of simple visual tasks are indeed early (Ramachandran and Braddick, 1973; Fiorentini and Berardi, 1980; Ball and Sekuler, 1987; Berardi and Fiorentini, 1987; Karni and Sagi, 1991; Poggio et al., 1992; Shiu and Pashler, 1992; see also Sagi, this volume).

If learning occurs at V1, the spatial location specificity is expected to be fine-grained due to the small size of receptive fields of neurons in this area (e.g., Dow et al., 1981). To test spatial specificity we modified the experimental paradigm in the following manner: The target was placed in only one of two positions symmetrically located about the fixation cross, and the array had a fixed location and was composed of 7 × 7 elements. We used two target locations rather than one to ensure proper fixation. We found that learning was location specific: Moving the target by only 1° (within one hemifield, while maintaining its distance from the fixation point at a constant value of 1.5°) reverted the threshold to its pretraining value, indicating that learning is confined to a very small region. Figure 19.3 demonstrates the average psychometric curves at the onset of training on targets "3" for two groups (filled symbols), where one of the groups was pretrained for other, adjacent, target locations (filled circles). Note that the two initial curves for locations "3" are almost overlapping (filled symbols). That is, subjects were nearly unaffected by prior experience with pop-out in nearby locations. The psychometric curve for the naive group following training (with target at locations "3") shows that, following specific practice, performance is substantially improved. Interestingly, the absolute performance is different at different locations, and is not only a function of eccentricity. There is also some transfer asym-

transfer across locations

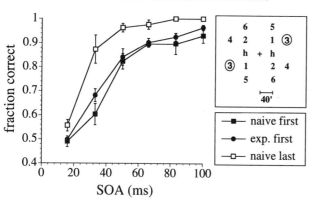

Figure 19.3

Example of location specificity: Subjects were trained on pop-out detection with target (when present) located in one of two locations (pairs of locations indicated by numbers of upper inset). Group one (*n* = 3) was trained for target at locations "3," and their psychometric curves in the initial and final sessions are shown by the filled and open squares, respectively. The shift in curve indicates the dramatic effect of training. A second group (*n* = 7) was trained with target at various adjacent locations (including 1, 2, h, and 5), and then tested at locations "3." The resulting psychometric curve (filled circles) is very similar to that of the naive group, indicating that training is location specific.

metry, which may be related to this a priori difference (Ahissar and Hochstein, 1994).

Next we tested orientation specificity. Neurons that respond to orientations that are remote from those presented will not have been activated during the training process. Thus, if following training, subjects are presented with the same stimulation paradigm, but with all the elements rotated, threshold is expected to increase greatly. Rotating all the elements by 90° indeed increased the threshold, as illustrated by the examples in figure 19.4A and B. Further practice reduced it to the same level as with the previously trained orientations. We then tested whether learning was specific to the presented orientations, regardless of their density or contextual role in the task, by swapping the orientations of the target and distractors. As illustrated in figure 19.4A and B, threshold was increased in a similar manner. We subsequently asked whether training was specific to the trained target or to the distractors. Rotating either only the target or only the distractors by 30° had a similar effect in increasing the threshold (see example in figure 19.4B). This suggests that strengthening of lateral inhibition between similar orientations is not sufficient to account for the training-induced decrease in threshold. Rather, specific two-dimensional interactions between target and distractors must contribute to the process.

transfer across orientations

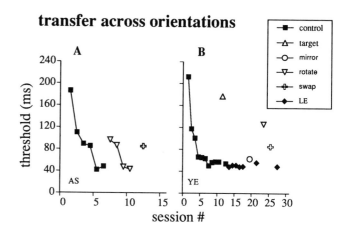

Figure 19.4

Orientation specificity. (*A*) An example of a subject who was trained with the original stimuli (distractor orientation at 60°, target at 30°), was then tested and further trained with all line bars rotated by 90° (*rotate*), and was then tested with target and distractor orientations switched (*swap*). (*B*) An example of a subject who practiced monocularly (right eye, distractors at 45°, target at 15°). He was then tested with the target rotated (to 75°, *target*), resulting in very little transfer. Following a repetition of the control test, this subject was tested with the original stimulus but with the other eye (*LE*). Complete transfer was found across eyes. Only a small increase in threshold was found when tested with a mirror symmetric image (distractors at 135°, target at 165°; *mirror*), though rotating all elements by 90° or swapping target and distractors had a far greater effect on performance.

How specific are these interactions? We tested the transfer to mirror symmetric orientations, and surprisingly we found nearly complete transfer (figure 19.4B). This indicates that learning involves units that are more complex than simply involving interactions between two specific orientations. These units may construct basic categorizations, perhaps, in our case, depending on the target orientation being steeper than that of the distractors (see Wolfe et al., 1992a). Interestingly this suggestion need not refute the hypothesis that these computations are part of V1 processing. In a recent study aimed at revealing the neural basis of pop-out, Knierim and Van Essen (1992) found units in V1 that responded according to categories of two-dimensional interactions. They found that some (less oriented) cells responded to stimuli with either of two orthogonal orientations while maintaining their preference for orientation-contrast stimuli rather than for fields of elements of similar orientations. Their findings support the suggestion that two-dimensional interactions aimed at forming ecologically significant categories may occur already at V1. Since their stimuli were not aimed at characterizing the range of physiologically represented categories, additional study is required to define their full range. This task may be as challenging as that undertaken by Bela Julesz in defining the range of textons.

The trained target has an additional consistently repeated feature—its size. Neuronal responses in V1 are size specific (compared with "size-constancy" maintaining responses in inferotemporal cortex; Gross and Mishkin, 1977). Thus, it was expected that changing the size of the elements in the display would also greatly affect the performance achieved by size-specific training. To examine that prediction, we tested trained subjects with a similar stimulus, only now width and height of the stimulus (including of the single elements and the interelement distances) were halved. Performance was greatly degraded as expressed by the increased threshold demonstrated in figure 19.5, top. Another group of subjects was trained in the reverse order: first with the half-sized stimulus, and then with the (original) larger size. We found that initial and asymptotic performance were very similar for both stimuli. However, for the group that started with the small stimulus, transfer to the big stimulus was nearly complete, as shown in the examples of figure 19.5, bottom. The asymmetry cannot be accounted for by a difference in difficulty since the initial and final performances of the two groups are similar. It would be of importance to study the range of size changes for which this asymmetry persists. Ecologically this asymmetry may be used for a "zoom-in" mechanism, whereby upon encountering a given visual stimulus at a distance the visual system is primed to its getting retinally bigger—correlated with its getting closer.

Strong support for the claim of plasticity within early visual cortex could derive from finding that improvement is eye specific. While changes in V1 do not necessarily imply eye specificity, eye specificity would constitute a strong indication that learning occurred in V1. (Only at the input levels of V1 are neuronal responses ocular specific while at subsequent V1 stages, neurons, though dominated by one eye, are generally activated by both; Hubel and Wiesel, 1968). We therefore tested ocular specificity. A group of seven subjects was trained with one eye covered. We found that on average both initial and final performance was poorer monocularly than binocularly (~185 msec → ~60 msec vs. ~135 msec → ~40 msec). We found nearly complete transfer across eyes (see example in figure 19.6 and figure 19.4B). In fact, a sub-

transfer across sizes

large ➔ small

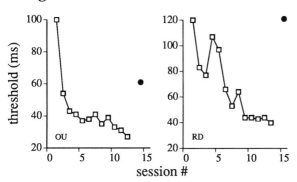

small ➔ large

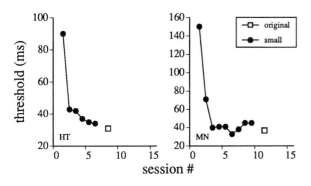

Figure 19.5

Size specificity, and its asymmetry. Examples of thresholds for four subjects are illustrated. Two practiced with the large (original) stimulus (squares), and were then tested with the small stimulus (circles). The other two subjects practiced with the small stimulus, and were then tested with the large stimulus. Note that while the effect of training with the large stimulus was specific to that stimulus, there was complete transfer from training with the small stimulus to subsequent testing with the large stimulus.

transfer across eyes

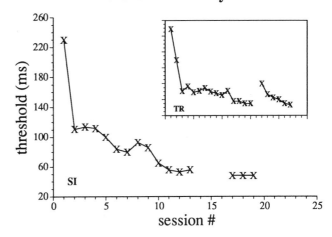

Figure 19.6

Monocular learning. Threshold for a subject who was trained monocularly and then tested and trained with the alternate eye. When switching eyes, no increase in threshold was found for this subject. Among seven subjects a large increase was found for only one (inset; scales are the same in both graphs.)

Ahissar & Hochstein: How Early Is Early Vision?

stantial increase in threshold upon switching eyes was evident only for one subject (figure 19.6, inset). Thus ocular specificity did not solve the question of physiological site. Our result is in agreement with the findings of Wolfe and Franzel (1988), which suggest that visual search is performed at a stage that utilizes binocular information.

Given these stimulus specificities, which are in agreement with those predicted by neuronal changes in area V1, and given the "preattentive" nature of the pop-out task, one might assume that improvement in this task would not require selective attention. To test this assumption, we trained another group of subjects on the same stimulation paradigm, but with a different task. Note that the group of four stimulus types, schematically illustrated in figure 19.1, denotes two possible discriminations, or tasks: The first (top versus bottom)—the pop-out task—

pop-out learning task-specificity

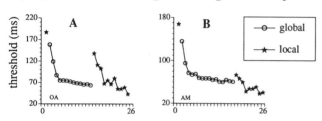

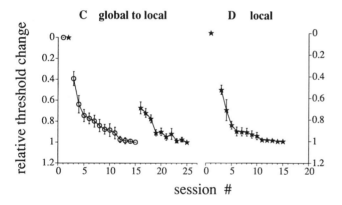

Figure 19.7
Substantial improvement in pop-out detection needs task-specific attention. (A–C) Each subject was first pretested with the local element pop-out task, then practiced global array orientation identification, and upon reaching asymptotic threshold was tested and further trained on the pop-out task. Threshold for local detection was somewhat reduced by global identification training but further reduced by subsequent pop-out detection practice. (A, B) Single subject examples. (C) Averaged, normalized data for six subjects (error bars are intersubject SE). (D) A control group of six subjects who practiced pop-out detection initially. Quantitatively the best test of transfer is comparison of the first sessions following the pretest with and without intervening training on the global determination (C and D, respectively). This comparison takes into account the training effect of the pop-out pretest session, which does not decay for many months.

and the second—(left vs. right)—determining the alignment of the entire array. The stimulus parameters were chosen so that the average threshold for both tasks (as found in pilot studies) would be very similar. The second group of subjects practiced determination of the global array orientation. The question was whether training with this set of stimuli for a very large number of trials (20,000 and more) would induce improvement in the pop-out task. Under these conditions, subjects are exposed to the stimuli while alert, and actively attending the very same spatial areas that were essential for the original detection task. The spatial windows of attention were overlapping since in both cases subjects had to attend to the entire array: array position was varied from trial to trial so that local determination of the array orientation would not be possible. Similarly, for the pop-out task, the odd element could be in any position besides the fixation point (except when testing for location specificity). We found that practicing the global task somewhat improved performance in the local task, but only to a small extent (figure 19.7). To achieve their best threshold, subjects had to specifically train on the pop-out task. This partial transfer across tasks is stimulus specific and does not transfer to the pop-out task performed with rotated elements.

Why did pop-out learning have no effect at all on the global discrimination task? Perhaps the latter is performed at a subsequent processing area (above V1). It would be of great interest to determine more fully the extent of specificity of attention required by utilizing more similar tasks.

Summary and Conclusions

How do we account for the composite specificity: On the one hand specificity to basic stimulus attributes, suggesting an early stimulus-determined processing site, and on the other hand, specificity to the given task-related attentional demand, suggesting a high-level cortical involvement? One possibility, suggested for the process of general improvement in perceptual and motor skills (Fitts, 1964), is that there are two learning stages with different time constants: an initial fast "cognitive" stage in which subjects "learn how to learn" the task, accompanied and followed by a slow, purely perceptual stage, which involves the peripheral processing level. Thus, the initial fast rate of improvement seen for our tasks may reflect mainly a cognitive, task-related, stimulus nonspecific, stage. However, if this hypothesis were true, then we would expect that following an initial pop-out session, training on a different task that uses the same spatial stimuli would be sufficient for the stimulus dependent improvement. Then, for the group described above, we would have expected that training the global task would have induced complete transfer to the pop-out task, which was not the case.

In summary, mechanisms that produce pop-out detection retain plasticity in adults and as such account for improved performance as a function of experience when task-specific practice is given. These mechanisms operate at a retinotopic stage (resolution of at least 1° at 1.5° from fixation), which is also size and orientation specific. However, these mechanisms are two-dimensional and involve interactions between differently oriented elements. They transfer across mirror transformations, indicating that this two-dimensional stage involves more than the actually presented orientations, possibly basic categorization.

This combination of learning specificities indicates that complex computations and top-down control are operating at a level at which computations are performed separately for adjacent locations. It thus questions the current hierarchical view based on different characteristics of single neuronal responses in the various visual areas, which associates processing hierarchy with spatial convergence and increasing attentional control (see review by Desimone and Ungerleider, 1989). However, it does not indicate a unique solution. Changes may involve neuronal assemblies in the primary visual cortex. This interpretation implies that learning in early processing networks is selectively controlled by top-down task-related mechanisms, and includes a more elaborate two-dimensional processing than commonly suggested. The other alternative, that changes are at a higher processing stage (Logan, 1988), means that there is a coding that maintains fine spatial resolution. This coding may be expressed either in a reduced functional size of single neuronal receptive fields (Moran and Desimone, 1985), or through interactions within neuronal assemblies. The third possibility claims that current physiological findings regarding single unit properties indeed describe an existing distributed processing. Learning may involve both early bottom-up and higher, task-related processes associated with different cortical areas. However, behavioral improvement requires both. Thus the actual performance is achieved by some intercortical binding mechanism. Judging among these alternatives may help us understand how the separate parts interact in order to produce the whole. However, this will require a multidisciplinary approach involving psychophysics, single-unit recordings at different loci, and noninvasive imaging techniques that will assess the contribution of the different areas preferably in behaving humans.

Acknowledgments

We thank the organizers of the Bela Julesz Workshop for inviting us to contribute this chapter and take this opportunity to extend to Bela Julesz best wishes for many more active fruitful enjoyable years. We thank the U.S.–Israel Binational Science Foundation (BSF), the Israel Academy of Sciences and Humanities (BRF), and the Hebrew University Center for Neural Computation for support.

References

Ahissar, E., Vaadia, E., Ahissar, M., Bergman, H., Arieli, A., and Abeles, M. (1992). Dependence of cortical plasticity on correlated activity of single neurons and on behavioral context. *Science* 257, 1412–1415.

Ahissar, M., and Hochstein, S. (1993). The role of attention in early perceptual learning. *Proc. Natl. Acad. Sci. U.S.A.* 90, 5718–5722.

Ahissar, M., and Hochstein, S. (1994). Spatial anisotropy in feature search performance and learning. *Invest. Ophthalmol. Visual Sci.* 35, 4.

Ball, K., and Sekuler, R. (1987). Direction specific improvement in motion perception. *Vision Res.* 27, 953–965.

Berardi, N., and Fiorentini, A. (1987). Interhemispheric transfer of visual information in humans: Spatial characteristics. *J. Physiol.* 384, 633–647.

Bergen, J. R., and Julesz, B. (1983a). Parallel versus serial processing in rapid pattern discrimination. *Nature (London)* 303, 696–698.

Bergen, J. R., and Julesz, B. (1983b). Rapid discrimination of visual patterns. *IEEE Trans. Syst. M.* 13, 857–863.

Desimone, R., and Ungerleider, L. G. (1989). Neural mechanisms of visual processing in monkey. In F. Boller and J. Grafman (Eds.), *Handbook of Neuropsychology* (Vol 2, pp. 267–299). Amsterdam: Elsevier Science Publishers.

Dow, B. M., Snyder, A. Z., Gautin, R. G., and Bauer, R. (1981). Magnification factor and receptive field size in foveal striate cortex of the monkey. *Exp. Brain Res.* 44, 213–228.

Fahle, M. (1991). A new elementary feature of vision. *Invest. Ophthalmol. Visual Sci.* 32(7), 2151–2155.

Fiorentini, A., and Berardi, N. (1980). Perceptual learning specific for orientation and spatial frequency. *Nature (London)* 287, 43–44.

Fitts, P. M. (1964). Perceptual-motor skill learning. In A. W. Melton (Ed.), *Categories of Human Learning* (pp. 243–285). New York: Academic Press.

Gilbert, C. D., and Wiesel, T. N. (1989). Columnar specificity of intrinsic horizontal and corticocortical connections in cat visual cortex. *J. Neurosci.* 9, 2432–2442.

Gross, C. G., and Mishkin, M. (1977). The neural basis of stimulus equivalence across retinal translation. In S. Harned, R. Doty, J. Jaynes, L. Goldberg, and G. Krauthamer (Eds.), *Lateralization in the Nervous System* (pp. 109–122). New York: Academic Press.

Haenny, P. E., and Schiller, P. H. (1988). State dependent activity in monkey visual cortex. I. Single cell activity in V1 and V4 on visual tasks. *Exp. Brain Res. 69*, 225–244.

Haenny, P. E., Maunsell, J. H., and Schiller, P. H. (1988). State dependent activity in monkey visual cortex. *Exp. Brain Res. 69*, 245–259.

Hubel, D. H., and Wiesel, T. N. (1968). Receptive fields and functional architecture of monkey striate cortex. *J. Physiol. (London) 148*, 574–591.

Julesz, B. (1981). Textons, the elements of texture perception and their interactions. *Nature (London) 290*, 91–97.

Julesz, B. (1984). A brief outline of the texton theory of human vision. *Trends Neurosci. 7*, 41–45.

Julesz, B. (1986). Texton gradients: The texton theory revisited. *Biol. Cybern. 54*, 245–251.

Karni, A., and Sagi, D. (1991). Where practice makes perfect: Evidence for primary visual cortex plasticity. *Proc. Natl. Acad. Sci. U.S.A. 88*, 4966–4970.

Knierim, J. J., and Van Essen, D. C. (1992). Neuronal responses to static texture patterns in area V1 of the alert Macaque monkey. *J. Neurophysiol. 67*, 961–980.

Logan, G. D. (1988). Towards an instance theory of automatization. *Psychol. Rev. 95*, 492–527.

Maunsell, J. H. R., and Newsome, W. T. (1987). Visual processing in monkey extrastriate cortex. *Annu. Rev. Neurosci. 10*, 363–401.

Maunsell, J. H. R., and Hochstein, S. (1991). Effects of behavioral state on the stimulus selectivity of neurons in area V4 of the macaque monkey. In B. Blum (Ed.), *Channels in the Visual Nervous System: Neurophysiology, Psychophysics and Models* (pp. 447–470). London: Freund Publ.

Merigan, W. H., Nealey, T. A., and Maunsell, J. H. R. (1992). Qualitatively different effects of lesions of cortical areas V1 and V2 in macaques. *Perception 21*, Suppl. 2, 55–56.

Moran, J., and Desimone, R. (1985). Selective attention gates visual processing in the extrastriate cortex. *Science 229*, 782–785.

Nothdurft, H. C. (1992). Feature analysis and the role of similarity in preattentive vision. *Percept. Psychophys. 52*(4), 355–375.

Nothdurft, H. C., and Li, C. Y. (1985). Texture discrimination: Representation and luminance differences in cells of the cat striate cortex. *Vision Res. 25*, 99–113.

Poggio, T., Fahle, M., and Edelman, S. (1992). Fast perceptual learning in visual hyperacuity. *Science 256*, 1018–1021.

Quick, R. F. (1974). A vector magnitude model of contrast detection. *Kybernetic 16*, 65–67.

Ramachandran, V. S., and Braddick, O. (1973). Orientation specific learning in stereopsis. *Perception 2*, 371–376.

Recanzone, G. H., Merzenich, M. M., and Schreiner, C. E. (1992). Changes in distributed temporal response properties of S1 cortical neurons reflect improvement in performance on a temporally based tactile discrimination task. *J. Neurophysiol. 67*, 1071–1091.

Sagi, D., and Julesz, B. (1987). Short range limitation on detection of feature differences. *Spatial Vision 2*, 39–49.

Shiu, L., and Pashler, H. (1992). Improvement in line orientation discrimination is retinally local but dependent on cognitive set. *Percept. Psychophys. 52*, 582–588.

Treisman, A., and Gelade, G. (1980). A feature integration theory of attention. *Cog. Psychol. 12*, 97–136.

Wolfe, J. M., and Franzel, S. L. (1988). Binocularity and visual search. *Percept. Psychophys. 44*, 81–93.

Wolfe, J. M., Friedman-Hill, S. R., Stewart, M. I., and O'Connel, K. M. (1992a). The role of categorization in visual search for orientation. *J. Exp. Psychol. Human Percept. Perform. 18*, 34–49.

Wolfe, J. M., Yee, A., and Friedman-Hill, S. R. (1992b). Curvature is a basic feature for visual search tasks. *Perception (England) 21*(4), 465–480.

Wurtz, R., Goldberg, M., and Robinson, D. L. (1982). Brain mechanisms of visual attention. *Sci. Am. 246*(6), 100–107.

20

Toward a Computational Model of Visual Attention

John K. Tsotsos

The Need for Attentional Processing in Vision

In principle, it seems possible to model visual perception computationally (Tsotsos, 1993a). If a vision system knows which subset of an image corresponds to an object and the object type is known, the task of matching image subset to object model is straightforward. In fact, this is a subarea of computational vision in which successful algorithms exist (e.g., Dickinson et al., 1992). The trick is to quickly determine which is the image subset of interest and the corresponding object model. However, far too much computation is required to solve this problem in its general form, guaranteeing that the optimal solution is found in all cases. There is an exponential number of possible image subsets against which to match each potential object model. This conclusion can be proved formally using the methods from theoretical computational complexity. Optimal solutions seem computationally intractable in any implementation, machine or neural (see Tsotsos, 1988, 1989, 1990, 1992, 1993a).

The prevailing argument for why the brain needs visual attention is that there is insufficient neural machinery to deal with all stimuli equally. Broadbent (1971, p. 147), for example, points out "The obvious utility of a selection system is to produce an economy in mechanism. If a complete analysis were performed even on neglected messages, there seems no reason for selection at all." Given the mismatch between brain capacity and complete analysis of all input stimuli, the task facing perceptual theorists is to discover the balance that Nature has achieved among at least three competing requirements: how much information to process and to what degree, how much brain capacity can be devoted to the task, and how quickly must an organism respond to perceptual stimuli.

The remainder of this chapter is devoted to presenting a theoretical foundation for modeling visual attention, followed by descriptions of three current computational hypotheses for modeling attention. For additional background, the reader is referred to Allport (1989) and Colby (1991).

A "First Principles" Argument

The first principles required are straightforward: images, a model base of known objects and events, and an objective function to be optimized that reflects how well an image subset matches a particular member of the model base. One common experimental paradigm, visual search, has been cast into a formal framework using these primitive elements. In Tsotsos (1989), it was proven that visual search, in the case where explicit targets are given in advance, has time complexity which is linear in the size of the image (and this linear response time vs display size is verified experimentally in a large body of work). If, on the other hand, no explicit target is provided, the task is NP-Complete; it is currently believed that such problems are computationally intractable regardless of the implementation, whether it be neural or machine. The intractability is due solely to the combinatorial nature of selecting which parts of the input image are to be processed; there are an exponential number of such image subsets. Since those proofs are based on more abstract yet equally difficult computational problems, it is instructive to consider how the computer science community deals with such combinatorial problems.

For such problems, algorithms have been developed that are not guaranteed to always find the best solution, but can find solutions quickly given some error tolerance. The goal is to find the subset of the input that maximizes an objective function. Strategies for developing partial solutions are exploited to guide search through the space of possibilities so that as few solutions are generated as possible before the best one is located. The intractability of these problems is not due to the computation of the objective function; rather the problem is so difficult only because there is an exponential number of possible solutions to explore. The best of the algorithms are ones that exploit parallel processing; even so, all of them require some serial search through a set of possible solutions (Tsotsos, 1992).

What could the objective function for vision be? Whether a given neuron computes a response that represents a specific object, a specific scene, or a portion of a code as part of a distributed representation is not relevant to this discussion. What is important is that for any particular natural scene a potentially large number of neurons will initially respond with some degree of strength simply because the receptive fields of neurons in higher level areas are so large they will contain elements that might be part of the selectivity profiles of many cells. This large initial set of responding neurons may be considered as a "first guess" as to the contents of a scene. The mapping from image subset to responding neurons is one-to-many; similarly, there are 2^R image subsets within any neuron's receptive field where R is the number of receptors in the receptive field, and thus the mapping from neuron to image subset is also one-to-many. Thus, there is no unique one-to-one mapping between image subsets and neurons. How can this ambiguity be corrected? An objective function is required that reflects this ambiguity and provides a measure for its reduction.

In the formulation of the visual search problem such an objective function was proposed (Tsotsos, 1989). There is one objective function for each known object or image event. The best match is the image subset and model that exhibits the smallest matching error and the model must explain (or cover) as much of the image subset as possible. The brute-force search strategy then is to match each objective function against all possible image subsets. Given formally, the best fit of model to data is sought such that the following is satisfied:

$$\sum_{x \in M, j_x \in I'} |x - j_x| < \theta \quad \text{and} \quad \sum_{x \in M, j_x \in I'} x \cdot j_x > \phi \quad (20.1)$$

The first term is the error measure while the second is the cover measure. The input is the set I, I' is a subset of I, and M is a set of values corresponding to a particular object or event in the model base. θ and ϕ are two thresholds. I is not necessarily the image itself but may be a collection of all features computed from a given image. A correspondence between elements of M and elements of I' can be hypothesized where element j_x in I' is the element corresponding to x in M. Each possible combination of correspondences may be considered as a separate hypothesis.

Suppose a test image is made up of 256 pixels and a target image has 64 pixels. The correspondence required above is for each element of the target image (each pixel) to be mapped onto a unique pixel of the test image. This forms a hypothesis about where exactly in the test image the target image is believed to be represented. The spatial organization of the mapping need not preserve the structure of the target stimulus, that is, pixels chosen for the mapping may be arbitrarily distributed throughout the image. In the Marr view of the vision, this is necessarily the case since he did not believe there was a role for task (target) directed computations (Marr, 1982). So for this example, there are $\binom{256}{64}$ such possible, bottom-up mappings ($256!/64! \, 192!$ is approximately 10^{56}; in general if α is the size of the test image and β is the size of the target image both in pixels, then the number of combinations can be given by a polynomial function of the image size whose highest order term is α^β). If spatial structure is preserved and there is no rotation or scaling of the target in the test image, then there are only 64 possibilities such that the target image is entirely within the test image. Attentional selection may determine which mapping to attempt to verify first; if the first such mapping selected is a good one, a great deal of search can be avoided, otherwise there is the potential for a very inefficient search process. For sufficiently small images and/or massive computational power, this brute force concept will work perfectly well without attention. For the brain, this approach fails.

It is easily shown that equation (20.1), is optimized, that is,

$$\theta = 1 \quad \text{and} \quad \phi = \left(\sum_{x \in M} x^2 \right) - 1$$

if and only if the set I' is identical to the set M. That is, the set of features or computations that is represented by I' is of the same type and value as those represented by M. I' is a set of features at the same level of abstraction as M and spatially organized in the same manner as M. The role of attention in the image domain is to localize this set I' in a way such that any interfering or corrupting signals are minimized. In doing so, attention also seeks to increase the discriminability over other such objective functions as quickly as possible. Note that any error and cover functions may be used; they would all behave in the above fashion. The only constraint on these functions is that they lead to convex solution landscapes.

Thus, the central thesis of this chapter is that attention acts to optimize the search procedure inherent in the above "in principle" solution to vision. The main effect of attention is to reduce the number of candidates that is considered in matching, both of image subsets as well as object or event models. Attention operates continuously and automatically: without attention, vision in general is not possible. The models described in this chapter deal only with the localization of the image subset and not with model selection.

Pyramid Processes

Analysis at the complexity level (Tsotsos, 1988) confirms what several have suggested (Uhr, 1972; Burt, 1988; Anderson and Van Essen, 1987; Nakayama, 1991): the computational complexity of vision necessitates pyramidal processing. Although pyramids solve the complexity problem by reducing the size of the representations to be processed, they introduce others. Consider the simple three-level pyramid shown in figure 20.1 where each node computes some possibly non-linear weighted sum of its inputs as its output value in a feedforward manner.

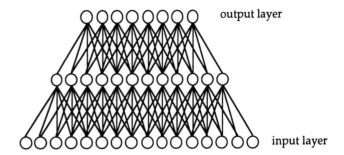

Figure 20.1
A simple pyramidal processing architecture.

Suppose that the input stimulates only one of the centrally located input layer units. That single unit will cause a response in all the units of the output layer simply due to its connectivity. This causes the input to be blurred across the output layer. Similarly, a given unit in the output layer is activated by several units of the input layer, thus responses exhibit a dependence on spatial context. If there are two separate units active in the input layer, they will both activate large parts of the output layer and will overlap for a large portion of the pyramid. This can lead to serious interpretation ambiguities. The examples described all assume that information flow is from input to output layer (data driven). However, information flow in the visual cortex appears to be bidirectional. It is easy to see that the same kinds of problems arise if information flows from top to bottom (task driven). Although pyramid structures help reduce the computational complexity of information processes via convergence of information, they corrupt the signals flowing through them unless some additional mechanisms are included. Each of the following proposals for modeling visual attention provides different solutions to these problems of information flow as well as to the problem of attentional selection.

The Major Computational Hypotheses

There are several major classes of hypotheses for the computational modeling of visual attention, described by the terms *selective routing*, *temporal tagging*, and *selective tuning*.

The Selective Routing Hypothesis

Several models fall into the *selective routing hypothesis* category. The first is that of Koch and Ullman (1985). The idea has found wide acceptance and is used as part of a number of models. The model includes the following elements: (1) an early representation, computed in parallel, permitting separate representations of several stimulus characteristics; (2) a selective mapping from these representations into a central nontopographic representation such that this central representation at any instant contains only the properties of a single location of the visual scene; (3) a winner-take-all (WTA) network implementing the selection process based on one major rule: conspicuity of location (minor rules of proximity or similarity preference are also suggested); and (4) inhibition of this selected location causes an automatic shift to the next most conspicuous location. The other models in the selective routing category and the models in the temporal tagging category share these basic elements. The selective tuning model includes elements 1, 3, albeit with an entirely new formulation, and 4.

Feature maps code conspicuity within a particular feature dimension. The saliency map combines information from each of the feature maps into a global measure where points corresponding to one location in a feature map project to single units in the saliency map. Saliency at a given location is determined by the degree of difference between that location and its surround (as suggested by Julesz and Bergen, 1983, with their texton difference idea and further explored by Nothdurft, 1993, who showed that feature contrast is the major determinant in speed of visual search and not feature values per se). Different features may be weighted differently or their contribution may be modulated by higher-order computations. Details on the construction of this representation are not given. The WTA network implements a parallel computation based on the values in the saliency map localizing the most conspicuous location. Due to biological constraints on connectivity as well as theoretical convergence difficulties, the WTA takes a particular form; it requires a tree of intermediate nodes breaking up the computation into smaller subtasks and permitting better convergence properties. If the size of the saliency map is n units, and the branching factor of the intermediate tree is m, then the network requires $\log_m n$ comparisons to determine the globally most salient item. Then, a second pyramid marks the location of the most salient item and through another $\log_m n$ steps the most salient item reaches the output of the system. The WTA will not converge if there are two equally strong items. A shift of attention thus requires at most $2 \log_m n$ time steps. Faster convergence can be achieved if locations are physically closer to each other.

The WTA algorithm may no longer be considered biologically plausible because its time course does not agree with current observations. Kröse and Julesz (1989) show that shifts of attention do not take time proportional to the distance between items but rather are accomplished in constant time; also Remington and Pierce (1984) report no topographic relationship on time to shift attention. The intermediate tree of computations has yet to find an anatomical correlate, but perhaps most importantly, the mechanism does not immediately yield the kinds of attention-related receptive field changes observed in areas such as V4 (Moran and Desimone, 1985).

The shifter circuit model, the second in this category, presented a strategy for information flow in stereopsis, visual attention, and motion perception (Anderson and Van Essen, 1987). The model enables the realignment of successive representations in the processing stream starting in the lateral geniculate nucleus and the input layers of area V1. The realignment is based on the preservation of spatial relationships, thus the name "shifter" circuits. The shift is accomplished by a succession of stages linked by diverging excitatory inputs. Control of the direction of shift is accomplished at each stage by inhibitory neurons that selectively suppress sets of ascending inputs. For visual attention, the routing stages are grouped into small and large scale shifts. Control signals are generated externally to the main processing stream. If shifts are assumed to be contiguous it is straightforward to show that this strategy requires many thousands more connections per neuron than the accepted average figure of 1000 for each of fan-in and fan-out.

The Olshausen, Anderson, and Van Essen (1994) model is an elaboration of the shifter circuit idea; a partial implementation with simulation results is also included. The problem described above with the original shifter circuits model is remedied via a clever restructuring of the connectivity patterns between layers. By allowing the spacing between neighboring connections to increase in successively higher layers, the routing network has early layers that are well suited for small-scale shifts while the higher layers can implement larger-scale shifts. The key goal of the Olshausen et al. mechanism is to form position- and scale-invariant representations of objects in the visual field. This is accomplished via a set of control neurons, originating in the pulvinar, that dynamically modifies synaptic weights of intracortical connections so that information from a selected region of primary visual cortex is routed to higher areas. The topography of the selected portion of the visual field is preserved by the resulting transformations.

The dynamics of the control neurons are defined using simple differential equations and control neurons receive their input from a saliency map representation. They suggest that the posterior parietal areas act as the saliency map representation. Each node in the processing hierarchy performs a simple linear weighted sum operation.

Selected objects in the visual field are found by the Koch and Ullman mechanism, then routed to the top layer of the processing pyramid (inferotemporal cortex, IT). The selected object is transformed by the routing so that it spans the top-level representation. There, a Hopfield associative memory is used for recognition (Hopfield, 1982).

This model is presented in detail and the results of the computer simulations show performance as expected. Rotations are not handled and it does not seem that the shifter kinds of connectivities are sufficient to ensure rotation-invariant representations. Finally, there is no evidence yet that area IT is an image-centered representation of only a subset of the retinal image.

The Temporal Tagging Hypothesis

The *temporal tagging hypothesis* proposes that selected items are distinguished as they flow through the processing system because they are tagged by superimposing a frequency modulation of 40 Hz on the signal. Crick and Koch (1990) suggest that an attentional mechanism binds together all those neurons whose activity relates to the relevant features of a single visual object. This is done by generating coherent semisynchronous oscillations in the 40–70 Hz range. These oscillations then activate a transient short-term memory. These suggestions are not fully developed computationally in that paper. However, in a subsequent effort, Niebur, Koch, and Rosin (1993) detail a model based on those suggestions.

Niebur et al. (1993) assume that salient objects have been selected in the visual field by the Koch and Ullman mechanism. The saliency map is claimed to be found in subcortical areas (superior colliculus or the dorsomedial region of the pulvinar). That is where the attentional modulation is added and this modulation occurs only at the level of primary visual cortex V1. The modulation affects only the temporal structure of the spike trains of V1 neurons but not their mean firing rate. The existence of frequency-selective inhibitory interneurons is assumed in V4. These are required to act as bandpass filters selective to spikes arriving every 25 msec or so. Thus, they would pass temporally tagged spike trains and block other non-frequency-modulated signals. Both Crick and Koch (1990) and Niebur et al. (1993) assume that selective attention activates competition within a stack or microcolumn of neurons in V4. In the presence of multiple stimuli, neurons will compete with each other. Since the outputs of V1 neurons are tagged, their postsynaptic targets in V4 will win in the V4 level competition. They go on to say that there are no attentional effects on firing rates in V1, only in V4 or higher areas.

The model is quite detailed and provides for quantitative single-cell performance predictions; results of their simulations are in terms of firing rates. The agreement with the relevant experimental data is good. Several major issues arise from this model. First, because the model assumes the selection mechanism of Koch and Ullman, it inherits the timing problems described above. Second, if attentional modulation originates in the subcortical areas, then it is difficult to see how the effects of targets or memory items can be accounted for (Haenny, and Schiller, 1988; Chelazzi et al., 1993). In those studies, single V4 and IT neurons were found that seemed to code the target stimulus and effect the execution of the task. Within both the routing and tagging models, the path lengths required for communication with external gating control in order to affect this influence seem to be wasteful; a closer locus of attentional control seems more likely on this basis.

The Selective Tuning Hypothesis

The *selective tuning hypothesis* claims attention is used to tune the visual processing architecture in order to overcome the problems with pyramid computation and to permit task-directed processing. Selective tuning takes two forms: spatial selection is realized by inhibition of irrelevant connections and feature selection is realized by inhibition of the units that compute nonselected features. The limited space allows only a brief summary in this review article. The interested reader can refer to more detailed accounts (Tsotsos, 1990, 1993b; Culhane and Tsotsos, 1992a,b). The starting point for the model has been described. The search process that localizes the image subset I' is as follows. A winner-take-all process operates across the entire visual field at the top layer: it computes the global winner. The search process then proceeds to the lower levels. The WTA can accept guidance for areas or stimulus qualities to favor if that guidance were available but operates independently otherwise. To localize the global winner in the visual field, a hierarchy of WTA processes is activated. The global winner activates a WTA that operates only over its direct inputs. This localizes the winner within the top-level winning receptive field. In this way, all of the branches of the hierarchy that do not contribute to the winner are pruned. This pruning idea is then applied recursively to successively lower layers. The end result is that from a globally strongest response, the cause of that largest response is localized in the sensory field at the earliest levels. The paths remaining may be considered the pass zone while the pruned paths form the inhibitory zone of an atten-

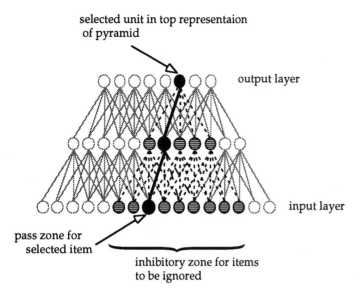

selected unit in top representaion of pyramid

output layer

input layer

pass zone for selected item

inhibitory zone for items to be ignored

Figure 20.2
An illustration of the inhibitory beam of the selective tuning model. The black solid nodes and connections are those selected; the gray open nodes and gray connections are those that are "don't cares," and the dashed connections between the striped nodes are the connections that are inhibited.

tional beam (see figure 20.2). The WTA does not violate biological connectivity constraints. A formal relationship exists between this model and the adaptive beamforming concept of adaptive filter theory used for antenna arrays (Haykin, 1991).

Due to the localizing action of top-down pruning described above, if one were to "record" the output of a unit at the top of the processing pyramid, the time course of the response would show an initial high value, then gradually decrease over time as successively lower layers are pruned away. The decrease would not be due to any suppressive effects acting on this unit; rather, the pruning action of removing parts of its supporting subpyramid leads to a reduction in response over time (qualitatively agreeing with the time course of IT neuron responses as observed by Chelazzi et al., 1993; Gochin et al., 1991; Oram and Perrett, 1992).

The process of selection requires two traversals of the pyramid; the overall time course is consistent with that observed in Chelazzi et al. (1993) (more on this later). These traversals involve

1. Computing pyramid representation in a bottom-up fashion, modified by the biases if available

2. Detecting and localizing the most salient item in a top-down manner, pruning parts of the pyramid that do not contribute to the most salient item, and continuously propagating changes upward

The remainder of this section provides some detail on how this may be accomplished.

The model requires several different types of computing units. Interpretive units compute the visual features. Gating units compute the WTA result across the inputs of a particular interpretive unit and gate winning input through to the next higher interpretive units. Gating control units control the downward flow of selection through the pyramid and are responsible for the signals, which either activate or shut down the WTA processes. Bias units provide top-down, task-related selection via multiplicative inhibition. Figure 20.3 gives the overall architecture that ties these basic units types together. A grouping consisting of one interpretive unit, its associated gating control and bias unit, the set of WTA gating units on the inputs of the interpretive unit, and associated connections will be termed an assembly.

The notation to be used below is now introduced; the figure should be used as a supplement to this description. Physical units are distinguished from their value by the use of a "hat" ("^") where the hatted variable represents the unit, and the same variable without the hat represents the value of the unit. The first subscript gives the layer of the hierarchy in which the unit is found; the second subscript gives the assembly in which the unit is found; the third subscript represents an identifier used to distinguish units within a set. Superscripts always refer to time, in particular, time within the iterations of a given WTA process. Further,

$\hat{I}_{l,k}$ is the interpretive unit in assembly k in layer l; $I_{l,k}$ is its positive real value representing its response;

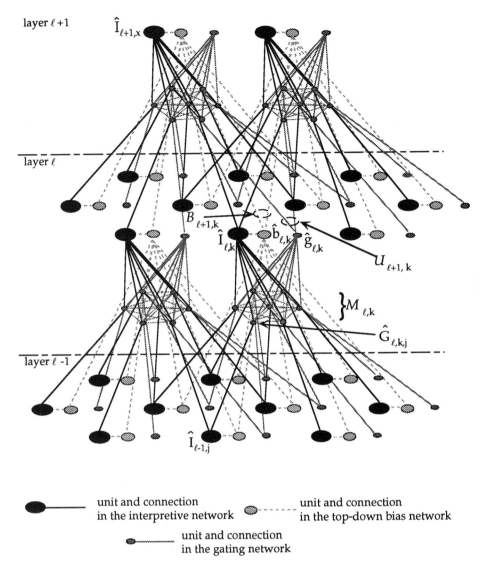

layer ℓ +1 $\hat{I}_{\ell+1,x}$

layer ℓ

$B_{\ell+1,k}$

$\hat{I}_{\ell,k}$ $\hat{b}_{\ell,k}$ $\hat{g}_{\ell,k}$

$U_{\ell+1,k}$

$\}M_{\ell,k}$

$\hat{G}_{\ell,k,j}$

layer ℓ -1

$\hat{I}_{\ell-1,j}$

●——— unit and connection in the interpretive network

◌ - - - - - unit and connection in the top-down bias network

●‧‧‧‧‧‧ unit and connection in the gating network

Figure 20.3
Three layers of the processing pyramid showing the details of the unit and connection types for the selective tuning model. Refer to the text for further description.

$\hat{G}_{l,k,j}$ represents the jth WTA gating unit, in assembly k in layer l linking $\hat{I}_{l,k}$ with $\hat{I}_{l-1,j}$;

$\hat{g}_{l,k}$ is the gating control unit for the WTA over the inputs to $\hat{I}_{l,k}$;

$\hat{b}_{l,k}$ is the bias unit for $\hat{I}_{l,k}$;

$M_{l,k}$ is the set of gating units for unit $\hat{I}_{l,k}$;

$U_{l+1,k}$ is the set of gating units in layer $l + 1$ making efferent connections to $\hat{g}_{l,k}$;

$B_{l+1,k}$ is the set of bias units in layer $l + 1$ making efferent connections to $\hat{b}_{l,k}$.

The standard iterative formulation for a WTA process is (having its roots in Feldman and Ballard, 1982):

$$C_k^t = C_k^{t-1} - \sum_{\substack{i \in V \\ i \neq k}} w_{i,k} C_i^{t-1} \qquad (20.2)$$

where the values of the units in the WTA process ($C_j \in V$ for all defined j) at time t are given by C_k^t, all units are connected to all others, and the relative amount of influence of unit i on unit k is reflected by the weight $w_{i,k}$. All units decay in value with time; the process terminates when all units but one have value of 0.0. In the new formulation of the WTA for the selective tuning model, winning units (there may be more than one) maintain their actual response strength while other units decay. In this way the instantaneous representation of winners in the hierarchy always reflects the actual input. This is accomplished using a simple observation: if the inhibitory signal is based on the response differences, then an implicit but global ordering of response strengths is imposed on the network. The largest item will thus not be inhibited, but will participate in inhibiting all other units. The smallest unit will not inhibit any other units but will be inhibited by all. $\Delta_{i,j}$ represents this contribution based on response differences. The contribution in the WTA from unit i to unit j is set such that

if $0 < \theta < G_{l,k,i}^{t-1} - G_{l,k,j}^{t-1}$ then

$$\Delta_{i,j} = G_{l,k,i}^{t-1} - G_{l,k,j}^{t-1}, \qquad \text{else } \Delta_{i,j} = 0 \qquad (20.3)$$

$G_{l,k,j}^{t}$ is the positive real-valued response of gating unit $\hat{G}_{l,k,j}$ at time t, such that $0 \leqslant G_{l,k,j}^{t}$. θ is a threshold set to

$$\theta = \frac{Z}{2^{\gamma} + 1} \qquad (20.4)$$

assuming that at least one of the values in the competition has value greater than θ and that Z is their maximum possible value. This setting guarantees convergence within at most γ iterations (Tsotsos, 1993b). The WTA stops once the gating units in the competition are partitioned into two classes: those with value zero, and those with value greater than θ but within θ of each other (the winners). Thus, the term $w_{i,k} C_{i}^{t-1}$ is equation (20.2) is replaced by $\Delta_{i,j}$.

The second component of the new WTA rule is the signal for providing top-down bias. $\hat{b}_{l,k}$ is the bias unit for $\hat{I}_{l,k}$ with real-value $b_{l,k} \geqslant 0$ defined by

$$b_{l,k} = \min_{\hat{a} \in B_{l+1,k}} \{a\}. \qquad (20.5)$$

$B_{l+1,k}$ is the set of bias units in layer $l + 1$ making efferent connections to $\hat{b}_{l,k}$. The nature of the bias computation is to inhibit any nonselected units allowing the selected ones to pass through the pyramid without interference. The default value of bias units is 1.0; this value changes only if some other value is inserted at the top of the pyramid due to task information. Since it is assumed that the inhibitory effect is multiplicative, the simplest policy is for bias units to compute the minimum over all top-down bias signals received. Those interpretive units that compute quantities that are not selected are inhibited allowing the selected ones to pass. So, for example, if red items are being sought, the interpretive units that are selective for red stimuli would be unaffected while all other color-selective units would be biased against to some degree.

The WTA is initialized at time t_0 by setting the values of each gating unit to the output of the biased interpretive unit to which it is connected in the layer below

$$G_{l,k,j}^{t_0} = b_{l-1,j} I_{l-1,j} \qquad (20.6)$$

These values are computed on the first traversal of the pyramid (the bottom-up traversal).

The next important component of the new WTA rule is the control signal, which turns the selection process on and off. $\hat{g}_{l,k}$ is the gating control unit for the WTA over the inputs to $\hat{I}_{l,k}$ and has value defined by

if $\sum_{\hat{a} \in U_{l+1,k}} \{a\} > 0$ then $g_{l,k} = 1$,

else $g_{l,k} = 0 \qquad (20.7)$

where the sum is computed after the networks involved have converged. $\hat{g}_{l,k}$ provides top-down control of the WTA processes by selecting the path of the beam's pass zone depending on the winning WTA units in the next higher layer. If the gating control unit has value one, then the WTA process is turned on; otherwise it is turned off. This is implemented by multiplicatively modifying the iterative rule so that if the WTA is off, all updated values are zero. Using this signal at the top of the pyramid, the entire process is controlled. In this way, the gating units are affected but not the interpretive units; only a pathway is closed down. The value of $\hat{g}_{l,k}$ is zero for all units during the first phase of the process (points 1 and 2 of the three-stage algorithm given earlier). During this first phase, the gating units (all the $\hat{G}_{l,k,j}$) are open and the WTAs are all disabled so that the responses computed by the interpretive units based on the stimulus in a bottom-up fashion can pass through the pyramid. Then the value of $\hat{g}_{l,k}$ becomes one for all the units at the top layer turning on the top-most WTA process. The results of this WTA process then determine the values of $\hat{g}_{l,k}$ for the successively lower layers through the application of equation (20.7) for each lower layer in order.

To enforce stability and so that no oscillations occur, the overall result is rectified (negative new unit values are set to zero) by passing the entire right side of equation (20.2) through a rectifying function $\mathbf{R}$ such that

$$\mathbf{R}[x] = x \text{ if } x > 0, \qquad \text{else } \mathbf{R}[x] = 0 \qquad (20.8)$$

Each of the preceding functionalities, including the control signals and the WTA action, are incorporated into a new updating rule so that after the stimulus is presented to the input layer and top-down biases are presented to the top layer, no further actions are required. The rule is given by

$$G_{l,k,j}^{t} = g_{l,k} R\left[G_{l,k,j}^{t-1} - \left(\sum_{\substack{i \in M_{l,k} \\ i \neq j}} \Delta_{i,j} \right) \right] \qquad (20.9)$$

The most important consequence of this new rule is that convergence properties are guaranteed. It was proved in Tsotsos (1993b) that this WTA is guaranteed to converge and to not oscillate. This is possible only because the iterative update is based on differences of units and thus only the largest and second largest values need be considered; a two-unit network is thus easy to characterize. There is no logarithmic dependence on either topographic distance or numbers of competitors, thus providing a much better match to experiments (Kröse and Julesz, 1989; Remington and Pierce, 1984). The actual convergence time is dependent only on differences between strengths of signals in the same sense as that observed by Duncan and Humphreys (1989).

Because of the time course of the gating control signals, they, and in turn the units of the pyramid as well, exhibit an oscillatory pattern in time. If attention can shift every 20–50 msec or so [the time between shifts varies with experiment: Sagi and Julesz (1985) found some inspection times to be as short as 17 msec; Saarinen and Julesz (1991) found good performance at 33 msec; Bergen and Julesz (1983) noted 50 msec], then this is the cycle time of the gating control signal as well. Since gating control is set to 0.0 for part of each selection and to 1.0 for the remainder, the signal is periodic in nature with a frequency of 20–50 Hz. This may be considered as an alternative explanation for the oscillations that motivate the temporal tagging model. This gating signal may be

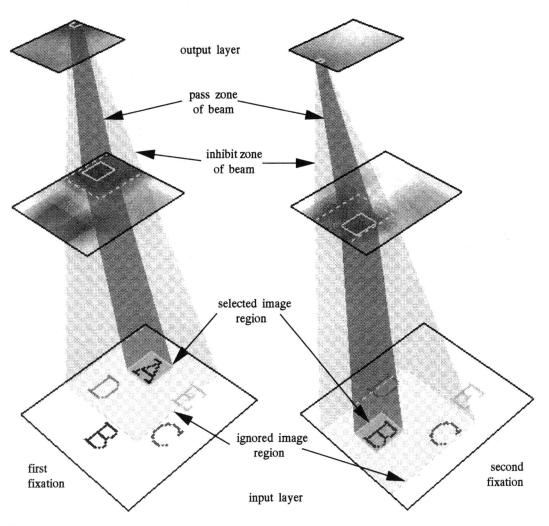

Figure 20.4
A hypothetical pyramid of three layers and a representation of shapes (letters) each with a different luminance. In other words, each letter is made up of pixels all of which are a uniform level of brightness and each letter is of a unique brightness. The selective tuning algorithm finds each in luminance order using the strategy described in the text.

The inhibitory and pass zones of the inhibitory beam are clearly seen in the first two attentional fixations shown (first fixation is on the left). The computations of each of the two layers above the input layer is a simple average luminance.

considered as a sort of system clock to use a computational metaphor.

Finally, it is important to note that this algorithm, under biological connectivity constraints, very closely approximates the provably optimal parallel time complexity for finding the maximum value of a given set (Karp and Ramachandran, 1990).

The computer implementations have successfully tested many components of this mechanism (Culhane and Tsotsos, 1992a,b). An example is shown in figure 20.4 where a hypothetical test network of three layers shows the structure and successive shifts of attention for the inhibitory beam for a representation of saliency that incudes only luminance.

Conclusions

This chapter reviews the major computational hypotheses for the modeling of visual attention. They are all based on similar principles: there is insufficient brain capacity to process all visual stimuli to the same degree of detail; early representations of the scene are computed in parallel and these representations are further inspected by a serial process; selection of items to process is implemented by a winner-take-all mechanism using a representation of saliency based on the early representations; the problem of information flow through a processing pyramid must be solved. Yet, the models accomplish these tasks in very different ways. The main conclusion that can be drawn is that although there seems to be broad agreement regarding the basic foundations of modeling, insufficient biological experimentation has been done at this point that might distinguish one model from another in terms of biological realism. In addition, the functionality of all of the models is limited.

The models have much in common in terms of their performance. For example, each of the models offers a believable explanation for the observations of Moran and Desimone (1985). Each can provide accounts of a variety of human visual search experiments in that serial search processes can be simulated. However, a number of important open questions remain that may help to differentiate the models from one another.

The selective routing and temporal tagging models all assume that control of the process that distinguishes selected signals from the others has a source external to the main processing stream (V1 → V2 → V4 → IT, for example). Although the pulvinar has been implicated as playing a role in visual attention, it is by no means clear that its role is that of producing control signals (see Desimone

et al., 1990). In contrast, the selective tuning model has control originating within the processing stream itself. An argument may be made supporting the latter scheme on the basis of length of connections; computationally, an argument may be made that minimization of overall connection length is important (Tsotsos, 1990).

Further distinguishing characteristics include the following:

1. The Olshausen et al. model assumes that spatial relationships must be preserved (in the topographic sense) while the temporal tagging and selective tuning models do not. These latter models permit spatial abstraction while the former does not, i.e., single units in IT seem to represent complex objects (as observed by Tanaka et al., 1991) as opposed to pixel-like retinal image copies. Spatial abstraction is a major contributor to the reduction of computational complexity (Tsotsos, 1990).

2. Only the selective tuning model explicitly includes top-down bias.

3. Each model comments on the location of saliency representations. Olshausen et al. suggest that the posterior parietal areas act as the saliency map. Niebur at al. claim it is found in superior colliculus or the dorsomedial region of the pulvinar. The selective tuning model assumes each processing layer is its own representation of what is salient.

4. Miller et al. (1993) observed suppression of response in IT neurons in a matching task that occurs within 10 msec of response onset. They conclude that the source of this suppression must be within or before IT. Chelazzi et al. (1993), in a different matching task for IT neurons, observed a first spike after 60–80 msec; 100–120 msec for full strength; 130–200 msec for full inhibitory attentional effect. Both of these works support a top-down version of attention and recognition. The routing and tagging models are bottom-up: only the attended signals ever reach the top. The tuning model relies on the initial signals to reach the top where they are used to guide further processing.

5. Although until very recently it was generally thought that attentional effects were not seen earlier than in V4 neurons (but see Haenny and Schiller, 1988), Motter (1993) has provided evidence to the contrary. This was predicted in the initial description of the selecting tuning model in Tsotsos (1990). Using an experimental paradigm that involved competing stimuli and directed attention, Motter showed that attentional effects are observed in V1, V2, as well as V4 neurons when targets were presented outside the receptive field of the neuron being

recorded. Distance was an important variable; this is the reason for the apparent difference between these results and those of Moran and Desimone (1985). The effect varies depending on the number of competing stimuli and usually manifested itself as a reduction in response if attention is directed away from the recorded neuron. There was no effect for single stimulus displays. These experiments point to a context-dependent view of attentional processing. The selective tuning model is a top-down model, and such effects arise naturally. The routing and tagging models are bottom-up models and it is not obvious how they may account for these results. The Niebur et al. model exhibits no attentional effects before area V4.

6. Schiller (this volume) presents neurophysiological evidence (which is supported by psychophysical evidence in Braun, 1994) that shows that V4 plays a significant role in the selection of less prominent stimuli from the visual scene and that this role is distinctly different than that of area MT. If V4 is lesioned, this function is destroyed for images where the target is a small item in a field of large ones in an odd-man-out task, but only little impairment is observed when the target is large in a field of small items. An MT lesion does not lead to the same effect. Such an observation is a natural one within the selective tuning model. For the large target-small distractors image the large item dominates responses at the top of the pyramid. It is the winner of the top-level WTA. If the target is small in a field of large distractors, however, the large units are the first winners; the small items would never be found unless the selective tuning is operational due to the characteristics of pyramid computation described previously. If V4 is on the path of the inhibitory beam, and it is lesioned, then the beam cannot operate correctly. In the other models, selection of the winner is made from early representations, and the difference between large and small targets would not be seen in this experiment.

The Olshausen et al. version of selective routing requires spacing of connections between layers to double with each layer; otherwise the model violates connectivity constraints. The Niebur et al. temporal tagging model requires the existence of inhibitory frequency-selective interneurons in V4. The selective tuning model requires the existence of local gating networks in each processing layer. It seems that the experimental verification of each of these points is critical for each of the models.

The models collectively form an interesting account of progress in the development of computational models of visual attention; it is clear that much research, both theoretical and experimental, remains.

Acknowledgments

Sean Culhane provided the examples of figure 20.4 with help from Eyal Shavit. I also thank Sean Culhane, Neal Davis, and Winky Wai for manuscript comments. The author is the CP-Unitel Fellow of the Canadian Institute for Advanced Research. This research was funded by the Information Technology Research Center, one of the Province of Ontario Centers of Excellence, the Institute for Robotics and Intelligent Systems, a Network of Centers of Excellence of the Government of Canada.

References

Allport, A. (1989). Visual attention. In M. Posner (Ed.), *Foundations of Cognitive Science* (pp. 631–682). Cambridge, MA: MIT Press.

Anderson, C., and Van Essen, D. (1987). Shifter circuits: A computational strategy for dynamic aspects of visual processing. *Proc. Natl. Acad. Sci. U.S.A. 84*, 6297–6301.

Bergen, J., and Julesz, B. (1983). Parallel versus serial processing in rapid pattern discrimination. *Nature (London) 303*, 696–698.

Braun, J. (1994). Visual search among items of different salience: Removing visual attention mimics a lesion in extrastriate area V4. *J. Neurosci. 14*, 554–567.

Broadbent, D. (1971). *Decision and Stress*. London: Academic Press.

Burt, P. (1988). Attention mechanisms for vision in a dynamic world. *Proc. Int. Conf. Pattern Recognition*, 977–987.

Chelazzi, L., Miller, E., Duncan, J., and Desimone, R. (1993). A neural basis for visual search in inferior temporal cortex. *Nature (London) 363*, 345–347.

Colby, C. (1991). The neuroanatomy and neurophysiology of attention *J. Child Neurol. 6*, S90–S118.

Crick, F., and Koch, C. (1990). Towards a neurobiological theory of consciousness. *Semin. Neurosci. 2*, 263–275.

Culhane, S., and Tsotsos, J. K. (1992a). A prototype for data-driven visual attention. *Proc. 11th Int. Conf.* Pattern Recognition, The Hague, August, 36–40.

Culhane, S., and Tsotsos, J. K. (1992b). An attentional prototype for early vision. *Proc. Second Eur. Conf.* Computer Vision, Santa Margherita Ligure, Italy, May, 551–560.

Desimone, R., Wessinger, M., Thomas, L., and Schneider, W. (1990). Attentional control of visual perception: Cortical and subcortical mechanisms. *Cold Spring Harbor Symp. Quant. Biol. LV*, 963–971.

Dickinson, S., Pentland, A., and Rosenfeld, A. (1992). From volumes to views: An approach to 3-D object recognition. *CVGIP: Image Understanding 55(2)*, 130–154.

Duncan, J., and Humphreys, G. (1989) Visual search and stimulus similarity, *Psychol. Rev. 96(3)*, 433–458.

Feldman, J., and Ballard, D. (1982). Connectionist models and their properties. *Cog. Sci. 6*, 205–254.

Gochin, P., Miller, E., Gross, C., and Gerstein, G. (1991). Functional interactions among neurons in inferior temporal cortex of the awake monkey. *Exp. Brain Res. 84*, 505–516.

Haenny, P., and Schiller, P. (1988). State dependent activity in money visual cortex I. Single cell activity in V1 and V4 on visual tasks. *Exp. Brain Res. 69*, 225–244.

Haenny, P., Maunsell, J., and Schiller, P. (1988). State dependent activity in monkey visual cortex II. Retinal and extraretinal factors in V4. *Exp. Brain Res. 69*, 245–259.

Haykin, S. (1991). *Adaptive Filter Theory*, 2nd ed. Englewood Cliffs, NJ: Prentice Hall.

Hopfield, J. (1982). Neural networks and physical systems with emergent collective computational abilities. *Proc. Natl. Acad. Sci. U.S.A. 79*, 2554–2558.

Julesz, B., and Bergen, J. (1983). Textons, the fundamental elements in preattentive vision and perception of textures. *Bell Syst. Tech. J. 62(6)*, Part II: 1619–1645.

Karp, R., and Ramachandran, V. (1990). Parallel algorithms for shared-memory machines. In J. van Leeuwen (Ed.), *Handbook of Theoretical Computer Science: Vol. A: Algorithms and Complexity* (pp. 871–941). Cambridge, MA: MIT Press.

Koch, C., and Ullman, S. (1985). Shifts in selective visual attention: Towards the underlying neural circuitry. *Human Neurobiol. 4*, 219–227.

Kröse, B., and Julesz, B. (1989). The control and speed of shifts of attention. *Vision Res. 29(11)*, 1607–1619.

Marr, D. (1982). *Vision*. San Francisco: W.H. Freeman.

Miller, E., Li, L., and Desimone, R. (1993). Activity of neurons in anterior inferior temporal cortex during a short-term memory task. *J. Neurosci. 13(4)*, 1460–1478.

Moran, J., and Desimone, R. (1985). Selective attention gates visual processing in the extrastriate cortex. *Science 229*, 782–784.

Motter, B. (1993). Focal attention produces spatially selective processing in visual cortical areas V1, V2 and V4 in the presence of competing stimuli. *J. Neurophysiol. 70(3)*, 909–919.

Nakayama, K. (1991). The iconic bottleneck and the tenuous link between early visual processing and perception. In C. Blakemore (Ed.), *Vision: Coding and Efficiency* (pp. 411–422). Cambridge: Cambridge University Press.

Niebur, E., Koch, C., and Rosin, C. (1993). An oscillation-based model for the neuronal basis of attention. *Vision Res. 33(18)*, 2789–2802.

Nothdurft, H.-C. (1993). Saliency effects across dimensions in visual search. *Vision Res. 33(5/6)*, 839–844.

Olshausen, B., Anderson, C., and Van Essen, D. (1993). A neurobiological model of visual attention and invariant pattern recognition based on dynamic routing of information. *J. Neurosci. 13(11)*, 4700, 4719.

Oram, M., and Perrett, D. (1992). Time course of neural responses discriminating different views of the face and head. *J. Neurophysiol. 68(1)*, 70–84.

Remington, R, and Pierce, L. (1984). Moving attention: Evidence for time-invariant shifts of visual selective attention. *Percept Psychophys. 35(4)*, 393–399.

Saarinen, J., and Julesz, B. (1991). The speed of attentional shifts in the visual field. *Proc. Natl. Acad. Sci. U.S.A. 88*, 1812–1814.

Sagi, D., and Julesz, B. (1985). "Where" and "What" in vision, *Science 228*, 1217–1219.

Tanaka, K., Saito, H., Fukada, Y., and Moriya, M. (1991). Coding visual images of objects in the inferotemporal cortex of the macaque monkey. *J. Neurophysiol. 66(1)*, 170–187.

Tsotsos, J. (1988). A 'complexity level' analysis of immediate vision. *Int. J. Comput. Vision 1(4)*, 303–320.

Tsotsos, J. K. (1989). The complexity of perceptual search tasks. *Proc. Int. J. Conf. Artificial Intelligence*, Detroit, 1571–1577.

Tsotsos, J. K. (1990). Analyzing vision at the complexity level. *Behav. Brain Sci. 13(3)*, 423–469.

Tsotsos, J. K. (1992). Is complexity theory appropriate for analyzing biological systems? *Behav. Brain Sci. 14(4)*, 770–773.

Tsotsos, J. K. (1993a). The role of computational complexity in understanding perception. In S. Masin (Ed.), *Foundations of Perceptual Theory* (pp. 261–296). Amsterdam: North-Holland.

Tsotsos, J. K. (1993b). An inhibitory beam for attentional selection. In L. Harris and M. Jenkin (Ed.), *Spatial Vision in Humans and Robots* (pp. 313–331). Cambridge: Cambridge University Press.

Uhr, L. (1972). Layered 'recognition cone' networks that preprocess, classify and describe. *IEEE Transact. Comput. C-21*, 758–768.

21

Neuronal Mechanisms of Visual Attention

Robert Desimone,
Leonardo Chelazzi, Earl K. Miller,
and John Duncan

Over the past two decades, research in visual neuroscience has established that the visual cortex has a massively parallel architecture, with feature-analyzing modules replicated throughout the cortical representation of the visual field, in each of several visual areas (for a review, see Desimone and Ungerleider, 1989). Yet, during this same time period, work in human vision by Julesz, Treisman, Posner, Sperling, and other psychologists (e.g., Posner, 1978, 1982; Sperling and Melchner, 1978; Bergen and Julesz, 1983; Julesz, 1990, 1991a, 1991b; Treisman and Souther, 1985; Treisman, 1986, 1988; Reeves and Sperling, 1986) demonstrated that the visual system is severely limited in its capacity to fully process and recognize more than one object in the visual field at a time. Instead, objects in the visual field must compete for focal attention, and the winner of this competition is determined by both bottom-up and top-down mechanisms. In this chapter, we will briefly review the role of attention in the neural systems for object recognition, we will then describe how mechanisms for visual memory may influence attentional systems, and, finally, we will describe some recent results on the neural mechanisms for visual search, which is a task in which memory and attention interact in a cooperative fashion.

Neurophysiological studies in monkeys are beginning to reveal how attention controls visual processing in the "ventral processing stream," which subserves object recognition in the cortex (Ungerleider and Mishkin, 1982), particularly extrastriate area V4 and the inferior temporal (IT) cortex. In both of these areas, when attention is directed at one location within the receptive field of a neuron, responses to stimuli at other locations within the receptive field are suppressed (Moran and Desimone, 1985). The cells act as though their receptive field "shrinks" around the attended location, with unattended stimuli being filtered out. This presumably explains why we have little awareness of unattended stimuli.

How does this attentional control over neurons come about? Recent work suggests that the competitive interactions among objects in a crowded scene are paralleled by competitive interactions among neurons within the visual system (Desimone et al., 1990; Desimone, 1992a). This competition can be biased in various ways, such that the neurons processing one object win out and that object becomes the primary recipient of cortical processing. One bottom-up neuronal mechanism that might tip the balance of processing toward one object is the interaction between the receptive field and its surround, a property of neurons in many parts of the visual system (Allman et al., 1985; Desimone et al., 1985; Desimone and Schein, 1987; Schein and Desimone, 1990; Knierim and Van Essen, 1992). Such cells have large suppressive regions surrounding their receptive fields, and the sensory properties of the surround and receptive field are matched. Thus, cells give their largest response to an optimal stimulus within the field that differs from stimuli in the surround (e.g., a red spot on a green surround, or a vertical bar on a field of horizontal bars). These mechanisms almost certainly contribute to preattentive image segmentation, or "pop-out," described by Julesz (1981, 1986, 1990, 1991b), Treisman and her colleagues (Treisman and Souther, 1985; Treisman, 1986; Treisman and Gormican, 1988), and others. The other way competition among neurons can be biased is by top-down selection mechanisms, in which objects are voluntarily selected for focal attention on the basis of their spatial location or their features.

Most neurophysiological work on the control of attention has been concentrated on spatially directed attention. Many of the structures associated with spatial attention are part of the "dorsal" processing stream in the cortex, which subserves spatial vision (Ungerleider and Mishkin, 1982). Because the targets of our gaze and our attention are usually linked, it is not surprising that many of the structures implicated in spatial attention are also implicated in the control of gaze, including the superior colliculus, posterior parietal cortex, the striatum, the pulvinar, and portions of prefrontal cortex (for reviews, see Robinson and McClurkin, 1989; Posner and Petersen, 1990; Desimone et al., 1990; Colby, 1992). Neurons in most of these structures are preferentially activated when attention is directed to points in their receptive fields. These structures presumably send (directly or indirectly) the appropriate spatial control signals to areas such as V4 and IT cortex, biasing cells in these areas so that any object at the attended location is processed preferentially over others and becomes the object of focal attention.

Recently, direct neural evidence for these biasing signals has been found in area V4 (Luck et al., 1993). Whenever attention is directed to a location within the receptive field of a neuron in this area, that neuron shows an increase in its maintained level of discharge, even in the absence of any sensory stimulus. The amount of change in activity appears to be roughly proportional to the dis-

tance from the focus of attention to the center of the receptive field. When a stimulus subsequently occurs at the attended location, the neuron is primed to respond to it, responses to stimuli at unattended locations in the receptive field being reduced.

Whether the suppression of unattended stimuli results from local competitive interactions among cells in V4 itself, or among the inputs to V4 cells, is still not known. The fact that the biasing mechanism works at a higher spatial resolution than the size of V4 receptive fields (since it is strongest when attention is directed to the center of the receptive field) suggests it may affect the inputs into V4, although one can imagine schemes achieving high spatial resolution through interactions among cells with partially overlapping receptive fields. It has recently been reported that attention affects the responses of cells in both V1 and V2, although the evidence for at least V1 is controversial (Motter, 1993; but cf. Moran and Desimone, 1985). Several neural models have been proposed to explain this gating of response with attention (Crick and Koch, 1990; Desimone, 1992a; Niebur et al., 1993; Olshausen et al., 1993; Tsotsos, this volume), but there is currently insufficient physiological data to distinguish among them.

Memory and Attention

Although spatially directed attention has proven to be an excellent model system for investigating attentional mechanisms, objects can also be selected for attention based on nonspatial features. Recent work indicates that this sort of attention depends, in part, on neural mechanisms for memory, since it is what we learn and remember of objects that determines their behavioral relevance, their familiarity and novelty, how well they segregate from background elements, and so on. When we attentively search a scene for a particular object (such as searching for the face of our friend in a crowd of people), it is our memory of the object that guides our attention. In this context, "working memory" and "attentive selection" may be just two aspects of the same neural mechanism, as will be clear from the descriptions below (in the same spirit, the neural system for spatial attention mentioned above involves working memory for spatial location as well, but we will not consider this here).

Neurophysiological studies have revealed a wide range of neural mechanisms underlying memory formation, any of which might influence attention and the competition among objects in the visual field in a bottom-up and top-down manner. Some of these memory mechanisms are

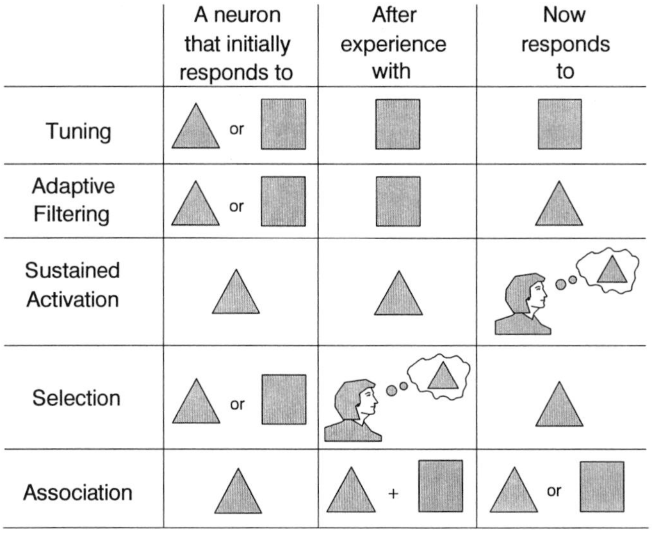

	A neuron that initially responds to	After experience with	Now responds to
Tuning	△ or ▢	▢	▢
Adaptive Filtering	△ or ▢	▢	△
Sustained Activation	△	△	(thinking) △
Selection	△ or ▢	(thinking) △	△
Association	△	△ + ▢	△ or ▢

Figure 21.1

Five of the ways in which neuronal activity is modified during the formation or expression of memory traces. (Adapted from Desimone, 1992b.)

explicit, or cognitive, whereas others are probably implicit and underlie noncognitive memory such as priming and perception learning. We have divided these memory mechanisms into five classes, which we will refer to as tuning, adaptive filtering, sustained activation, selection, and association (Desimone, 1992b).

The five mechanisms are illustrated in figure 21.1, which shows the response of hypothetical neurons to hypothetical stimuli before, during, and after an organism has had some type of experience with them. We will briefly review all five mechanisms in order of increasing "cognitive" involvement, with an emphasis on the three mechanisms that touch most closely on our own work, namely adaptive filtering, selection, and sustained activation.

Tuning

Tuning mechanisms come into play as a result of sensory experience or perceptual learning. Neurons in the auditory cortex of animals classically conditioned to specific tones, for example, tend to shift their preferred tone frequency to that of the conditioned stimulus (Bakin and Weinberger, 1990). Likewise, animals taught tactile discriminations develop enlarged representations of the relevant portion of their body in somatosensory cortex, and, in some cases, the receptive fields of neurons in that region sharpen (Merzenich et al., 1990). So far, the evidence for tuning mechanisms in adult animals comes from sensory systems other than vision, but there is no reason to suppose that they do not occur in vision as well.

Because tuning shifts the weight of cortical processing toward the learned item, it is likely to cause a shift in attentional weighting as well. If we practice finding a visual stimulus composed of a particular texture gradient, for example, that stimulus will tend to "pop out" from a texture field and will be found in shorter and shorter time (Shiffrin and Schneider, 1977; Karni and Sagi, 1991, 1993; Sagi, this volume).

Adaptive Filtering

In adaptive filtering, incoming sensory information is filtered by neurons according to how similar it is to information already held in either short- or long-term memory. In monkeys, for example, some of the neurons in IT cortex that respond selectively to particular object features, such as a specific color or shape, give their best response to objects that contain those features but that are new, unexpected, or not recently seen (Baylis and Rolls, 1987; Riches et al., 1991; Miller et al., 1991, 1993; Eskandar et al., 1992). As new stimuli become familiar, synaptic weights in the cortex appear to adjust so that the neuronal response is dampened, a case of "familiarity breeding contempt" at the neuronal level. As a result, increasing familiarity causes a "focusing" of activity in the cortex, such that familiar objects cause the most restricted activation (Miller et al., 1991; Li et al., 1993). The neurons remaining within this new focus of activation are presumably those that communicate the most critical information about the object, the noncritical neurons having been weeded out of the pool of highly activated cells.

Although identifying novel objects in the environment is probably not the primary function of these "adaptive filter" neurons, they may nonetheless serve this purpose for attentional control. The enhanced activation of these cells to novel stimuli will presumably give those cells (and the cells receiving their outputs) an advantage in any neural competition, shifting the attentional focus to the new items in the scene (figure 21.2). As the organism increases contact with the item, the memory will be strengthened, synaptic weights will adjust, and the activation of the adaptive filter cells will decrease, reducing the drive on attentional systems in turn. This will free the system to shift attention to the next new item.

Based on this work, one could view memory as an early filter that influences the processing of stimuli throughout the visual field, including their ability to compete for focal attention. Evidence for preattentive segregation of items based on their novelty and familiarity was recently found by Wang et al. (1992), who report that subjects can find a novel letter on a background of familiar ones with a reaction time that is nearly independent of

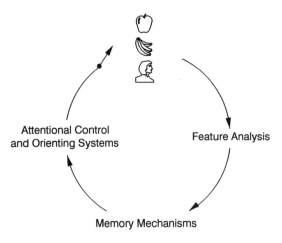

Figure 21.2
Interaction between systems for memory and attention. Information from multiple objects in a scene enters the visual system in a parallel fashion. These inputs may engage at least two cortical memory mechanisms, adaptive mnemonic filtering and selection. The adaptive mnemonic filter cells will respond preferentially to stimuli that are new or that have not been recently seen. This leads to increased attention and, typically, foveation of the new stimulus. As the stimulus becomes familiar, activation of the adaptive memory cells decreases, reducing the drive on the attentional systems and freeing the system to process other, competing stimuli. The cells engaged in selection may be preset to detect a specific relevant stimulus. When the stimulus appears, these cells are preferentially activated, causing attention to be directed to the relevant item. The interplay between the two mechanisms will determine the object that is attended and foveated.

the number of background elements (also see Reicher et al., 1976).

Selection

While adaptive filtering mechanisms may bias the organism toward novel items, often we must suppress orienting to novel items and attend to a familiar, relevant, one. Attention to relevant items appears to involve selection mechanisms, which are called into play when neurons are prepared, or primed, to respond to an expected stimulus that is behaviorally relevant.

This mechanism has been revealed in a particular variation of the delayed matching to sample task (Miller and Desimone, 1994). In this task, monkeys were instructed to signal when a particular object was repeated in a temporal sequence, ignoring other, irrelevant, stimulus repetitions. A subpopulation of IT neurons selective for object features such as shape, color, or texture gave enhanced responses to objects that both contained those features and also matched the item that the animal was searching for in the sequence. These cells appeared to be primed, or preset, to give an enhanced response to just the one object that the monkey was searching for and not to other, irrelevant, stimulus repetitions.

This population of enhanced cells was a separate population from the adaptive filter cells, which exist in the same cortex. In the same delayed matching task, the adaptive filter cells were suppressed by any stimulus repetition in the sequence, behaviorally relevant or not. Thus, there appear to be two parallel mechanisms for short-term memory in IT cortex, an automatic one that may bias the organism toward novel or unexpected stimuli and an active one, or "working memory," that may bias the organism toward a particular important or relevant stimuli. The interplay between these two mechanisms may determine the objects that we attend to (see figure 21.2).

Sustained Activation

Sustained activation appears to be closely related to the selection mechanism. In sustained activation, neurons are activated when previously stored stimuli are needed for working memory, but the stimuli are no longer available. For example, in parts of ventral prefrontal cortex, neurons that respond to specific objects may remain activated when the object is no longer present, as long as the monkey must hold that object "in mind" (Fuster, 1973; Fuster et al., 1982; Wilson et al., 1993; Chelazzi et al., 1993b). Comparable results have been reported for other parts of prefrontal cortex when monkeys hold a particular spatial location in mind (Fuster, 1973; Fuster et al., 1982; Funahashi et al., 1989) and in several sensorimotor structures when animals must delay a particular behavioral response.

The sustained activation mechanisms in prefrontal cortex may be one source of the neural bias signal that prepares IT neurons for expected visual objects, i.e., the cells showing enhanced responses to expected stimuli described earlier. A likely scheme is that the process of keeping an object in mind is associated with prefrontal activation, which in turn biases specific visual neurons in IT cortex and elsewhere to respond to specific expected stimuli in a scene, improving the chances of these biased cells winning in any neural competition. In some tasks, IT cells themselves show evidence of maintained activation in the absence of any stimuli (Fuster and Jervey, 1981; Miyashita and Chang, 1988; Miller et al., 1993) but unlike in prefrontal cortex it is easily disrupted when the animal views other stimuli (Miller et al., 1993; Chelazzi et al., 1993b).

Association

Finally, associative mechanisms are engaged as a result of pairings of different sensory stimuli. If two arbitrary visual stimuli occur repeatedly within a short time of each other, neurons in IT cortex will tend to respond to both of them more commonly than would be expected by chance pairings of responses (Miyashita, 1988). Associative mechanisms may also interact with sustained activation ones. When monkeys are taught that a picture of an apple is always followed by a picture of a banana, for example, presentation of the apple causes a sustained activation of some of the IT neurons that would normally respond only to the banana (Sakai and Miyashita, 1991). It is as though the occurrence of one stimulus automatically brings to mind the other. This suggests a role for these associative and sustained mechanisms in associative recall from long-term memory.

Visual Search

The interaction of neural systems for attention and memory is nowhere more apparent than in visual search. In the type of visual search we are considering, a representation of an object stored in memory is used to guide search of an external array of objects—like searching for a face in a crowd. Because the visual search task raises so many questions that are central to understanding attention, we will consider one recent study of ours in some detail (Chelazzi et al., 1993a).

We tested monkeys in a visual search task and recorded from IT neurons in the same region in which we found evidence for adaptive mnemonic filtering and selection mechanisms in memory tasks. The monkey was first shown a digitized picture of an object, briefly presented as a cue at the center of gaze. After a short, blank, delay period, an array of two to five stimuli was presented a few degrees from fixation and the monkey was rewarded for making a saccadic eye movement to the object (target) that matched the previous cue. The other array elements were also digitized objects, which were similar enough to the target that the latter did not "pop out."

For each cell, at least one of the array elements was chosen to be a "good" stimulus for the cell (i.e., one that would elicit a good response if presented alone), and at least one was chosen to be a "poor" stimulus (i.e., one that would elicit little or no response if presented alone). We asked how both the cue and target were represented in IT cortex, when either the good or poor stimulus was used as the cue and target.

As shown in figure 21.3, the good cue elicited a good response from the cells and the poor cue elicited little or no response, on average, as expected. Following the good cue, many cells had higher maintained activity during the delay than following the poor cue. This is the same sustained activation phenomenon found in memory studies

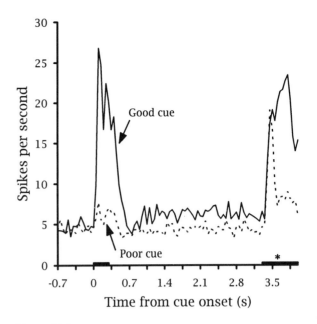

Figure 21.3

Graphs show average firing rates of a population of 22 cells recorded from anterior inferior temporal cortex while monkeys performed a visual search task. The cue was chosen to be either a good or a poor stimulus for the recorded cell and was presented at the center of gaze. After a delay, an array of two choice stimuli was presented peripherally, one of which was a good stimulus and one a poor stimulus for the cell. The animal made a saccadic eye movement to the stimulus (target) that matched the cue. The dark line shows responses on trials in which the good stimulus was the cue-target, and the dashed line shows responses on trials with the poor stimulus. The two dark horizontal bars indicate when the cue stimulus and choice array were presented. The average saccadic latency to the target was 300 msec, indicated by the asterisk. Cells had a higher maintained firing rate in the delay preceding the choice array when their preferred stimulus was the cue. Following the delay, cells were equally activated, on the average, by their preferred stimulus in the choice array, regardless of whether it was the target. However, 200 msec later (or about 100 msec before the eye movement was made), responses diverged depending on whether the target was the good or the poor stimulus.

and presumably reflects the animal's active maintenance of the memory trace of the cue.

When the choice array appeared, it initially activated IT cells regardless of whether the good or poor stimulus was the target, on the average. Thus, it seems as though all of the items in the array initially activate whatever cells in IT cortex are selective for their properties. However, by about 200 msec after array onset, responses to the array diverge depending on whether a good or poor stimulus for the recorded neuron is the target on that trial. If the good stimulus is the target, the response of the cell remains high (continuing through the time that the eye movement is made), but if the poor stimulus is the target, the response is suppressed down to nearly the baseline firing rate. It is as though 200 msec after array onset, the

Desimone et al.: Neuronal Mechanisms of Attention

target "captures" the responses of IT cells, so that they carry information about this stimulus alone. Since this divergence precedes the eye movement to the target by about 100 msec, IT cortex is potentially the source of the target information for the oculomotor system (Glimcher and Sparks, 1992; Schall and Hanes, 1993).

What is the cause of the divergence in IT response, leading to suppression of nontarget information? Although we cannot be sure of the cause, we find during the search task all of the mnemonic mechanisms at play in IT cortex that we find in our studies of memory.

First, as mentioned above, we see information about the cue-target reflected in the maintained firing rate of cells during the delay, presumably reflecting active maintenance of the memory trace. This higher maintained activity during the delay persists into the response to the choice array itself, presumably giving the cells coding the target a competitive advantage.

Second, we find cells showing adaptive mnemonic filtering. These cells show reduced activation by the choice array when the good stimulus is the target (compared to when it is a nontarget), presumably because the good target stimulus was recently seen in this case (as the cue). These cells may be helpful in grouping the nontargets.

Finally, we find cells showing evidence of the selection mechanism. The response of these cells to the choice array is potentiated at the very onset of the response when the good stimulus is the target, presumably because the cells were biased, or preset, to respond to it. The initially suppressed responses of the adaptive filter cells and the initially enhanced responses of the selection cells cancel each other out in the population average histogram shown in figure 21.3. Nonetheless, the information is present in the activity of individual cells in the population as soon as the choice array is presented and presumably affects competition among neural elements in IT cortex.

A critical question is whether the late suppression of IT responses to nontargets is the cause or the effect of focal attention being attracted to the target. According to some accounts of search, focal attention is used to "scrutinize" the elements in the array serially, locking onto the target when it is recognized (e.g., Bergen and Julesz, 1983; Treisman and Souther, 1985; Treisman, 1986, 1988; Julesz, 1990, 1991a). According to other accounts, the array elements are processed in parallel by a competitive network, and prior information about the target (i.e., the cue) is used to bias the competition toward the neural elements that represent it (e.g., Duncan and Humphreys, 1989; Bundesen, 1992). The winner of the competition then becomes the object of focal attention. Unfortunately, our data do not allow us to decide between these possibil-

ities conclusively. We can say only that the three memory effects in IT described above seem to be sufficient to identify the target element without invoking an external mechanism that serializes the process. In fact, our neural results may represent the actions of both serial and parallel processes—early selection of the target based on parallel processing of memory mechanisms within the first 200 msec or so, and later suppression of nontargets based on inputs from a focal attention system.

Acknowledgment

This work was supported in part by the Human Frontiers Science Program Organization.

References

Allman, J., Miezin, F., and McGuinness, E. (1985). Stimulus specific responses from beyond the classical receptive field: Neurophysiological mechanisms for local-global comparisons in visual neurons. *Annu. Rev. Neurosci. 8*, 407–430.

Bakin, J. S., and Weinberger, N. M. (1990). Classical conditioning induces CS-specific receptive field plasticity in the auditory cortex of the guinea pig. *Brain Res. 536*, 271–286.

Baylis, G. C., and Rolls, E. T. (1987). Responses of neurons in the inferior temporal cortex in short term and serial recognition memory tasks. *Exp. Brain Res. 65*, 614–622.

Bergen, J. R., and Julesz, B. (1983). Parallel versus serial processing in rapid pattern discrimination. *Nature (London) 303*, 696–698.

Bundesen, C. (1992). A theory of visual attention. *Psychol. Rev. 97*, 523–547.

Chelazzi, L., Miller, E. K., Duncan, J., and Desimone, R. (1993a). A neural basis for visual search in inferior temporal cortex. *Nature (London) 363*, 345–347.

Chelazzi, L., Miller, E. K., Lueschow, A., and Desimone, R. (1993b). Dual mechanisms of short-term memory: Ventral prefrontal cortex. *Soc. Neurosci. Abstr. 19*, 975.

Colby, C. L. (1992). The neuroanatomy and neurophysiology of attention. *J. Child Neurol. 6*, s90–s118.

Crick, F., and Koch, C. (1990). Some reflections on visual awareness. *Cold Spring Harbor Symp. Quant. Biol. 55*, 953–962.

Desimone, R. (1992a). Neural circuits for visual attention in the primate brain. In G. A. Carpenter and S. Grossberg (Eds.), *Neural Networks for Vision and Image Processing* (pp. 343–364). Cambridge: MIT Press.

Desimone, R. (1992b). The physiology of memory—Recordings of things past. *Science 258*, 245–246.

Desimone, R., and Schein, S. J. (1987). Visual properties of neurons in area V4 of the macaque: Sensitivity to stimulus form. *J. Neurophysiol. 57*, 835–868.

Desimone, R., and Ungerleider, L. G. (1989). Neural mechanisms of visual processing in monkeys. In F. Boller and J. Grafman (Eds.), *Handbook of Neuropsychology* (Vol. 2, pp. 267–299). New York: Elsevier.

Desimone, R., Schein, S. J., Moran, J., and Ungerleider, L. G. (1985). Contour, color and shape analysis beyond the striate cortex. *Vision Res.* 25, 441–452.

Desimone, R., Wessinger, M., Thomas, L., and Schneider, W. (1990). Attentional control of visual perception: Cortical and subcortical mechanisms. *Cold Spring Harbor Symp. Quant. Biol.* 55, 963–971.

Duncan, J., and Humphreys, G. W. (1989). Visual search and similarity. *Psychol. Rev.* 96, 433–458.

Eskandar, E. E., Richmond, B. J., and Optican, L. M. (1992). Role of inferior temporal neurons in visual memory: I. Temporal encoding of information about visual images, recalled images, and behavioral context. *J. Neurophysiol.* 68, 1277–1295.

Funahashi, S., Bruce, C. J., and Goldman-Rakic, P. S. (1989). Mnemonic coding of visual space in the monkey's dorsolateral prefrontal cortex. *J. Neurophysiol.* 61, 331–349.

Fuster, J. M. (1973). Unit activity in prefrontal cortex during delayed-response performance: Neuronal correlates of transient memory. *J. Neurophysiol.* 36, 61–78.

Fuster, J. M., and Jervey, J. P. (1981). Inferotemporal neurons distinguish and retain behaviorally relevant features of visual stimuli. *Science* 212, 952–955.

Fuster, J. M., Bauer, R. H., and Jervey, J. P. (1982). Cellular discharge in the dorsolateral prefrontal cortex of the monkey in cognitive tasks. *Exp. Neurol.* 77, 679–694.

Glimcher, P. W., and Sparks, D. L. (1992). Movement selection in advance of action in the superior colliculus. *Nature (London)* 355, 542–545.

Julesz, B. (1981). Textons, the elements of texture perception, and their interactions. *Nature (London)* 290, 91–97.

Julesz, B. (1986). Texton gradients: the texton theory revisited. *Biol. Cybern.* 54, 245–251.

Julesz, B. (1990). Early vision is bottom-up, except for focal attention. *Cold Spring Harbor Symp. Quant. Biol.* 55, 973–978.

Julesz, B. (1991a). Some strategic questions in visual perception. In A. Gorea (Ed.), *Representations in Vision: Trends and Tacit Assumptions in Vision Research* (pp. 331–349). Cambridge, England: Cambridge University Press.

Julesz, B. (1991b). Early vision and focal attention. *Rev. Modern Phys.* 63, 735–772.

Karni, A., and Sagi, D. (1991). Where practice makes perfect in texture discrimination: Evidence for primary visual cortex plasticity. *Proc. Natl. Acad. Sci. U.S.A.* 88, 4966–4970.

Karni, A., and Sagi, D. (1993). The time course of learning a visual skill. *Nature (London)* 365, 250–252.

Knierim, J. J., and Van Essen, D. C. (1992). Neuronal responses to static texture patterns in area V1 of the alert macaque monkey. *J. Neurophysiol.* 67, 961–980.

Li, L., Miller, E. K., and Desimone, R. (1993). The representation of stimulus familiarity in anterior inferior temporal cortex. *J. Neurophysiol.* 69, 1918–1929.

Luck, S. J., Chelazzi, L., Hillyard, S. A., and Desimone, R. (1993). Effects of spatial attention in area V4 of the macaque. *Soc. Neurosci. Abstr.* 19, 27.

Merzenich, M. M., Recanzone, G. H., Jenkins, W. M., and Grajski, K. A. (1990). Adaptive mechanisms in cortical networks underlying cortical contributions to learning and nondeclarative memory. *Cold Spring Harbor Symp. Quant. Biol.* 55, 873–887.

Miller, E. K., and Desimone, R. (1994). Parallel neuronal mechanisms for short-term memory. *Science* 263, 520–522.

Miller, E. K., Li, L., and Desimone, R. (1991). A neural mechanism for working and recognition memory in inferior temporal cortex. *Science* 254, 1377–1379.

Miller, E. K., Li, L., and Desimone, R. (1993). Activity of neurons in anterior inferior temporal cortex during a short-term memory task. *J. Neurosci.* 13, 1460–1478.

Miyashita, Y. (1988). Neuronal correlate of visual associative long-term memory in the primate temporal cortex. *Nature (London)* 335, 817–820.

Miyashita, Y., and Chang, H. S. (1988). Neuronal correlate of pictorial short-term memory in the primate temporal cortex. *Nature (London)* 331, 68–70.

Moran, J., and Desimone, R. (1985). Selective attention gates visual processing in the extrastriate cortex. *Science* 229, 782–784.

Motter, B. C. (1993). Focal attention produces spatially selective processing in visual cortical areas V1, V2, and V4 in the presence of competing stimuli. *J. Neurophysiol.* 70, 909–919.

Niebur, E., Koch, C., and Rosin, C. (1993). An oscillation-based model for the neuronal basis of attention. *Vision Res.* 33, 2789–2802.

Olshausen, B. A., Anderson, C. H., and Van Essen, D. C. (1993). A neurobiological model of visual attention and invariant pattern recognition based on dynamic routing of information. *J. Neurosci.* 13, 4700–4719.

Posner, M. I. (1978). *Chronometric Explorations of Mind.* Englewood Cliffs, NJ: Erlbaum.

Posner, M. I. (1982). Cumulative development of attentional theory. *Am. Psychol.* 32, 53–64.

Posner, M. I., and Petersen, S. E. (1990). The attention system of the human brain. *Annu. Rev. Neurosci.* 13, 25–42.

Reeves, A., and Sperling, G. (1986). Attention gating in short-term visual memory. *Psychol. Rev.* 93, 180–206.

Reicher, G. M., Snyder, C. R. R., and Richards, J. T. (1976). Familiarity of background characters in visual scanning. *J. Exp. Psychol. Human Percept. Perform.* 2, 522–530.

Riches, I. P., Wilson, F. A., and Brown, M. W. (1991). The effects of visual stimulation and memory on neurons of the hippocampal formation and the neighboring parahippocampal gyrus and inferior temporal cortex of the primate. *J. Neurosci.* 11, 1763–1779.

Robinson, D. L., and McClurkin, J. W. (1989). The visual superior colliculus and pulvinar. In R. Wurtz and M. E. Goldberg (Eds.), *The Neurobiology of Sacadic Eye Movements* (pp. 337–360). New York: Elsevier.

Sakai, K., and Miyashita, Y. (1991). Neural organization for the long-term memory of paired associates. *Nature (London)* 354, 152–155.

Desimone et al.: Neuronal Mechanisms of Attention

Schall, J. D., and Hanes, D. P. (1993). Neural basis of target selection in frontal eye field during visual search. *Nature (London) 366*, 467–469.

Schein, S. J., and Desimone, R. (1990). Spectral properties of V4 neurons in the macaque. *J. Neurosci. 10*, 3369–3389.

Shiffrin, R. M., and Schneider, W. (1977). Controlled and automatic human information processing: II. Perceptual learning, automatic attending, and a general theory. *Psychol. Rev. 84*, 127–190.

Sperling, G., and Melchner, M. J. (1978). The attention operating characteristic: Examples from visual search. *Science 202*, 315–318.

Treisman, A. (1986). Features and objects in visual processing. *Sci. Am. 255*, 114–125.

Treisman, A. (1988). Features and objects: The fourteenth Bartlett memorial lecture. *Quart. J. Exp. Psychol. 40*, 201–237.

Treisman, A., and Gormican, S. (1988). Feature analysis in early vision: Evidence from search asymmetries. *Psychol. Rev. 95*, 15–48.

Treisman, A., and Souther, J. (1985). Search asymmetry: A diagnostic for preattentive processing of separable features. *J. Exp. Psychol. [Gen.] 114*, 285–310.

Ungerleider, L. G., and Mishkin, M. (1982). Two cortical visual systems. In J. Ingle, M. A. Goodale, and R. J. W. Mansfield (Eds.), *Analysis of Visual Behavior* (pp. 549–586). Cambridge: MIT Press.

Wang, Q., Cavanagh, P., and Green, M. (1992). Familiarity and pop-out in visual search. *Assoc. Res. Vision Ophthamol. Abstr. 33*, 1262.

Wilson, F. A. W., O Scalaidhe, S. P., and Goldman-Rakic, P. S. (1993). Dissociation of object and spatial processing domains in primate prefrontal cortex. *Science 260*, 1955–1958.

22

Perceptual Correlates of Neural Plasticity in the Adult Human Brain

V. S. Ramachandran

In this chapter, I present some findings that suggest we need to radically revise two of the basic concepts in neuroscience: the concept of the receptive field as a set of receptors funneling in information onto single sensory neurons and the idea of fixed topography, or "maps," in the adult brain.

My interest in these topics began nearly 20 years ago when I encountered my first random-dot stereogram portraying a square in depth. I looked intently at the stereogram for 2 or 3 min and was about to give up in frustration when the square suddenly emerged. I noticed, also, that with repeated exposures to the same pattern, there was a progressive reduction in perception time until I started seeing stereopsis almost immediately. Indeed, using naive subjects, I was even able to obtain "learning curves" for seeing random-dot stereograms (Ramachandran, 1976; Ramachandran and Braddick, 1973).

Just 5 years earlier, Barlow et al. (1967) had discovered neurons in area 17 of the cat that were sensitive to retinal disparity and, therefore, to stereoscopic depth. It occurred to me that if these neurons were indeed the basis of stereoscopic depth perception in humans, then the stereoscopic learning effect I had observed may be actually taking place at this very early stage, perhaps in area 17 itself. If so, the learning ought to be specific to certain elementary stimulus dimensions such as *retinal location* and *orientation* since topography and orientation selectivity are two of the basic characteristics of neurons in area 17.

Position and Orientation Specificity of Perceptual Learning

In my first experiment, I had 16 naive subjects viewing a cyclopean "hyperbolic paraboloid and torus." The cyclopean figure eventually emerged to the immediate left (or right) of the central fixation spot. As soon as they saw the stereoscopic figure they pressed a key that recorded their latency or reaction time (RT) for seeing the figure and simultaneously switched off the pattern. After 10 sec, the pattern appeared again in the same location and the whole procedure was repeated once more. As shown in figure 22.1, there is a progressive reduction in perception

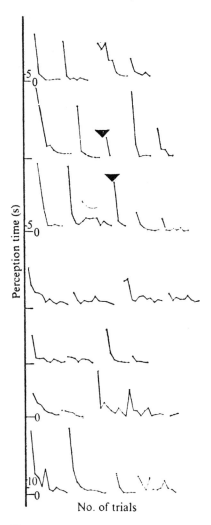

Figure 22.1
Perception time on successive trials for 14 subjects (after Ramachandran, 1976). Each point refers to a single trial. On some trials the perception time was too long to be included in the graph; for these the line ending at the top of the plotting area points to the position of the data point. Data for each subject are plotted to the same scale. The line connecting the dots is broken where the pattern was shifted between trials. Two of the subjects were switched back again to the original position of the stereogram after they had reached an asymptote on the second position: arrowhead indicates point where this change was made. They apparently retained very little of the training they had acquired on the first position.

time and one can obtain a "learning curve" by plotting RT against number of trials. We also verified that after the last trial stereo could be seen even in a 150 msec flash, without requiring eye movements.

After the learning had occurred, we simply shifted the entire stereogram during the 10 sec intertrial interval so that the cyclopean figure came to occupy the opposite hemifield. Remarkably, we found that the subject had to "learn" to see stereo all over again! There was usually some reduction in latency on the very first trial, but the

surprising thing was that there was a significant failure of transfer. We concluded from this experiment that stereoscopic learning is specific to *retinal location*. These results have recently been confirmed and significantly extended by O'Toole and Kersten (1992).

In a second experiment, which I did in collaboration with Dr. O. J. Braddick (Ramachandran and Braddick, 1973), I used a stereogram component of tiny needles tilted 45° instead of dots, i.e., a random-line stereogram. After learning had occurred, we found that it failed to transfer to stereograms that were identical to the first but were composed of needles tilted in the opposite direction. The conclusion from this experiment was that stereoscopic learning was also selective to orientation.

These two experiments implied that stereoscopic learning was specific to two primitive stimulus dimensions— orientation and retinal location. We concluded, somewhat reluctantly at that time, that perhaps the learning was actually taking place in the primary visual areas. I was therefore quite delighted to see the elegant experiments of Dov Sagi and his co-workers presented in this volume —that a completely different type of perceptual learning was also specific to retinal location and to stimulus element orientation. They too conclude, like we did, that such learning effects may actually involve the primary sensory areas (see also the chapter by Ahissar and Hochstein, this volume).

I turn now to a different set of experiments that also suggest, quite clearly, that rapid changes can occur in the receptive field structure of neurons in the primary visual areas. These experiments concern the "filling in" of scotomas in the visual field.

Scotomas

My interest in scotomas began over 15 years ago when, as a student in neurology clinics, I encountered patients with focal lesions in the visual cortex. Such patients usually have what is described as a scotoma—a region in the visual field within which nothing can be consciously perceived (Teuber et al., 1960). Remarkably, the patients themselves are often unaware of this gaping hole in the visual field. When they look at a colored wall or a regular pattern of any kind (e.g., a carpet or a tile floor), the scotoma gets "filled in" by the surrounding color or pattern. Or if they gaze at a companion seen against a background of wallpaper, the companion's head may vanish and be "replaced" by the wallpaper pattern. According to folklore, King Charles II used to decapitate his ladies-in-waiting using this benign procedure, although he used his natural blind spot rather than a scotoma. (I have personally found the procedure to be very effective at faculty meetings.)

Of the natural blind spot (corresponding to the optic nerve head), Sir David Brewster (1832) has written: "We should expect, whether we use one or both eyes, to see a black or dark spot upon every landscape within 15° of the point which most particularly attracts our notice. The Divine Artificer, however, has not left his work thus imperfect ... the spot, in place of being black has always the same colour as the ground." (Sir David was apparently not troubled by the question of why the Divine Artificer should have created an imperfect eye to begin with!)

Does the filling in of scotomas involve "referring" a *sensory representation* of the surrounding pattern to the region of the scotoma, or is there simply a failure to notice the absence of signals from this region of the visual field? Indeed, is the phenomenon any more mysterious than the fact that we do not ordinarily notice the gap behind our heads or the tiny gaps between individual retinal receptors? This distinction is not merely semantic.

For events behind our heads, we have what might be loosely called a conceptual (or "propositional") representation akin to a logical inference. But for the region corresponding to the scotoma, there may be an actual perceptual representation in the visual pathways. How can we distinguish between these possibilities without getting tangled up in an obscure philosophical conundrum?

We know surprisingly little about the nature of the neural representation that corresponds to the filling in of scotomas and blind spots. Unfortunately, observations on the natural blind spot are difficult to make because it is so far from the center of gaze, and patients with small, well-circumscribed scotomas of cortical origin are not easy to come by. In an effort to overcome these difficulties, Richard Gregory and I recently developed a novel technique for creating an artificial blind spot or scotoma that is closer to the center of gaze (Ramachandran and Gregory, 1991). The filling in of such an artificial scotoma, we found, was just as vivid as the filling in of the natural blind spot, and the technique has the additional advantage of facilitating careful observations.

Figure 22.2
Stimulus used to study perceptual fading and filling in (after Ramachandran and Gregory, 1991). The background consisted of twinkling spots of eight different gray levels. The square subtended 1.5° × 1.5° and it had the same mean luminance (60 cd m⁻²) as the twinkling texture. The fixation spot was about 6° away from the border of the square. On steady fixation, the square vanished in about 5 sec and was filled in by the twinkling noise in the surround. Also, if the square was very small (<0.2°), it could be seen to vanish even if it was very bright or dark, that is, nonequiluminous with the surround. (The effect could then be seen even if the fixation spot was only 2° from the square.) The fading occurred even more quickly (<2 sec) if the square was in a different stereoscopic plane (nearer or further) than the twinkling texture. This finding was confirmed by four subjects.

Artificial Scotomas

To create an artificial scotoma, we used a twinkling pattern of dots that resembles the "snow" seen on a detuned television set (figure 22.2). You can repeat our experiment by using your own television set at home. Pick a channel on which you can see only "snow"—no picture. In the middle of the screen, stick a small, circular gummed label with a tiny black dot on its center. (The purpose of the black dot is to ensure steady fixation.) About 7 or 8 cm from this black dot, stick a 1-cm-square piece of gray paper (pick a gray that has roughly the same mean luminance as the twinkle on the television screen). If you view the display from a distance of about 1 m and fixate the central dot very steadily for 5 to 10 sec, you will find that the square vanishes completely and gets replaced by the twinkle invading from the surround. This filling in with the twinkle is obviously analogous to the filling in of scotomas and blind spots and may be based on similar neural mechanisms.

But what causes the square to fade in the first place? The effect is vaguely reminiscent of *Troxler fading*, the tendency for small, stationary objects in the peripheral visual field to disappear completely on steady, prolonged fixation. However, unlike Troxler fading, the effect that we have observed cannot be due to local adaptation (e.g., in the retina) to the luminance edges that define the square because these edges are being refreshed constantly on the screen. Indeed, the fading is actually enhanced if dynamic noise background is used instead of static, two-dimensional noise. We would argue, therefore, that the fading is caused by adaptation or fatigue of neural detectors that are specialized for extracting texture borders and kinetic edges. Such neurons have been described in both area 17 and the middle temporal (MT) area.

We noticed that the fading of the square was especially pronounced with eccentric viewing. This finding may simply reflect the progressive increase in receptive field size with retinal eccentricity. If the fading occurs as a result of fatigue of neurons that extract the border of the gray square, then even a tiny eye movement will restore the square by stimulating a new set of neurons. Because the receptive fields are smaller near the fovea, a smaller eye movement will be sufficient to restore the square near the center of gaze, and this might explain why the square does not fade as easily in central vision. Gregory and I tested this hypothesis directly by waiting until the square disappeared and then moving it to see how large a displacement would be needed to make it reappear (figure 22.3). We found, as expected, that much greater

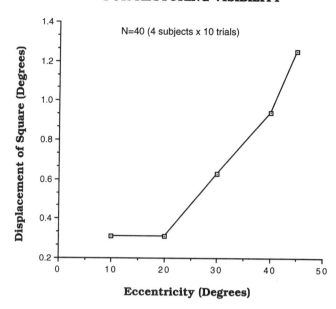

DISPLACEMENT OF SQUARE FOR RESTORING VISIBILITY

Figure 22.3

Displacement thresholds for restoring visibility of the square as a function of eccentricity. Notice that smaller displacements will restore visibility near the center of gaze than in peripheral vision. (Each datum point represents the mean of 40 trials: 4 subjects × 10 trials each.)

displacements were required in peripheral vision than near the center of gaze.

A New Visual Aftereffect

Obviously, one can ask questions about artificial scotomas analogous to the ones I asked about the blind spot in the introduction. Do we really need to speak of filling in, or does the process merely involve ignoring the absence of signals from that region of the retina? And at what stage in visual processing does the filling in occur? In an attempt to answer the first question, Gregory and I waited until the square faded and had been filled in completely with twinkle from the surround. We then switched off the entire display and replaced it with a homogeneous gray screen. To our surprise, we found that there was now a square-shaped patch of twinkling dots in the region corresponding to the square, and this twinkly patch persisted for as long as 10 sec! What is truly surprising about this percept is its dynamic nature—that it is actually seen to twinkle. One wonders whether the numerous reciprocal connections and feedback pathways that exist between different cortical visual areas are somehow involved in maintaining this dynamic representation.

There are at least two equally plausible interpretations of this aftereffect that are not mutually exclusive. First, it is possible that whatever neural process initiates the filling in continues to remain active even after the display is switched off. In other words, the aftereffect might represent a persistence of the neural representation corresponding to the filling in. A second, more likely interpretation is that the dynamic noise creates a peculiar state of adaptation in the surround that subsequently "induces" a twinkling patch of noise in the region of the square, i.e., the effect may arise from "renormalization" in the visual areas of the brain. Additional evidence for the second hypothesis has been obtained by Tyler et al. (1993).

The Physiological Basis of Filling in

What are the physiological mechanisms underlying the filling-in process described above? A partial answer comes from the experiments of De Weerd et al. (1993) who have recently explored the "filling in" of artificial scotomas by training monkeys to look at stimuli such as the ones we used in our psychophysical study (figure 22.2). First, they had the monkey fixate on a central spot on the screen and recorded from a single neuron in V2. Next, they plotted the classic receptive field of the neuron and then covered it with an "occluder" that was much larger than the receptive field and extended well beyond its margins. (The neuron stopped firing, of course, since the occluder had no contours on it that could excite the classical receptive field.) Finally, they introduced twinkling visual noise around the occluder to mimic our "artificial scotoma" stimulus and found, to their surprise, that after 10 sec the neuron began to fire as though it was responding to the "filled in" twinkle! (Recall that our perceptual filing in effect also took 5–10 sec to occur.) They concluded that the receptive field must have expanded two or three times its original size so that it now included regions outside the occluder.

These observations are important for two reasons. First, they imply that the "classic receptive field" is just the tip of the iceberg and that ongoing visual stimulation can change even the basic structure of the receptive field by disinhibiting silent surrounds. Second, this observation provides an explanation for our perceptual filling in effect. Since these cells were originally responding to stimuli inside the scotoma, perhaps higher brain centers are "fooled" into thinking that stimuli immediately outside the scotoma are now inside it. This would correspond roughly to what I am calling filling in.

Scotomas of Cortical Origin

So far, I have considered the filling of artificial scotomas, but do similar principles hold also for scotomas caused by cortical damage? The filling-in phenomenon is usually taken for granted by neurologists, even though there have been few systematic studies on it and the clinical literature on the subject is characteristically vague. Indeed, even the very existence of the phenomenon has been questioned recently. Sergent (1988), for example, presented semicircles and other geometric figures to patients with hemianopia (blindness in an entire half of the visual field) and commissurotomy ("split brain") and found that very little perceptual filling in occurred. More recently, Dennett and Kinsbourne (1992) have argued on philosophical grounds that filling in does not "really" occur and may merely amount to an inappropriate metaphor that requires the assumption of an audience in a Cartesian theater. To resolve these issues empirically, rather than philosophically, Diane Rogers-Ramachandran and I recently examined two patients who had damage to the right occipital pole (visual cortex) producing a small 6°-diameter scotoma to the immediate left of the center of gaze. The scotoma was of relatively recent onset (about 8 months) in both patients and was caused by lesions in the posterior poles of the right occipital lobe.

To begin with, we tried presenting the two halves of a vertical white line on either side of the scotoma (figure 22.4a) and found that the line was completed, but, intriguingly, the process took 4 or 5 sec to occur. (A time delay of this kind is never seen for bridging lines across the natural blind spot.) Furthermore, if the lines were switched off after completion had occurred, one of the two patients reported that he could clearly see a persisting white phantom of the completed part of the line lingering inside the scotoma for several seconds. Finally, when we deliberately misaligned the two segments by about 2° so that they were no longer collinear, both patients reported that the lines started moving horizontally (figure 22.4b) toward each other until they were perfectly lined up and connected across the scotoma. The sensation of movement was reported to be very vivid, and the whole process took several seconds to occur. (This effect was also seen with horizontal lines but was reported to be "less vivid" and occurred only over a much smaller distance—about 0.5°.) One possible interpretation of this curious illusion is that the two segments might be "seen" by a single large receptive field of a cell in one of the "form" areas (e.g., V4) higher upstream. In the absence of conflicting information from area 17 (which is damaged)

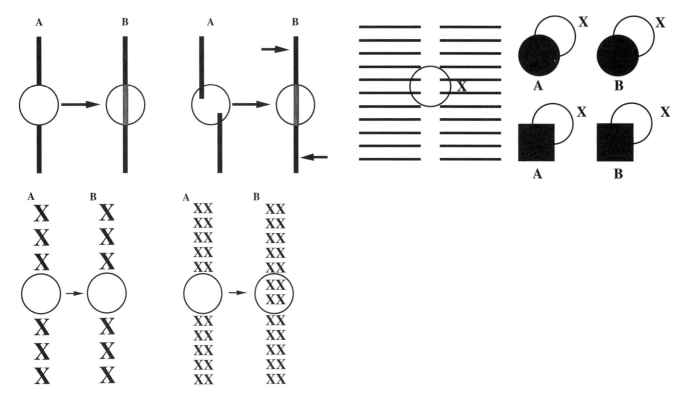

Figure 22.4

Schematic illustration of stimuli that were shown to the patients. The X represents the fixation spot and the circle on the left represents the scotoma. In each figure the drawing on the left (marked A) depicts what was shown to the patient and the drawing on the right (marked B) depicts what the patient saw. The "completion" of the figures usually took 5 or 6 sec (see text) to occur. (*a*) Two white bar segments were presented on either side of the scotoma (each segment was about 6° long and 1/2° wide). The bar was completed quite vividly, but the process usually took 4 or 5 sec. (*b*) The two vertical bar segments were misaligned horizontally. Subjects report that the lines moved vividly toward each other (arrows) until they became collinear. We also tried presenting a small "reference" spot about 2° to the right of the upper line so that the spot was collinear with the bottom line. Intriguingly, the spot was "pushed" to the right so that it was no longer collinear with the bottom line! On the other hand, when we presented the

reference spot about 2° *above* the upper end of the upper line segment, then the upper line moved horizontally as before leaving the reference spot behind, i.e., the spot did not move with the line. (*c*) A column of large Xs was not completed across the scotoma. (*d*) If the Xs were small, completion occurred. A similar effect was also seen if the vertical bar was composed of tiny horizontal line segments. (The subject then saw horizontal lines inside the scotoma.) (*e*) An illusory vertical strip was displayed so that it fell on the scotoma. The patient reported that completion of the illusory strip occurred rather than completion of the horizontal lines. If all the horizontal lines (except the middle two) were removed, then patients saw completion of the horizontal lines. (*f*) A circle with a missing segment was placed on the scotoma. The circle was "completed" in 7 or 8 sec. A similar effect was observed when the corner of a square fell on the scotoma (*g*).

about the tips of the lines, the visual system may simply interpret the signals as coming from a single vertical object.

Interestingly, a similar effect can be observed even in normal vision. To demonstrate this, we began with two vertical line segments that were separated vertically by 4° and misaligned horizontally by about 1° (as in figure 22.4b). We then had four naive subjects stare at a fixation spot placed about 8° away from the two lines. The subjects reported that after steady fixation for 10 to 15 sec, the lines became perfectly collinear in a manner analogous to what had been observed by the two patients. (The illusion could be enhanced considerably by blurring the line tips that were close to each other.) However, when

we moved the lines close to the center of gaze, the effect became very weak and occurred only over misalignment of up to 1°, whereas in the patients the horizontal separation could be as great as 3°. Also, normal subjects rarely report the very vivid sensation of movement that was clearly experienced by the patients. Nevertheless, it is tempting to speculate on the possibility that both effects have a similar origin and that the reason the effect is amplified considerably in the patients is because the damaged part of area 17 fails to signal the misaligned terminators that fall inside the scotoma.

Instead of using a continuous vertical line, what if one were to use a more complex pattern, such as a vertical column of Xs (figure 22.4c and d) or tiny triangles? Would the subject then actually see Xs or triangles inside the scotoma? To our surprise, both subjects reported that this was indeed the case—especially when the Xs and triangles were sufficiently small (0.3°). If the Xs or triangles were large (> 1°), however, they were clearly reported to be missing from the region of the scotoma. This failure to complete large Xs is important, for it implies that the other completion effects observed in these patients are probably not confabulatory in origin.

We then presented an illusory vertical strip (figure 22.4e) to patient R.J. so that it passed through the region corresponding to his scotoma. Interestingly, he reported completion of the illusory strip rather than completion of the horizontal lines. If all the horizontal lines except the middle two were removed, however, he saw completion of the lines.

We also tried presenting a "counterphase" flickering checkerboard pattern to patient R.J. and found that the filling in occurred in two distinct stages. First, he reported seeing inside his scotoma a stationary, nonflickering check surrounded by the flickering checks; later, after a few seconds, the flicker also seemed to fill in so that the whole field looked uniform. Similarly, when he stared at a field of flickering red dots, the red color seemed to bleed into the scotoma and fill it completely first, so that it looked homogeneously red for several seconds before it became filled in with the pattern as well. These remarkable effects suggest that there may be parallel fill mechanisms for colors, motion, and texture corresponding, perhaps, to higher brain areas that are specialized for these attributes. The fact that filling in can occur in distinct stages provides additional evidence for the existence of these areas in the human visual system.

Finally, we tried presenting a square or a circle to one of the patients (B.M.) so that a portion of the figure fell inside the scotoma (figure 22.4f and g). When one corner of the square was inside the scotoma, he initially reported that the corner was missing, but he claimed that it emerged gradually over a period of 6 or 7 sec. A similar gradual completion occurred when an arc of a circle fell on the scotoma. The effects occurred whether or not the relevant part of the figure (corner of the square or arc of the circle) was deleted physically from the display. These effects contrast sharply with observations on the natural blind spot. When the corner of a square or arc of a small circle falls on the blind spot, no perceptual completion occurs.

Why is there a difference? One possibility is that there is a normal patch of visual cortical cells in area 17 in the region corresponding to the blind spot—cells that receive an input from the other eye. These cells could signal the absence of a corner or arc, thereby preventing perceptual completion by higher extrastriate visual areas. (This argument holds whether or not the other eye is closed.) In patient B.M., however, the relevant part of 17 is simply missing, and in the absence of conflicting signals, the higher visual areas are allowed to complete the figure without interference.

We also repeated these experiments on two patients with paracentral retinal scotomas (produced by a laser) and found that gaps in lines were not completed even with prolonged viewing; there was no motion or completion of misaligned bars; there was no completion of coarse checkerboards; and two-dimensional textures and homogeneous colors were completed perceptually without any difficulty. (Interestingly, if the homogeneous color was luminance modulated at speeds higher than 6 to 7 Hz, subjects exclaimed that they could see the outline of their own scotoma. Chromatic modulation did not produce this effect.) We may conclude, therefore, that more sophisticated types of perceptual interpolation can occur across scotomas of cortical origin than across scotomas of retinal origin.

Taken collectively, these findings suggest that the visual system uses information from the region surrounding the scotoma to interpolate perceptually across the gap, that is, the process is very different from (say) one's failure to notice the "gap" behind one's head. (The difference is that in the latter case, you have an inference or guess about what is behind your head, but there is not true perceptual representation in the visual areas of the brain.) Also, I believe these effects provide us with a window into normal visual processes because it is unlikely that the brain has evolved a mechanism for the sole purpose of filling of scotomas. A more likely possibility is that filling in is a manifestation of a process known as surface interpolation, which occurs regularly when we view ordinary visual scenes. If so, studying the filling in of cortical scotomas may give us novel insights into the neural mechanisms underlying other types of *normal* surface interpolation such as amodal completion (i.e., the apparent completion of an object that is partially occluded), an effect that has been explored extensively by Kanizsa (1979) and Nakayama and Shimojo (1992).

Filling in the Blind Spot

What does it feel like to have a scotoma and yet be unaware of it? You can get some idea by examining your own blind spot corresponding to the optic disc—the place where the optic nerve exits from the back of the eyeball. To demonstrate the blind spot, shut your right eye and hold figure 22.2 about 10 inches away from your face while looking at a small fixation spot on the extreme right edge using your left eye. Now move the page toward or away from you very slowly, and you will find that there is a critical distance at which the square on the left disappears completely. Notice, however, that when the square disappears, it does not leave a gap or a dark hole behind in the visual field. Indeed, the entire field looks homogeneous, and the region corresponding to the blind spot has the same texture as the background. Curiously, the blind spot remains invisible even when you look at a complex repetitive visual pattern such as wallpaper; this fact has led many authors to suppose that the pattern from the surround somehow mysteriously fills in the gap corresponding to the blind spot.

We may now ask, What types of patterns can be completed across the blind spot? How sophisticated is the process? What are the spatial and temporal constraints on the process? And what does it have in common with other types of perceptual interpolation such as the filling in of artificial scotomas and scotomas of cortical origin, and amodal completion?

The reader can answer these questions by using a felt pen and a piece of paper. The results may be summarized as follows (Ramachandran, 1992, 1993):

1. Straight lines can be completed readily across the blind spot.

2. If there are two collinear segments, one on either side of the blind spot, and if the upper line segment is red and the lower segment is green, you still see the line as continuous and yet, paradoxically, you cannot discern a border between the two colors. The paradox arises, presumably, because although somewhere in the visual pathways there are nerves signaling that the line is continuous (or, at least, not discontinuous), there are no nerves signaling the red-green color border that falls on the blind spot.

3. There are also clear limits to the filling-in process. For example, if you aim the blind spot on the corner of a square or the arc of a small circle, these figures do not appear complete. They are clearly chopped off by the blind spot (Ramachandran, 1992, 1993). The implication of these observations is that the filling in of the blind spot is a primitive process that occurs at a relatively early stage in visual processing.

4. What if there are two separate lines running through the blind spot, one black and the other white? Would you see a grayish smear at the center of the cross? If you try this experiment you will find that the two lines *compete* for completion. Typically, the line you are paying attention to seems to be complete and seems to partially oc-

clude the other line. If the two lines are of unequal length, however, the longer line seems to complete more readily than the shorter one. This observation is important, for it implies that the filling-in mechanism must use information from an extended distance rather than just from the area immediately surrounding the blind spot.

What Exactly Does "Filling in" Mean?

As we have emphasized in previous papers (e.g., Ramachandran, 1993; Churchland and Ramachandran, 1993), we use the phrase "filling in" in a strictly metaphorical sense. We certainly do not wish to imply that there is a pixel-by-pixel rendering of the visual image or some internal neural screen (or "Cartesian theater") and we are in complete agreement with Dennett's views on this (Dennett, 1992). We disagree, however, with his specific claim that there is no "neural machinery" corresponding to the blind spot. (There is, in fact, a patch of cortex corresponding to each eye's blind spot that receives input from the other eye as well as from the region *surrounding* the blind spot in the same eye; see Fiorani et al., 1992; Churchland and Ramachandran, 1993; Ramachandran, 1993). There is, however, so much confusion associated with the exact meaning of the phrase "filling in" that I would like to take this opportunity to clarify the terminology.

What we mean by filling in is simply this: that one quite literally *sees* visual stimuli (e.g., patterns or colors) as arising from a region of the visual field where there is actually no visual input. This statement applies to both blind spot filling in as well as filling in of artificial scotomas (an analogous definition can be provided for cortical scotomas). In neural terms what this means is that a set of neurons is being activated in such a way that a visual stimulus is perceived *as arising* from a location in the visual field where there is, in fact, no visual stimulus (physiologists call this "local sign"). This is a purely descriptive "theory neutral" definition of filling in and one does not have to invoke—or debunk—little homunculi watching screens or Cartesian theaters, or whatever, to accept this definition. In this respect, our view of filling in is also inconsistent with Dennett's claim that filling in is the same as "finding out" (e.g., I can find out what is behind my head by asking someone, but I can't *see* what is behind my head unless I use a periscope). We would add, however, that this minor point of disagreement does not in any way detract from the importance and originality of Dennett's central thesis. The homunculus comes in many disguises and Dennett has, on the whole, done a marvelous job in exorcising it from neurology and cognitive science.

Blind Spot Filling In: Similarities with Amodal Completion

As noted earlier, it is very unlikely that the visual system has evolved dedicated neural machinery for the specific purpose of filling in the blind spot. What we are seeing here, instead, may be a manifestation of a very general visual process—one that we call surface interpolation (Ramachandran, 1992, 1993). Hence, it is very likely that the process may have much in common with—and may show some of the same neural machinery as—certain other types of perceptual filling in such as the perceptual continuity of occluded objects (amodal completion, Kanizsa, 1979). If this conjecture is correct, then it would be instructive to look for similarities and differences between blind-spot completion and a variety of other perceptual completion effects that have been reported in the literature (e.g., cortical scotomas, artificial scotomas, illusory contours, amodal completion).

We are currently in the process of tabulating these similarities and differences (Ramachandran, Rogers-Ramachandran, and Damasio, 1995) but in this chapter I will just consider similarities with amodal completion—a striking perceptual illusion that has been studied extensively by Kanizsa (1979), Bregman (1981), and Nakayama and Shimojo (1992).

There are clearly similarities between amodal completion (i.e., completion behind occluders) and blind-spot filling in. For example, one can readily see continuity of lines behind occluders and perhaps continuity of some types of visual textures as well. Even the "lining up" of non-collinear line segments seems to occur behind occluders in the peripheral vision (Durgin et al., 1994) just as it does across the blind spot (Lettvin, 1976; Ramachandran, 1992, 1993).

There are, however, important differences between completion across the blind spot vs. amodal completion, which implies that, although the two processes are similar, they are *not* identical (contrary to the views of Durgin et al., 1994). Consider the following differences:

1. The most important difference, of course, is that filling in across the blind spot is *modal*; whereas filling in behind occluders is, by definition, *amodal* (to use Kanizsa's terminology). What this means is simply that in one case you literally see the filled-in section, in the other case you don't! (This distinction will not appeal to behaviorists but should be obvious to anyone who has carefully observed such stimuli and is not wholly devoid of common sense.)

2. The corner of a square or the arc of a circle will get completed amodally behind an occluder but will *not* get completed modally across the blind spot (Ramachandran, 1992; 1993). In fact, subjects sometimes report the corner or arc being completed amodally behind an "imaginary" occluder corresponding to the blind spot; the occluder is usually reported to resemble an opaque smudged "cloud."

3. If a vertical line is moved horizontally so that its central portion traverses the blind spot, it is simply seen to move continuously. There is no perceptual change or glitch during the moment of crossing the blind spot. On the other hand, if a vertical column of dots (each dot being 1° and the separation between them being 6°) is moved across the blind spot, the middle spot seems to disappear and reappear behind a smudged circular occluder corresponding to the blind spot, i.e., it is completed amodally not modally (whereas a line is completed modally rather than amodally).

In spite of the differences, it is very likely that the two processes—modal vs amodal completion—share some neural activity *up to a certain stage* in visual processing. Evidence for this comes from the work of Fiorani et al. (1992). They found that a neuron in the patch of area 17 corresponding to (say) the left eye's blind spot responds not only to the right eye (as expected) but also to two collinear line segments lying on *either side* of the left eye's blind spot—as though it was filling in this segment. (The effect must imply a nonlinear interaction between ordinarily silent inputs from the retina surrounding the blind spot since very little response was seen to either line segment alone. This is about as close as you can get to finding a neural correlate of filling in.) Intriguingly, they also noted that similar effects could sometimes be seen in the rest of the normal visual field if an occluder was used instead of the blind spot. The implication is that, at least in the early stages of processing, both modal completion across the blind spot and amodal completion behind occluders may be based on similar neural mechanisms. But if so, why is there such a compelling phenomenological difference between the two? One possibility is that the presence of the occluder itself (as indicated by T-junctions, say) might be signaled by a *different* set of neurons that vetoes the modal completion. The net result may be a total pattern of neural activity that is different in detail from modal completion although there may be a shared subset of neurons that is active in both cases.

Plasticity in the Adult Somatosensory Pathways

I have until now considered filling in of scotomas in vision. Are there similar effects in other sense modalities such as touch and hearing?

It is known that a complete somatotopic map of the entire body surface exists in the somatosensory cortex of primates (Merzenich et al., 1983; Kaas et al., 1981, 1983, 1990; Jones, 1982). In a series of pioneering experiments. Merzenich et al. (1984) amputated the middle finger (3) of adult primates and found that within 2 months the area in the cortex corresponding to this digit starts to respond to touch stimuli delivered to the adjacent digits, i.e., this area is "taken over" by sensory input from adjacent digits.

Merzenich et al. (1983) also made two other important observations:

1. If a monkey "uses" one finger excessively (e.g., if that finger is placed on a revolving corrugated drum) for an hour and a half each day, then after 3 months the area of cortex corresponding to that finger "expands" at the expense of adjacent fingers (Merzenich et al., 1988), that is, there is an increase in the cortical magnification factor for the overstimulated finger. Also, the receptive fields of neurons in this area were found to have shrunk so that they were unusually small. Hence these effects are unlikely to be "epiphenomenal"—they must be *functionally* important.

2. If more than one finger was amputated there was no "takeover" beyond about 1 mm of cortex. Merzenich et al. (1983) concluded from this that the expansion is probably mediated by arborizations of thalamocortical axons that typically do not extend beyond one mm.

This figure—1 mm—was often cited as the fixed upper limit of reorganization of sensory pathways in adult animals (Calford, 1991). A remarkable experiment performed by Pons et al. (1991), however, suggests that this view might be incorrect. They found that after long-term (12 years) deafferentation of one upper limb the cortical area originally corresponding to the hand gets taken over by sensory input from the face. The cells in the "hand area" now start responding to stimuli applied to the lower face region! Since this patch of cortex is over 1 cm in width, we may conclude that sensory reorganization can occur over at least this distance—an order of magnitude greater than the original 1 mm "limit."

Immediate Unmasking

In addition to these long-term changes that are typically seen several weeks after deprivation or stimulation, Calford and Tweedale (1990) recently reported short-term changes that are based, presumably, on the unmasking of preexisting connections rather than anatomical "sprouting." They anesthetized the digital nerve supplying the middle finger of a flying fox and found that the

cortical neurons in S1 that originally subserved that digit could now be activated by touching the adjacent digits as well, i.e., the receptive fields had expanded to include adjacent digits. This short-term expansion of receptive fields—seen as little as 20 min after nerve block—is analogous to the artificial scotomas of De Weerd et al. (1993) and should be contrasted with the *shrinkage* of receptive fields and changes in topography observed by Merzenich et al. (1984). We must bear in mind, however, that although such effects have often been lumped together under the heading "plasticity," they may, in fact, be based on very different underlying mechanisms.

Curiously, Calford and Tweedale (1990) also found that this short-term receptive field expansion is seen for neuron in the mirror symmetric locations on the other hemisphere. Following digital nerve block of the middle finger in the left hand, for example, the neurons of the left hemisphere corresponding to the *right* middle finger also show an expansion of receptive fields. Such effects were observed in flying foxes as well as in primates.

It might be interesting to look for psychophysical correlates of these effects. One prediction would be that after digital nerve block during routine hand surgery in humans there should be changes in two-point discrimination and touch thresholds on the corresponding finger in the contralateral hand.

Perceptual Correlates of Plasticity in Humans

Despite the wealth of physiological experiments demonstrating striking plasticity in the primary sensory areas of primates, there has been almost no attempt to directly look for the behavioral consequences of this reorganization. Pons et al.'s (1991) observation, for example, makes the curious prediction that if one were to touch a monkey's face after long-term deafferentation, the monkey should experience the sensations as arising from the *hand* as well as from the face. To test this prediction, we recently studied the localization of sensations in several adult human subjects who had undergone amputation of an upper limb. Two of these (V.Q. and W.K.) have been described in detail elsewhere (Ramachandran et al., 1992a,b; Ramachandran, 1993a,b). In this chapter, I will just briefly summarize our findings for these two patients and will also describe some preliminary results from a third patient (FA).

Patient V.Q.

Patient V.Q. was an intelligent alert 17-year-old whose left arm was amputated 6 cm above the elbow about 4 weeks prior to our testing him. He experienced a vivid

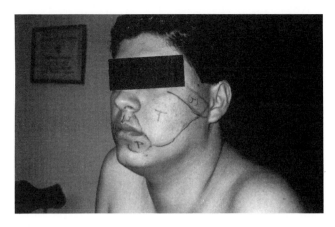

Figure 22.5
Regions on the left side of the face of patient V.Q. that elicited precisely localized referred sensations in the phantom digits. "Reference fields," regions that evoke referred sensations, were plotted by brushing a Q-tip repeatedly on the face. The region labeled "T" always evoked sensations in the phantom thumb, "P" from the "pinkie," "I" from the index finger, and "B" from the ball of the thumb. This patient was tested 4 weeks after amputation.

phantom hand that was "telescoped," i.e., it felt like it was attached just a few centimeters below his stump and pronated. We studied localization of touch (and light pressure) in this patient using a Q-tip that was brushed at various randomly selected points on his skin surface. His eyes were shut during the entire procedure and he was simply asked to describe any sensations that he felt and to report the perceived location of these sensations. Using this procedure, we found that even stimuli applied to points remote from the amputation line were often systematically mislocalized to the phantom arm (figure 22.5). Furthermore, *the distribution of these points was not random* (Ramachandran et al., 1992b). There appeared to be two clusters of points with one cluster being represented on the lower part of the face ipsilateral to the amputation. There was a systematic one-to-one mapping between specific regions on the face and individual digits (e.g., from the cheek to the thumb, from the philtrum to the index finger, and from the chin to the fifth finger or "pinkie"). Typically, the patient reported that he simultaneously felt the Q-tip touching his face and a "tingling" sensation in an individual digit. By repeatedly brushing the Q-tip on his face we were even able to plot "receptive fields" (or "reference fields") for individual digits of the (phantom) left hand on his face surface (figure 22.5). The margins of these fields were remarkably sharp and stable over successive trials. Stimuli applied to other parts of the body such as the tongue, neck, shoulders, trunk, and axilla were never mislocalized to the phantom hand and no referred sensations were ever felt in the other (normal)

hand. There was, however, one specific point on the contralateral cheek that always elicited a tingling sensation in the phantom elbow.

The second cluster of points that evoked referred sensations was found about 7 cm above the amputation line. Again there was a systematic one-to-one mapping with the thumb being represented medially on the anterior surface of the arm and the pinkie laterally, as if to mimic the pronated position of the phantom hand.

We repeated the whole procedure again after 1 week and found a very similar distribution of points. We conclude, therefore, that these one-to-one correspondences are stable over time—at least over the 1-week period that separated our two testing sessions.

Patient W.K.

In testing the second patient (W.K.) we found a very similar pattern of results although there were some interesting differences as well. This patient had a right "forequarter" disarticulation, that is, his entire right arm and right scapula were removed. We tested him exactly 1 year after amputation.

We had WK close his eyes and firmly rubbed the skin of his right lower jaw and cheek with one of our fingers or the tip of a ball-point pen. A representation of the entire phantom arm was found on the ipsilateral face with the hand being represented on the anterior lower jaw, the elbow on the angle of the jaw, and the shoulder on the temporamandibular joint. Again, as in patient V.Q., there appeared to be a precise and stable point-to-point correspondence between points on the lower jaw and individual digits.

A second cluster of reference fields representing the hand was found just below the axilla. Since this region is close to the line of amputation it may be analogous to the cluster of points we found on V.Q.'s upper arm. In this region even a Q-tip was effective in eliciting referred sensations in the thumb, forefinger, pinkie, or palm. And lastly, there was also a third cluster of points near the right nipple and the arrangement of these points also showed some hint of topography. Thus it would appear that there is a tendency toward the spontaneous emergence of multiple somatotopically organized maps even in regions remote from the line of amputation. The exact mechanism by which such maps are formed remains an interesting question for future research.

We have now studied seven patients after upper limb amputation and found that sensations were referred from the face to the phantom arm in only three of them. The cluster(s) of points just proximal to the line of amputation, on the other hand, was seen in all seven patients. We shall discuss the reason for this variability in a later section.

Patient F.A.

Mr. F.A. lost his right arm as a result of an accident on a fishing boat in 1982. (His arm has been amputated about 8 cm below the elbow crease.) He experienced a very vivid phantom hand that was usually "telescoped"; the hand felt like it was directly attached to the stump with no intervening forearm. He could, however, voluntarily extend his hand so that it acquired a subjectively normal length and indeed could even attempt to grasp objects, fend off blows, or break a fall with his phantom.

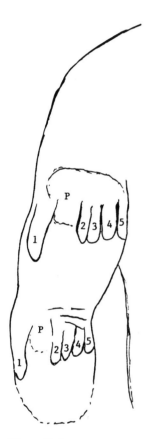

Figure 22.6
Somatotopic maps of referred sensations in patient F.A. Notice that there are two distinct maps—one close to the line of amputation and a second one 6 cm above the elbow crease. The maps are almost identical except for the absence of fingertips in the upper map. When patient F.A. imagined he was pronating his phantom, the entire upper map shifted in the same direction by about 1.5 cm (see text). 1, thumb; 2, index finger; 3, middle finger; 4, right finger; 5, pinkie. These reference fields usually elicited sensation in the *glabrous* portions of these digits. The dorsal surface of the hand was represented on the dorsolateral part of the upper arm lateral to the palm (P) and thumb (2) representations. No referred sensations in the phantom could be elicited by stimulating the skin region in between these two maps.

F.A. was one of the subjects we examined who did not initially have a map on his face (but see below). As in the other patients, however he had points near the amputation line that elicited referred sensations. After carefully mapping these points, we established that there were *two* distinct somatotopic representations that were almost completely identical to each other (figure 22.6). One of these extended from the amputation line to about 3 cm below the elbow, while the second one extended from about 6 cm above the crease to about 14 cm. Stimuli applied points in between these two maps were completely ineffective in producing referred sensations even though skin sensitivity was normal in this region. Note that the two maps are very similar except for the absence of finger tips in the second map.

Modality-Specific Effects

The neural pathways that mediate the sensations of pain, warmth, and cold are quite different from those that carry information about touch from the skin surface to the brain (Kenshalo et al., 1971; Landgren, 1960; Kreisman and Zimmerman, 1971). We wondered whether the remapping effects reported by Pons and his collaborators occur separately in each of these pathways or only in the touch pathways. To find out, we tried placing a drop of warm water on V.Q.'s face. He felt the warm water on his face, of course, but remarkably he reported (without any prompting) that his phantom hand also felt distinctly warm. On one occasion when the water accidentally trickled down his face, he exclaimed, with surprise, that he could actually feel the warm water trickling down the length of his phantom arm! We have now seen this effect in three patients, two patients after upper limb amputation and one after an avulsion of the brachial plexus. The latter patient was better able to use his normal hand to trace out the exact path of the illusory "trickle" along his paralyzed arm as a drop of cold water flowed down his face. (The distance traversed by this illusory trickle was about five times the distance on the face as one might expect from the obvious differences in cortical magnification for the face and arm representations.) Finally, in one patient, a vibrator placed on the jaw evoked a compelling sensation of "vibration" in the phantom hand.

How does the point-to-point referral of temperature sensations compare with that of touch? To explore this, we tried applying a drop of warm (or cold) water on different parts of the face and found that the heat or cold was usually referred to individual fingers so that there was a sort of crude "map" of referred temperature that was roughly superimposed on the touch map (e.g., touching the "thumb" reference field on the face with warm water evoked warmth in the thumb alone, whereas touching the pinkie part of the map evoked a warm sensation confined to the pinkie). To make sure that these effects were not simply due to simultaneous activation of touch receptors, we also tried touching the thumb reference field on the face with warm water while simultaneously applying tepid water to the pinkie region of the map. The patient then reported that he could feel the touch in both digits—as expected—but that the warmth was felt *only* in the thumb. We conclude that there are independent modality-specific "reference fields" for touch, heat, and cold on the face and that these reference fields are usually in approximate spatial registration.

Digit Amputation

We also examined a 45-year-old patient whose middle (third) finger had been amputated at the base when she was 16. Using a Q-tip, we found that touching either digit 2 or 4 on various points on the side that was adjacent to the amputated digit evoked referred sensations in roughly the corresponding locations on the phantom finger. Drops of warm or cold water at these sites evoked warmth or cold in the phantom finger, and when we tightly gripped and released her index finger, she felt her phantom finger being tightly gripped. (Interestingly, a "memory" of the gripping sensation persisted for 7 or 9 sec in the phantom but not the normal digit.) These findings are the first report of a direct perceptual correlate of the observations of Merzenich et al. (1983; also see Ramachandran et al., 1992b).

What would happen if *two* dissimilar sensations are referred simultaneously to the same location on the phantom? How would the two referred sensations interact with each other? To find out we applied a drop of warm water on digit 2 and cold water on digit 4 and asked the patient what she felt. After a short delay of 2 or 3 sec the patient reported that she experienced the two sensations clearly alternating in time—a wave of cold was followed by a wave of warmth and then again by a wave of cold. This alternation continued until the sensations eventually died out. When the drop of hot water and the drop of cold water were both placed on a single digit, however, she volunteered that a novel sensation was experienced —a kind of paradoxical "heat-cold"—as though the phantom was simultaneously warm and cold.

We then repeated these experiments on an additional seven patients with digit amputation. Systematic mislocalizations of sensations were seen in only three of the seven patients. The reason for this variability is unclear, but it may reflect the extent to which the patients learn to "ignore" the anomalous referred sensations from the adjacent digit. Alternately, it is possible that in some patients the weak referred sensations in the phantom are masked or inhibited by the stronger "real" sensations arising from the normal digit.

Memory-Like Effects

The upper limb amputees as well as the digit amputees spontaneously volunteered the following intriguing observation. When stimuli were applied on the face (or adjacent digit), there was often 2–3 sec latency before the sensation was referred to the phantom, and when the stimulus was removed the sensation usually persisted for 8–10 sec in the phantom but not in the site where the stimulus was delivered (Ramachandran et al., 1992b). These effects were especially pronounced for referral of temperature, but they also occurred for simple touch sensations.

The delay in experiencing the referred sensations suggests that the receptive field properties of neurons in the remapped cortical areas may not be entirely normal—a conjecture that can be verified experimentally. The reason for the echo-like persistence of the referred sensations, on the other hand, is far from clear, but the effect certainly deserves further study since it may be related to what psychologists call "short-term memory." One possibility is that the persistence is mediated by the numerous reciprocal pathways that are known to connect the different sensory maps in the thalamus and cortex—a process similar, perhaps, to the "reverberations" postulated by Hebb (1949).

"Learned" Paralysis of Phantom Limbs

Another puzzling observation we made also deserves mention. Most patients who have lost a limb experience very compelling phantom arm or leg, which they can "move" voluntarily. (As we shall see later, we have also studied a patient who was *congenitally* missing both arms, but nevertheless experienced vivid phantom arms.) Yet, we noticed that if patients had a preexisting *paralysis* of the arm caused by a peripheral nerve lesion (e.g., a brachial plexus avulsion or infiltration by carcinoma) they usually complained that although they experienced a phantom arm, they could not *voluntarily* move the phantom—it felt "paralyzed" and usually occupied the same position that the paralyzed arm had before amputation! This raises an interesting question. Why does the mere fact that a limb was paralyzed (say) a few months before amputation cause the phantom to be paralyzed whereas patients who have lost the whole limb and therefore never moved it for many years, can still "imagine" voluntary movement? How can a *phantom* be paralyzed?

The answer is surely that in the former case patients have *learned that the limb is paralyzed*, i.e., every time they tried to move their limb there was proprioceptive feedback from the limb muscles informing them that the limb was not following the command, i.e., the brain was receiving *evidence* that the limb was paralyzed. In the amputees, on the other hand, when the subject tries to move the limb, there is simply *no* feedback from the limb that either confirms or contradicts the command signals. Thus, it looks as though the contradictory signals that were sent to the brain during the months preceding the amputation were somehow "wired" into the brain so that there was a permanent memory trace of the paralysis left in place.

Discussion: The Remapping Hypothesis

The occurrence of "referred sensations" in the phantom limb is in itself not new. It has been noticed by many previous researchers (Mitchell, 1871; Cronholm, 1951) that stimulating points on the stump often elicits sensations from missing fingers, and the great American psychologist William James (1887) once wrote, "A breeze on the stump is felt as a breeze on the phantom." Unfortunately, since the results of Pons and his collaborators were not available at that time, such findings were often attributed to direct reinnervation of the stump by the severed axons. Even when points remote from the stump were found to be effective in producing referred sensations, the phenomenon was often attributed to "diffuse" connections in the nervous system. I would argue, instead, that the effects I have observed are a direct consequence of the remapping observed by Pons et al. (1991), which in turn is constrained by *proximity of maps in the brain*. The reason that there are two clusters of points, for example, one on the face and one near the upper arm, is that the hand area in the Penfield homunculus is flanked on one side by the face and on the other side by the upper arm, shoulder, and axilla (figure 22.7). If the sensory input from the face and from around the stump were to "invade" the cortical territory of the hand, one would expect precisely this sort of clustering (Ramachandran et al., 1992b) of points (figure 22.7). In the rest of this chapter I shall refer to this view as the "remapping hypothesis" of referred sensations (Ramachandran et al., 1992b).

With regard to our empirical results, what is novel may be summarized as follows: (1) There was a precise one-to-one correspondence between points on the face and

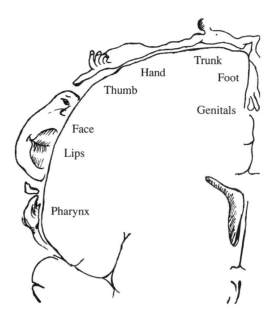

Figure 22.7
The Penfield "homunculus." Notice that the sensory hand area is flanked below by the face and above by the upper arm and shoulder—the two regions where we usually find reference fields in arm amputees. Also, note that the area representing the genitals is just below the foot representation—a fact that might explain the frequent occurrence of certain foot fetishes even among normal individuals.

individual digits. Also, the points were not distributed randomly; there were two clusters of points—one on the lower face region and one near the amputation. (2) The possible existence of topography. The very fact that adjacent points on the normal skin surface (e.g., the cluster of points on the lower face or near the amputation line) map onto adjacent points in the phantom limb (i.e., hand, digits, etc.) is in itself suggestive of topography, of course. Also, in two patients, when we moved the Q-tip from the TMJ along the mandible toward the symphysis menti, they experienced movement of referred sensation on their phantom arm. Furthermore, the perceived direction, distance, and speed of movement on the phantom closely followed the movement of Q-tip on the jaw—e.g., short excursion on the jaw produced equivalently short excursion on the phantom. This finding, again, is also suggestive of the occurrence at least of *patches* of topography even in regions remote from the stump. Our observations suggest, however, that the topography is always much more distinct in the second map near the stump (e.g., figure 22.6) than it is on the face. The reason for this difference is unclear. (3) The referral of even complex sensations from regions remote from the line of amputation, for instance, warm water trickling down the face was felt as a sensation of warm water trickling down the phantom hand; a grip applied to a normal finger was felt as the phantom finger being "tightly gripped." (4) Reorganization is relatively rapid; the study was carried out after 4 weeks rather than 12 years. This rapidity might suggest that the reorganization is based on the unmasking of silent synapses (e.g., through disinhibition) rather than on anatomical sprouting. Whatever the interpretation, however, these findings represent the first clear demonstration that highly organized, modality-specific "rewiring" of the adult mammalian brain can occur in as little as 4 weeks and that this rewiring can be *functionally effective*. It remains to be seen, of course, whether this latent capacity can be exploited for therapeutic purposes.

Sprouting or Unmasking?

What is the actual neural mechanism underlying the "expanded" hand representation in the Silver Spring monkeys (Pons et al. 1991) and in our patients? We need to consider two theories:

1. When a patch of sensory neurons (e.g., in the "hand area") is deprived of sensory input, it might begin to secrete some neurotrophic factors that provoke sprouting of new axon terminals from neurons supplying anatomically adjacent cortical areas. These same trophic factors might subsequently "attract" these terminals to the denervated zone.

2. Perhaps even in normal individuals any given point on the skin projects simultaneously to several locations, e.g., the sensory input from the face projects simultaneously to both the face and the hand neurons in the cortex (or thalamus). The unwanted input to the hand area, however, might be subject to tonic presynaptic inhibition (e.g., via an inhibitory interneuron) by the "correct" axons that arrive there from the hand. If the arm is amputated, on the other hand, this occult input is unmasked through disinhibition and this would lead to mislocalized sensations.

There is at present no strong reason for favoring one hypothesis over the other. There are some hints that rapid "unmasking" of synapses can occur in the visual system (De Weerd, 1993) as well as in the somatosensory system (Wall, 1971; Calford and Tweedale, 1990). Such short-term changes, however, usually result in an enlargement of receptive field size and there is no strong evidence that topography can be altered. Furthermore, the unmasking idea is rendered somewhat unlikely by the fact that neither the arborization of thalamocortical axon terminals nor corticocortical connections has been found spanning more than a few millimeters of the cortex (Calford, 1991; Pons, 1992).

Even if the sprouting hypothesis turns out to be correct, however, one would still have to account for the emergence of topography and modality specificity, i.e., the sprouting would have to be *organized* and the new axon terminals would have to find their appropriate targets. The guidance of such new terminals to appropriate targets would, if it occurred at all, have to depend on poorly understood mechanisms such as "chemoaffinity."

Site of Remapping: Thalamus or Cortex?

There is very little evidence from the physiological work on the question of whether the somatosensory remapping occurs in the thalamus or cortex (or indeed, the spinal cord). One way to answer this question would be to repeat our psychophysical experiments on neurological patients instead of amputees. One could select patients who have damage to the internal capsule causing loss of sensations (and/or movements) in the limbs (or just arm) *without a loss of sensation in the lower face*. If the remapping effects are cortical in origin then we would expect sensations from the face to be mislocalized or "referred" to the paralyzed arm. To our knowledge, there are no such effects reported in the clinical literature but they would be easy enough to look for.

Two-Point Discrimination

Teuber et al. (1949) and Haber (1958) have reported an enhancement of two-point discrimination and tactile sensitivity near the amputation line. At that time, they had no simple explanation for this, but the work of Pons et al. (1991) and Merzenich et al. (1984) suggests that the effect may arise from the increased cortical magnification produced by dual representation (e.g., the upper arm skin above the stump now projects to two cortical areas—the upper arm area over which it originally mapped as well as the new cortical area vacated by the hand).

The improvement seen near the actual amputation stump is, unfortunately, open to multiple interpretations (e.g., patients tend to *use* the stump much more extensively than the corresponding normal part of the other limb). One way to avoid this problem would be to measure two-point thresholds on the ipsilateral *face* region. We have preliminary results from one patient that such improvement in two-point thresholds on the face does indeed occur.

Recall that Merzenich (1989) and his collaborators also found that when monkeys frequently used one finger, for example, by placing it on a revolving corrugated drum for an hour and a half a day, there was an increase in the area of cortex devoted to that finger. To explore the perceptual correlates of this effect, Craig (1993) asked for human volunteers to wear vibrators on their forearm for several days and then studied localization of touch sensations in these subjects. He found that three out of the four subjects made errors in localization and often reported "diffuseness" of the tactile sensations. Although one cannot rule out the possibility that changes in the sensory receptors were produced by the vibrators, the most parsimonious interpretation of these effects would, again, be in terms of central reorganization. Craig's results are also consistent with observations made by our group (Ramachandran et al., 1993b) on two subjects who wore transcutaneous electrical neural stimulators (TENS)—units on the volar surface of the forearm for 3 months. In one subject we observed a 30% decrease in two-point thresholds and in both subjects there was a persistence of involuntary "muscle twitching" sensations for as long as a week after the units were removed! If these effects are repeatable, they might not only provide a promising technique for exploring the perceptual correlates of neural plasticity—both sensory and motor—in adult human subjects, but may also serve as an experimental model for an occupational disease known as "focal dystonia."

Phantom-Limb Pain

The remapping hypothesis may also help explain phantom-limb pain. Keeping in mind that the remapping is ordinarily modality specific—touching the face evokes "touch" in the phantom but cold water is felt as cold and hot water as warmth—we may conclude that the fibers concerned with each of these modalities must "know" where to go. But if there were a slight error in the remapping—a sort of "cross-wiring"—so that some of the touch input gets accidentally connected to the pain areas, the patient might experience severe pain every time regions around the stump or face were accidentally touched. (The provoking stimulus may be so trivial that the patient may not notice it at all while being overwhelmed by the pain.) Also, such "cross-wiring" might lead to subtle changes in gain control that may cause an amplification of pain signals in the somatosensory pathways.

But the experience of phantom-limb pain almost certainly involves the participation of more central mechanisms as well—as emphasized by Melzack (1992). Let me briefly mention two anecdotes that serve to illustrate this idea. First, patient V.Q. claimed that he would sometimes wake up at night with an excruciating pain in his phantom hand—a feeling that his fingers were clenching very tightly and "digging the nails into the palm." Oddly enough, he could often relieve the pain by the simple device of voluntarily *unclenching* the phantom fingers! (Other maneuvers such as flexing the phantom elbow or the contralateral normal fingers proved ineffective.) The second observantion was made on patient F.A. who had a vivid phantom after amputation of his right arm below the elbow crease. On questioning him I realized that although his phantom hand was usually "telescoped" (i.e., attached directly to the stump with no intervening arm), he could, if he wished, voluntarily extend his arm to reach out and "grab" objects that were apparently within his reach. But what if an object were well beyond his reach? Would his phantom be capable of reaching for that object too? Why should the physical limitations of flesh apply to a phantom? To find out, I waited until F.A. had pretended to reach out to "grab" a coffee cup that lay within his reach and then suddenly, without telling him, I pulled the cup away further. He shouted immediately in agony "ouch—don't do that—it hurts." Apparently, he had "seen" and felt the cup being wrenched away from his phantom fingers and this had produced severe pain in his missing fingers! Illusions such as this would be very hard to explain in terms of our current knowledge of pain pathways and, as emphasized by Melzack (1992), they serve to remind us that there is no direct "hot line" from pain receptors to "pain centers" in the brain.

Some Potential Problems

Intersubject Variability

How general are the findings we have reported here? Of the seven patients we have seen so far, the "map" on the face was seen in three. The second cluster of points near the line of amputation, on the other hand, was seen in all seven patients.

Why do some patients not have a cluster of points on the face? There are at least five possibilities that are not mutually exclusive. First, the brain maps themselves might vary slightly from patient to patient, and this, in turn, might influence the degree of remapping. Second, some patients may eventually "learn" to ignore the referred sensations from the face by using visual feedback. Third, even without visual feedback the plasticity exhibited by the afferent pathways may be propagated further along the pathways to perception so that the input gets correctly interpreted as originating from the face alone (i.e., the peripheral organ might "specify" the central connections as suggested by Weiss, 1939). Fourth, the aberrant connections that are formed may get deleted by the same genetic mechanism that causes their elimination in the embryo. And fifth, if the patient uses the stump constantly the skin corresponding to it may "regain" the territory that was initially lost to the face.[1] Obviously, more extensive testing of a large number of patients is needed before we can distinguish among these possibilities. It is worth noting, in this context, that at least in one patient (F.A.) who showed clear evidence of remapping as revealed by MEG (Yang et al., 1993a) did *not* refer sensation for his face to his hand suggesting that the second or third of these four hypotheses is correct, that is, the remapping in the primary sensory areas is not *sufficient* to guarantee the occurrence of referred sensations, although it may be necessary.

Halligan et al. (1993) have recently studied a patient whose arm had been amputated at the shoulder level. They were able to replicate our basic observation—the occurrence of a "map" on the ipsilateral lower face. Curiously, they found that although the map was nearly complete and was in many ways quite similar to the one we had observed, it lacked an index finger and thumb. Careful questioning of the patient revealed that she had completely lost sensations in her thumb and index finger for over a year preceding the amputation (she had suffered from carpal tunnel syndrome). It was as though this sensory loss had been "carried over" into her phantom! Halligan et al. (1993) also report that this patient often experienced excruciating pains in her "phantom" fifth digit and that massage applied to the representation of the pinkie on the jaw often relieved the pain (massage applied on the contralateral side proved ineffective). This observation is important and is quite consistent with a number of informal observations that we have also made on patient V.Q. who told us that rubbing or scratching his ipsilateral lower face often relieved itching in his phantom hand. We suggest that for every patient who experiences phantom-limb pain, one should perhaps begin by carefully mapping points on the normal body surface that elicits referred sensations in the phantom. One could then affix TENS units to these points on the map that corresponds to the painful location on the phantom. A carefully planned clinical trial along these lines might be quite worthwhile.

Multiple Maps

The "remapping" hypothesis predicts that two *clusters* of points should be seen—one near the face and one near the line of amputation. As we have seen, this is generally true (e.g., one hardly ever sees points on the ipsilateral leg, contralateral face, contralateral leg, abdomen, etc.). However, in two of our patients there were *more than one* map near the line of amputation and we have no simple explanation for this. For example, WK (whose arm had been disarticulated at the shoulder) had at least *two* maps proximal to the amputation line—one below the axilla and a second less distinct one near the ipsilateral nipple. Likewise, a patient, FA, described above, had two distinct maps—one that was 3 cm below the elbow crease and the second map (identical to the first) 6 cm above the crease—with nothing in-between! There are, of course, multiple representations of the body surface in both the thalamus and in S1, and one wonders whether the multiple maps that we observed reflects remapping occurring separately in each of these brain areas.

Contralateral Points

Points on the normal skin surface that elicited referred sensations in the phantom were usually clustered around regions proximal to the line of amputation and around the ipsilateral face as predicted by the remapping hypothesis, although the details of the maps varied considerably from patient to patient (e.g., in two patients the maps were on the lower jaw but in a third patient they were mainly clustered on and around the temperomandibular joint and pinna).

These observations are, on the whole, consistent with the remapping hypothesis, but mention must be made of the occasional presence of small maps in the *contralateral* limb at locations that were approximately mirror-symmetrical with the line of amputation. In one patient (R.W.), for example, in addition to the two clusters that are usually found (i.e., on the face and near the amputation line) a small (2-cm-diameter) well-circumscribed region of skin near the contralateral elbow was found that elicited referred sensations in the phantom hand. Moving a pencil in this region produced a vivid sensation of movement in an equivalent direction in the phantom and scratching it was effective in eliminating itch sensations in the phantom! (Other regions on the normal arm were completely ineffective in producing these effects.) In the second patient (F.A.) we found a clearly organized "map" on the normal arm that was an exact mirror image of the map that was above the line of amputation. The curious

---

1. If this argument is correct, then the "face map" should be seen much more consistently in patients with brachial plexus avulsion than in amputees and we have some evidence that this is indeed true. The reason for this difference is that in amputees the nerves that supply the arm can reinnervate the stump after an initial period of retrograde degeneration whereas in the avulsion cases, the roots degenerate permanently and there is no possibility of reinnervation.

thing about this map, however, was that the sensation was referred to the fingers of the *normal* limb. Again, no other areas of skin surface on the normal arm were effective in evoking referred sensations.

These effects are difficult to account for in terms of the remapping hypothesis as it currently stands, but they might be explicable in terms of the transcallosal effects reported by Calford and Tweedale (1990). These authors found that digital nerve block in flying foxes and primates produces the expected immediate expansion of receptive fields in the contralateral hemisphere, but there were also striking changes in the mirror symmetric locations of the ipsilateral hemisphere corresponding to the normal hand —changes that took less than 20 min to emerge. It is not known how long the changes last, but it is conceivable that remapping effects of the kind observed by Merzenich et al. and Pons et al. may also induce analogous *long-term* changes in the other hemisphere. If such changes were to occur, they would explain the maps we saw in the normal arms of our two patients.

Stability of Maps over Time

In patients W.K., V.Q., and F.A. the overall features of the map were remarkably stable with repeated testing across weekly intervals (for 4 weeks). In patient F.A., however, we made a very intriguing observation that suggests that the fine details of the map may be dynamically maintained.

Recall that F.A. lost his arm 10 years ago when the beam of a sailboat landed on his arm and crushed it. (His arm was subsequently amputated 8 cm below the elbow crease.) Upon careful questioning, we discovered that Mr. F.A.'s phantom hand usually occupied a position halfway between pronation and supination with the fingers slightly flexed as though he was holding an imaginary vertical staff. We were also struck by the fact that the topography of pain on the upper arm seemed to approximately "mimic" the position of the phantom fingers—a tendency that we had also previously noticed in other patients. Out of curiosity, we asked him to voluntarily pronate his phantom hand all the way and remapped the points on the upper arm while his hand was still pronated. To our astonishment, we found that the entire "map" had shifted systematically leftward by about 1 cm as if to partially "follow" the pronation (Ramachandran, 1993). Since the arm below the elbow was clamped, this shift in the map could not be attributed to accidental upper arm movements. Also, when he returned the phantom to its resting position, the map also shifted rightward and returned to its original location. A particularly convincing way of demonstrating this effect was to place a constant

stimulus such as a small drop of water on (say) the pinkie region of the map. When he was then asked to pronate his phantom, he reported that he very distinctly felt the drop of water moving from the pinkie to the ring finger.

These observations are quite remarkable for, although their functional significance is not obvious, they suggest that the fine details of the map may be dynamically maintained and that either the map in S1 itself or in subsequent "readout" can be profoundly modified by reafference signals from motor commands sent to the hand.

Long-Term Changes in Maps of Referred Sensations

As noted above, in patient FA, there were no reference fields on the face at all. This was true, however, only during the first three testing sessions. On a subsequent occasion when we repeatedly prodded his face for obtaining magnetoencephalographic (MEG) recordings (Yang et al., 1993a,b), he reported, with some surprise, that he had started to notice some sensations in his phantom hand. These referred sensations were more noticeable the following day when he was shaving, than during the actual MEG recording session. It was as though the repeated mechanical stimulation had somehow revived dormant connections that had always been there. Alternately, the sensations might have emerged spontaneously even without the prodding. This needs to be explored in additional patients. Interestingly, such sensations were now evoked for *both* sides of the face, although less reliably from the contralateral side than the ipsilateral side. (The contralateral effects may be based on callosal connections as noted above.) The reference fields were clearly defined on the ipsilateral face, especially for digits one and two but there was no discernable topography. Such long-term changes in the map on the face have also been recently observed by Halligan and Marshall (1994) who studied their patient on two successive occasions separated by a year.

The short-term and long-term changes may be based on very different mechanisms, but whatever the explanation might be, they are sure to have important implications for our understanding of brain function. They provide the first *behavioral* evidence for the views of Merzenich et al. (1983) and Jenkins et al. (1987, 1990) that even in the adult brain, neural connections are being modified all the time in the sensory pathways.

A Theory of Phantom Limbs

The remapping hypothesis not only explains referred sensations but may also provide a novel explanation for the very existence of phantom limbs. The old clinical explanation of phantom limbs is that the illusion arises from irritation of severed axon terminals in the stump by the presence of scar tissue and "neuromas." Unfortunately, as first pointed out by Melzack (1992), this explanation is quite inadequate since injecting local anesthetic into the stump or even removing the neuromas surgically often fails to abolish the phantom or to eliminate phantom-limb pain.

We would like to suggest, instead, that the phantom-limb experience arises because tactile and proprioceptive input from the face and tissues proximal to the stump "takes over" the brain in area 3B as shown by Pons et al., but possibly also in "proprioceptive" maps. Consequently, spontaneous discharges from these tissues would get misinterpreted as arising from the missing limb and might therefore be felt as a "phantom." This hypothesis is different from, although not incompatible with, the view that phantom limbs arise from the persistence of a "neuro-signature" in a "diffuse neural matrix" (Melzack, 1992). We would argue, however, that the effect arises from mechanisms of a more specific nature such as remapping.

The remapping hypothesis does not, however, explain all aspects of the phantom-limb experience. Consider, for example, the observation that phantom limbs are occasionally seen in patients who have *congenital* absence of limbs. We have recently studied one such patient (D.B.)—a 20-year-old lady whose arms had both been missing from birth. All she had on each side was the upper end of the humerus—there were no hand bones and no radius or ulna. Yet she claimed to experience very vivid phantom limbs that often gesticulated during conversation! It is unlikely that these experiences are due to confabulation or wishful thinking for two reasons. First, she claimed that her arms were "shorter" than they should be by about a foot. (She knew this because her hand did not fit into the prosthesis like a hand in a glove "the way it was supposed to.") Second, her phantom arms did not feel like they were swinging normally as she walked—they felt rigid! These observations suggest that her phantom limbs did not originate simply from her desire to be "normal." It is also difficult to see how the remapping hypothesis, in its simple form, can explain the vivid gesticulation and other spontaneous movements that both D.B. and other patients experience. We would suggest, instead, that the sensations arise from *reafference* signals derived from the motor commands sent to the phantom. What is remarkable, however, is that the neural circuitry generating these gesticulatory movements were "hard-wired" and had actually survived intact for 20 years in the absence of any visual or kinaesthetic reinforcement.

Based on these observations, we suggest that the phantom limb experience probably depends on integrating information from three different sources: first, from the spontaneous activity of tissues in the face and tissues proximal to the amputation, namely, the "remapped" zones; second, from reafferance signals that accompany motor commands sent to the muscles of the phantom limb; and third, to some extent even from the neuromas —as taught by the old textbooks. Information from these three sources is probably combined in the parietal cortex to create a vivid dynamic image of the limb—an image that persists even when the limb is removed. Indeed, there is at least one case on record of a patient actually *losing* his phantom (Sunderland, 1959) as a result of a stroke affecting his right parietal cortex, just as one would predict from our hypothesis.

Conclusions

Taken collectively, the findings on visual and somatosensory filling in that we have considered in this review challenge two of the most widely accepted dogmas in neuroscience: the concept of the receptive field as a set of receptors simply converging onto sensory neurons, and the concept of fixed maps, or topography. The results suggest, instead, that even in adults, the classical receptive field is just the tip of the iceberg—its profile can be altered by ongoing visual stimulation in the surround (as in artificial scotomas). And it appears that topography, too, can change over surprisingly short periods; shortly after arm amputation, a subject begins to feel sensations in the missing arm when stroked on the face. Although these findings should not force us to go all the way back to the eccentric ideas of Karl Lashley (1950), they do imply that we need to revise some of our views on the stability and functional significance of maps and receptive fields.

It is at present unclear whether the remapping effect we have seen in our patients is based on sprouting or unmasking. The fact that anatomical studies have repeatedly failed to reveal any preexisting long-range connections, however, suggests that the sprouting hypothesis is probably correct. If so, perhaps the single most important implication of our work is that the sprouting must be sufficiently "fine-grained" and precise that it permits the emergence of topography and the elaboration of even such sophisticated compound sensations such as "trickle" or "gripping," although, of course, the sensations are abnormally localized. The rapid occurrence of such precise, functionally effective sprouting has never before been documented in the adult human brain and it provides some grounds for optimism.

I would like to conclude by pointing out a more general implication of our work—the experiments on phantom limbs, artificial scotomas, and stereoscopic "learning." The results of these experiments suggest that we must give up thinking of the human brain as a digital computer and think of it, instead, as an extraordinarily dynamic biological system. In a computer, the input processing unit passively transmits the transduced sensory information on to the central processor. In the brain, on the other hand, it looks as though the structure of the input processing unit itself (e.g., receptive fields and topography) is modified continuously by changes in the sensory input—as revealed by our experiments on stereoscopic learning and artificial scotomas. And the rapid changes in topography exemplified by the work of Pons and Merzenich on monkeys and by our own work on phantom limbs imply that even in the adult human brain, the sensorium is continuously "updating" its model of reality as it encounters new evidence from the external world.

Acknowledgments

I thank F. H. C. Crick, V. Mountcastle, J. Bogen, E. Jones, P. Halligan, J. Marshall, H. Neville, J. Rauschaker, D. Rogers-Ramachandran, P. Churchland, C. Gallen, and R. L. Gregory for stimulating discussions, R. Abraham, M. Botte, H. Forney, and W. Vaughn for referring their patients to us, and S. Cobb, T. Young, M. Parsa, and L. Hustana for extensive assistance in testing the patients.

References

Barlow, H. B., Blakemore, C., and Pettigrew, J. (1967). The neural mechanism of binocular depth discrimination. *J. Physiol. (London) 193*, 327–342.

Bregman, A. (1981). Asking the "what for?" question in auditory perception. In M. Kubovy, and J. Pomerantz, (Eds.), *Perceptual Organization*. Hillsdale, NJ: Lawrence Erlbaum.

Brewster, D. (1832). *Letters in Natural Magic*. John Murray, London.

Calford, M. (1991). Neurobiology. Curious cortical change. *Nature (London) 352*, 759–760.

Calford, M. B., and Tweedale, R. (1990). Interhemispheric transfer of plasticity in the cerebral cortex. *Science 249*, 805–807.

Churchland, P., and Ramachandran, V. S. (1993). Why Dennett is wrong. In B. Dahlbom (Ed.), *Dennett and His Critics*.

Craig, J. (1993). Anomalous sensations following tactile stimulation. *Neuropsychologia 31*, 277–291.

Cronholm, B. (1951). Phantom limbs in amputees. A study of changes in the integration of centripetal impulses with special reference to referred sensations. *Acta Psychiatr. Neurol. Scand. Suppl. 72*, 1–310.

Denett, D. C. (1992). *Consciousness Explained*. New York: Random House.

Denett, D. C., and Kinsbourne, M. (1992). Time and the observer: The where and when of consciousness in the brain. *Behav. Brain Sci. 15*, 183–247.

De Weerd, P., Gattas, R., Desimone, R., and Ungerleider, L. G. (1993). Center-surround interactions in area V2/V3; A possible mechanism for filling in? *Soc. Neurosci. Abstr. 19*, 27.

Durgin, F., Tripathy, L., and Levi, D. (1995). *Perception*, in press.

Fiorani, M., Rosa, M. G. P., Gattass, R., and Rocha-Miranda, C. E. (1992). Dynamic surrounds of receptive fields in primates striate cortex: A physiological basis. *Proc. Natl. Acad. Sci. 89*, 8547–8551.

Haber, W. B. (1958). Reactions to loss of limb: Physiological and psychological aspects. *Ann. N.Y. Acad. Sci. 74*, 14–24.

Halligan, P., and Marshall, J. (1994). *Neuroreport*, in press.

Halligan, P., Marshall, J., and Wade, D. T. (1993). *Neuroreport 4(3)*, 223–236.

Hebb, D. O. (1949). *The organization of Behaviour*. New York: Wiley.

James, W. (1887). The consciousness of lost limbs. *Proc. Am. Soc. Psychic. Res. 1*, 249–258.

Jenkins, W. M., and Merzenich, M. M. (1987). In F. J. Seil, E. Herbert, and B. M. Carlson (Eds.), *Progress in Brain Research* (pp. 249–266). Amsterdam: Elsevier.

Jenkins. W. M., Merzenich, M. M., and Recanzone, G. (1990). Neocortical representational dynamics in adult primates: Implications for neuropsychology. *Neuropsychologia 28*, 573–584.

Jones, E. (1982). Thalamic basis of place- and modality-specific columns in monkey somatosensory cortex: A correlative anatomical and physiological study. *J. Neurophysiol. 48*, 546–568.

Kaas, J. H., Nelson, R. J., Sur, M., and Merzenich, M. M. (1981). *The Organization of the Cerebral Cortex* (pp. 237–261). Cambridge, MA: MIT Press.

Kaas, J. H., Merzenich, M. M., and Killacky, H. P. (1983). The reorganization of somatosensory cortex following peripheral nerve damage in adult and developing mammals. *Annu. Rev. Neurosci. 6*, 325–356.

Kaas, J. H., Krubitzer, L. A., Chino, Y. M., Langston, A. L., Polley, E. H., and Blair, N. (1990). Reorganization of retinotopic cortical maps in adult mammals after lesions of the retina. *Science 248*, 229–231.

Kanizsa, G. (1979). *The Organization of Vision*. New York: Praeger.

Kenshalo, D. R., Hensel, H., Graziade, I. P., and Fruhstorfer, H. (1971). In R. Dubner and Y. Kawamura (Eds.), *Oral-Facial Sensory and Motor Mechanisms* (pp. 23–45). New York: Appleton-Crofts.

Kreisman, N. R., and Zimmerman, I. D. (1971). Cortical unit responses to temperature stimulation of the skin. *Brain Res. 25*, 184–187.

Landgren, S. (1960). Thalamic neurons responding to cooling of the cat's tongue. *Acta Physiol. Scand. 14*, 255–267.

Lashley, K. (1950). In search of the Engram. *Society for Experimental Biology Symposium, No. 4*. Cambridge: Cambridge University Press.

Lettvin, J. (1976). A sidelong glance at seeing. *The Sciences 16*, 1–20.

Melzack, R. (1992). Phantom limbs. *Sci. Am. 266*, 90–96.

Merzenich, M. M., Kaas, J. H., Wall, J. T., Nelson, R. J., Sur, M., and Felleman, D. (1983). Topographic reorganization of somatosensory cortical areas 3b and 1 in adult monkeys following restricted deafferentation. *Neuroscience 8*, 33–55.

Merzenich, M. M., Nelson, R. J., Stryker, M. S., Cynader, M. S., Schoppmann, A., and Zook, J. M. (1984). Somatosensory cortical map changes following digit amputation in adult monkeys. *J. Comp. Neurol. 224*, 591–605.

Merzenich, M. M., Recanzone, G., and Jenkins, W. M. (1988). Cortical representational plasticity. In P. Rakic and W. Singer (Eds.), *Neurobiology and the Neocortex* (pp. 41–67), New York: John Wiley.

Mitchell, S. W. (1871). Lippincott's *Magazine of Popular Literature and Science 8*, 563–569.

Nakayama, K., and Shimojo, S. (1992). Experiencing and perceiving visual surfaces. *Science 257*, 1357–1362.

O'Toole, A. J., and Kersten, D. J. (1992). Learning to see random-dot stereograms. *Perception 21*, 227–243.

Pons, T. (1992). Perceptual correlates of massive cortical reorganization. *Science 258*, 1159–1160.

Pons, T. P., Preston, E., Garraghty, A. K. et al. (1991). Massive cortical reorganization after sensory deafferentation in adult macaques. *Science 252*, 1857–1860.

Ramachandran, V. S. (1976). Learning-like phenomena in stereopsis. *Nature (London) 262*, 382–384.

Ramachandran, V. S. (1992). Blind spots. *Sci. Am. 266*, 85–91.

Ramachandran, V. S. (1993a). Filling in gaps in perception II. Scotomas and phantom limbs. *Curr. Direct. Psychol. Sci. 2*, 36–65.

Ramachandran, V. S. (1993b). Behavioral and MEG correlates of neural plasticity in the adult human brain. *Proc. Natl. Acad. Sci. U.S.A. 90*, 10413–10420.

Ramachandran, V. S., and Braddick. O. (1973). Orientation-specific learning in stereopsis. *Nature (London) 350*, 699–702.

Ramachandran, V. S., and Gregory, R. L. (1991). Perceptual filling in of artificially induced scotomas in human vision. *Nature (London) 350*, 699–702.

Ramachandran, V. S., Rogers-Ramachandran, D., and Damasio (1995), in preparation.

Ramachandran, V. S., Rogers-Ramachandran, D., and Stewart, M. (1992a). Perceptual correlates of massive cortical reorganization. *Science 258*, 1159–1160.

Ramachandran, V. S., Stewart, M., and Rogers-Ramachandran, D. C. (1992b). Perceptual correlates of massive cortical reorganization. *NeuroReport 3*, 583–586.

Ramachandran, V. S., Gregory, R. L., and Aiken, W. (1993a). Perceptual fading of visual texture borders. *Vision Res. 33*, 717–722.

Ramachandran, V., Rogers-Ramachandran, D., and Grush, R. (1993b). Perceptual correlates of somatosensory plasticity in man. *Soc. Neurosci. Abstr. 19*, 1570.

Sergent, J. (1988). An investigation into perceptual completion in blind areas of the visual field. *Brain 111*, 347–373.

Suk, J., Ribary, U., Cappell, J., Yamamoto, T., and Llinas, R. (1991). Anatomical localization revealed by MEG recordings of the human somatosensory system. *Electroencephalogr. Clin. Neurophysiol. 78*, 185–196.

Sunderland, S. (1959). *Nerves and Nerve Injuries*. Philadelphia: Saunders.

Teuber, H. L., Krieger, H., and Bender, M. (1949). Reorganization of sensory function in amputation stumps: Two point discrimination. *Fed. Proc. 8*, 156.

Teuber, H. L., Battersby, W. S., and Bender, M. B. (1960). *Visual Field Defects after Penetrating Missile Wounds of the Brain*. Cambridge, MA: Harvard University Press.

Tyler, D. C., Tu, A., Douthit, J., and Chapman, C. R. (1993). Toward validation of pain measurement tools for children. A pilot study. *Pain 52*, 301–309.

Wall, P. (1971). The presence of inaffective synapses and the circumstances which unmask them. *Phil. Trans. R. Soc. London B278*, 361–372.

Weiss, P. (1939). *Principles of Development*. New York: Holt.

Yang, T., Gallen, C., Ramachandran, V. S., Cobb, S., and Bloom, F. (1993a). Noninvasive study of neural plasticity in the adult human somatosensory system. *Soc. Neurosci. Abstr.*

Yang, T. T., Gallen, C. C., Schwartz, B. J., and Bloom, F. E. (1993b). Non-invasive somatosensory homunculus mapping in humans by using a large-array biomagnetometer. *Proc. Natl. Acad. Sci. U.S.A. 90*, 3098–3102.

Some Afterthoughts

Bela Julesz

Two frogs accidentally fell in a jar of milk, and swam desperately to keep themselves afloat. The pessimist frog realized that it was impossible to climb out out the jar, stopped swimming, and drowned in the milk. The optimist frog, however, kept swimming until a miracle happened. The milk slowly solidified, became butter, enabling the frog to jump out of the jar.

An Aesop fable as told by my father

When I learned last year from my friend and close associate Thomas Papathomas that a Conference was planned to honor me on the occasion of my sixty-fifth birthday, my first reaction was to accept this celebration merely as a pretext for getting together some outstanding researchers, but otherwise I insisted on being left out of the scientific program in order to ensure the highest possible quality of its Proceedings. We decided to avoid the *Festschrift* format, because such an arrangement usually accepts all the papers from the participants. Instead, we wanted these conference papers both to reflect my personal interest in the topics and, more importantly, to be thoroughly refereed articles. I also decided to celebrate this occasion by writing a monograph of my own, *Dialogues on Perception*, as a gift to the participants and particularly to my many collaborators, students, and colleagues in visual perception. *Dialogues* contains 14 essays, heated debates between me and my critical self on some strategic problems of psychobiology that seem to be solved but, when more critically inspected, often turn out to be still unsolved. During the last few months I have finished the monograph and, now that I am reading the chapters in this volume, I am so glad that many of the strategic problems I discussed there are explored in these chapters. *Dialogues* has also been published by The MIT press.

During the conference I kept my vow and refrained from commenting on the papers, and I am also continuing to do so here. I enjoyed all the presentations, learned from each, and am greatly honored by all the authors who took so much effort to contribute to this volume.

Because each chapter is related to my interest—early vision—and because I eye-witnessed and contributed to its growth, I will make a few general comments, and also try to give the flavor of *Dialogues* in a few paragraphs.

It is my belief that psychobiology is still in a stage where molecular biology had been prior to the discovery of the double helical structure of DNA by Watson and Crick and the genetic code. Without knowing the code of the brain, it is hard to determine the strategic importance of any contribution in psychobiology made up to now. In light of this belief, I can sum up the essence of my main scientific contributions in two sentences without being able to evaluate their real significance: (1) I showed (by introducing random-dot stereograms and cinematograms) that—contrary to common belief—stereopsis and short-term motion perception are not local but global processes. Particularly, to solve the correspondence problem, one needs some global matching operation, similar to auto-correlation; and (2) I showed (by using texture pairs with controlled stochastic distributions) that—contrary to common belief—texture discrimination is not a global (statistical process), but instead is based on local conspicuous features, the textons. I regret that I did not name these textons (that pop out in iso-second-order texture pairs and resemble quasi-collinear structures, blobs, terminators, closed lines, etc.) using some noncommittal name such as "charm," "beauty," or "strangeness," as the physicists have named their quarks. Had I done so, much misunderstanding could have been avoided. I have a long chapter on textons and antitextons in my *Dialogues*. In both of my main contributions I emphasize that they were contrary to common beliefs. After all, science starts where common sense ends.

I have to confess that I regard my role as the inventor of the computer-generated random-dot methodology as —reportedly—Ravel regarded his as the composer of *Bolero*. The public mainly knows of him through this most popular musical piece, whereas Ravel was much prouder of his more sophisticated chamber music, known by only a few. Similarly, I regard my texton theory as a much more sophisticated scientific contribution than demonstrating that there is no camouflage in 3D (known in aerial reconnaissance, but unknown by psychologists until 1959). Alas, the world will probably remember me for a few more years for the latter, while my texton theory will be referred to by only a few specialists, if at all. I mention this merely to illustrate that my own scientific taste and pride differ from that of the majority of my colleagues and of the judgment of history, and therefore I am always cautious when commenting on other scientists' work.

I mentioned my work above with random-dot stereograms, cinematograms, and textures. I first became interested in these topics in the early 1960s, having begun my career at Bell Laboratories in machine vision trying in particular to remove the redundant information from images. This, in turn, required the segmentation of visual scenes into components. It was obvious to me from the start that, knowing whether the ears of a rabbit belong to the fence behind or to the rabbit, requires the enigmatic problems of semantics. On the other hand, knowing that the ears of the rabbit have the same depth, velocity, and texture as its body permits segmentation without semantics, provided I could show that the perception of depth, motion, and texture can be effortlessly obtained even for random textures, that is without the need of semantics. My earliest efforts along these lines, spanning the first decade, were collected in my first monograph, *Foundations of Cyclopean Perception* (1971). Its sequel—usually not realized—is my chapter (Julesz, 1978, "Global stereopsis: Cooperative phenomena in stereopsis depth perception," in *Handbook of Sensory Physiology, VIII: Perception*, Held. R., Leibowitz, H. W., and Teuber, H., Eds., Springer-Verlag). The rest is history, and most of the papers in this conference address some of these problems from this perspective. Of course, I would have never guessed in 1960–1962 that so much outstanding effort would go into these areas in the three decades since.

It is also interesting that some strategic demonstrations are fully understood only much later as the *Zeitgeist* matures. For instance, at the first international demonstration of the random-dot stereograms at the Fourth London Symposium on Information Theory in 1960, my claim that it proved that monocular pattern recognition was not necessary was debated. After all, there were some local shapes that looked identical in the two images that could be recognized prior to fusion. To prove my claim, I published in its Proceedings (Julesz, 1961) the demonstration shown in figure 1. Here the left and right images were a regular random-dot stereogram, but in the left image I broke the diagonal connections; whenever three adjacent dots along the diagonals were identical, I complemented

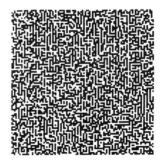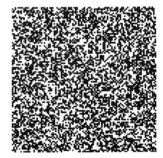

Figure 1
RDS with diagonal connectivity broken in one image. The stereo pair has 84% of their dots correlated (thus the low spatial frequencies are similar). (From Julesz, 1961, 1971.)

the contrast of the middle one. By this operation, the two stereograms retained 84% of their points to be correlated, so it is not surprising that they can be binocularly fused. Yet, when monocularly viewed, the two images appeared strikingly different.

When the images were blurred they looked very similar. So the coarse information has been retained in the two images. It took several years—after the concept of spatial-frequency channels became established and the use of such channels for stereopsis was shown (Julesz and Miller, 1975)—to understand that figure 1 was the first intimation that if some frequency bands overlapped in a stereopair, then some others could be in rivalry without disrupting stereopsis. Figure 1 also implied that "similarity" for stereopsis was based on correlation and not on some primitive notion of geometric congruency. Of course, this same figure, when presented monocularly in temporal succession, yielded good apparent movement for the center square. [By the way, in 1960 I tried all my random-dot stereograms as cinematograms with a special device constructed by my technician Richard Payne, and there was a great similarity between the two processes. However, since in my youth I concentrated on demonstrations, and cinematograms could not be printed in publications, it took me a decade when a computer-generated random-dot cinematogram movie was made to accompany my first monograph (FCP) in order to emulate the main cyclopean phenomena for stereo-blind observers.] This important insight of the very nature of "perceptual similarity" was somewhat ignored until Werkhoven showed it again for motion perception using his ingenious paradigm (Werkhoven et al., 1990). I quote this example merely to illustrate that pioneering experiments often require concepts added years later to be fully appreciated.

I was much aided in my early research by the epoch-making discoveries by the neurophysiologists. While our psychological findings with random textures implied that stereopsis and motion perception had to be rather early processes in the human brain, the pioneering work by Horace Barlow, Jerry Lettvin, David Hubel, and Gian Poggio, among others, even pinned down the processing sites of some of these processes in the earliest processing stages of the monkey's visual cortex. For me, it is a source of great satisfaction and pride that all four of these founders of modern neurophysiology came to the conference and actively participated in it. I was also very pleased that leaders of neurophysiology of the next generation, Robert Desimone, Peter Schiller, Jonathan Victor, and a close associate of mine, David Van Essen, also contributed to this volume. Here I single out only the neurophysiologists, since I regard the close collaboration between

psychologists and neurophysiologists as the essence of psychobiology. I feel a great pride that so many of the leading neurophysiologists found our work in psychology important enough to participate in this conference. It is this collaboration that led to the renaming of "cyclopean perception" as "early vision." For me the finding of Gian Poggio (1984) of cyclopean neurons in V1 layer IVB in the monkey cortex was of crucial importance. I knew from my psychological studies that stereopsis must be an early process, but that it can occur at the very input to the striate cortex was beyond my hopes.

I will not dwell on all my many friends, collaborators, and colleagues in psychology who contributed to this issue. After all, the Dialogues give tribute to most of them and their contributions. I make only one exception: I am most proud that so many of my former postdocs gave talks of the highest caliber, and that so many of them wrote articles that were selected to be included in this volume.

As I read the chapters in this volume and ruminate over the outcome of the many projects that I was so interested in during my scientific life, I feel an immense satisfaction. After all, it was worthwhile to select visual perception as my final career, one of the last intellectual frontiers in the last decades of our century. It was my good fortune to survive and arrive in the United States in this exciting period, witnessing and contributing to the birth of psychobiology. I used to wonder whether "cyclopean perception" would become a paradigm. It seems it did. As a matter of fact, several authors use random-dot stereograms, cinematograms, and textures matter of factly in their research, so I reached the highest distinction one can achieve during his lifetime: my work became a "scientific folksong" with its original composer assumed to be unknown.

As for the topics in this volume, they, indeed, reflect my primary interests. That psychology of early vision should be closely linked to neurophysiology and neuroanatomy has been my credo from the very beginning. I may add that in this symbiotic relationship I regard psychology as the leading discipline. After all, it is the intact human brain and its mental capabilities that have to be explained by neurophysiological findings, and the reverse seems much more speculative. As I discuss it in detail in Dialogues, my definition of a scientific psychology is similar to thermodynamics and physics. In thermodynamics, the impact of atoms and molecules with each other and the wall of the container on level I gives rise to emergent properties of temperature, pressure, entropy, enthalpy, etc., on level $I + 1$. Similarly, I regard a psychological paradigm scientific if on level I interacting neurons (by excitation and inhibition) in some area of the cortex yield some mental percepts of depth, motion, texture segregation, etc. on the next level $I + 1$. Of course, the metaphor to the thermodynamics of gases is crude. As the coupling between atoms and molecules becomes tighter, one can experience the many *cooperative phenomena* of liquid and solid physics with ever-increasing complexities. Similarly, I believe that the many cooperative phenomena of early vision will find some parallels in the workings of the neural level.

Whether level I could be substituted by artificial neurons, as modelers in AI and neural nets propose, remains to be seen. Perhaps, as the "code of the brain" will be known—if there is such a thing—models of machine vision and neurophysiological models might come closer. Of course, restricting psychology in the straitjacket of structuralism, believing that the prodigious feats of our mind could be explained by some thermodynamic model is a great oversimplification. Even though neurons can interact with their neighbors by both excitations and inhibitions, molecules in the thermodynamics interact merely by a single kind of interaction, just hitting each other. But more importantly, neurons in the brain can interact from *far distances*, which is probably the main reason why brains in general exhibit much more complex behavior than physical systems that are restricted to near interactions. I assume that early vision, such as stereopsis, motion perception, and texture discrimination, is being supported by neural processes that are restricted to nearby interactions alone. Of course, even in physics, as nearby molecules become strongly coupled, yielding liquid and solid states, phenomena of ever-increasing complexity emerge in these cooperative systems, from magnetism to high-temperature superconductivity. So my quest is to study psychology as an aggregate of cooperative systems in which neurons interact with their neighbors and try to exclude far interactions, except for one top-down process, I call—rather arbitrarily—focal attention.

The main sections on psychophysics are closely related to my own work on stereopsis, motion perception, texture discrimination, and focal attention. The first three topics were pioneered in *Foundations of Cyclopean Perception*, and I am elated by the sophisticated problems these fields have incorporated since 1971. I added focal attention to my interests somewhat later, although in my first paper on texture discrimination in 1962 I introduced the paradigm of distinguishing between effortless viewing and scrutiny that is now called preattentive (pop-out) versus attentive. It is my firm belief that much of vision can be explained by bottom-up processes and the only top-

down process to be evoked is focal attention. Of course, there are some interesting problems of visual cognition that are clearly top-down in nature, and I hope that they will be addressed during my lifetime. I am glad that at least two chapters in this volume are concerned with such processes. I am confident that as the technology progresses and huge memories become available in the next century, the study of semantic storage will come into age. Nevertheless, when I started some studies of learning phenomena in stereopsis and texture discrimination using random-dot textures (Julesz, 1984, p. 605), I did not expect to witness the remarkable learning phenomena for texture discrimination of Karni and Sagi (1990). The finding that learning and memory might be studied without semantics in early vision is, in my view, a very important event.

Next, I refer to three important contributions here too, even though I discussed them in detail in *Dialogues*. One is the work by Andrei Gorea and Thomas Papathomas. The second is the work by Ilona Kovacs in collaboration with me. The third is a new interpretation of the preattentive-attentive duality by Jochen Braun in a long cooperation with me. The reason to do so is as follows: Andrei and Thomas took a leading role in organizing this workshop (from selecting speakers to the reviewing process) and in their modesty they did not include a chapter of their own in this volume. Because I would like to see in this volume all the work that excites me, I decided to give a brief account of the flavor of their work with some references. Similarly, of the many excellent contributions that were made during the 5 years since we left Bell Labs and resumed work in the newly founded Laboratory of Vision Research at Rutgers University—discussed in great detail in *Dialogues*—the contributions by Ilona Kovacs stand out in their originality and promise as does the work with Jochen Braun, who was a postdoc with me for several years at Caltech.

Let me start first with the work with Ilona Kovacs that has just been published (Kovacs and Julesz, 1993; 1994b). Related issues are being pursued. Here I give only a brief account of the essence of our findings. The main finding is demonstrated in figure 2. Consider some adjacent Gabor patches that are of nearly collinear, but somewhat jittered orientations, in an array of randomly speckled Gabor patches. If these nearly collinear elements are not fully closed, then they blend with the background patches. However, if this "snake"-shaped curve "bites its tail," thus becoming a *closed* curve, it segregates vividly from the background, particularly when briefly presented. It is then possible to measure the detectability of some patches inside the closed curves as shown for a circle in figure 3 and

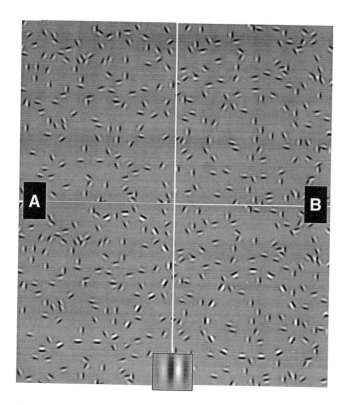

Figure 2
Superiority of closed versus open curves. (*Upper*) Two contours embedded in the background of randomly oriented elements. (*Lower*) The same contours are highlighted for didactic reasons. (*A*) A nonclosed contour composed of aligned Gabor patches (GPs) is only barely visible against the background. (*B*) A closed contour with the same angular difference and distance between elements is perceived much more easily. Perception of closed contours is best for brief presentations. For more than 180 msec duration, the observer starts to scrutinize other global structures at the expense of the primordial closed contour. (*Inset*): One GP element, which is a product of a sine wave luminance grating and a circular Gaussian envelope. GP wavelength (λ) was 0.12 arc deg; Gaussian envelope size was equal to λ; GP amplitude was 24% of mean luminance (30 cd/m²). (From Kovacs and Julesz, 1993.)

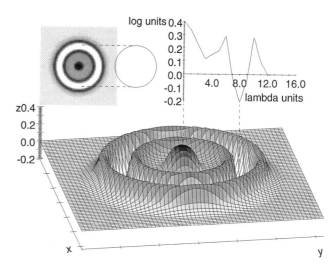

Figure 3
Sensitivity change for a single GP as a function of distance from the surrounding line (closed circle). Note the strong threshold enhancement effect inside the circle between 5 and 8 λ distance. $\lambda = 8$ represents the center of the circle. (From Kovacs and Julesz, 1993.)

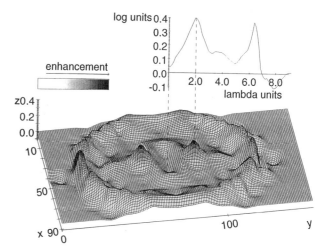

Figure 4
Similar to figure 3 but for a closed ellipse with 1.2 aspect ratio. (From Kovacs and Julesz, 1993.)

for an ellipse in figure 4. This is the "perceptual field" the Gestaltist psychologists were searching for in vain a generation ago. Perhaps they missed it because, in order to find a field, one has to have some "carriers of the field." Had we used just a homogeneous background without the speckled Gabor patches we also would have missed it. Perhaps one purpose of early vision is to find these global structures that we identified psychophysically.

These findings suggest that besides a collinear facilitatory mechanism that perceptually connects contour fragments, an orthogonal mechanism acts over larger distances and induces the segregation of the whole area surrounded by a closed contour.

I turn now to the influential paradigm of Andrei Gorea and Thomas Papathomas. They have developed a powerful methodology for examining the role of visual attributes (color, luminance, orientation, spatial frequency, etc.) for a variety of visual tasks. Their classes of multiattribute stimuli allow one attribute to elicit the percept simultaneously with, but independently of, other attributes. The main advantages of the stimuli are: (1) The interaction of attributes can be studied systematically. (2) The relative strength of two attributes can be compared directly when they are designed to elicit competing percepts. (3) Specific visual mechanisms can be selectively isolated by proper

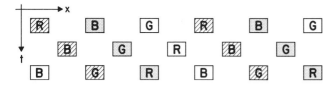

Figure 5
In this space-time (*x-t*) schematic diagram, chromatic and achromatic motion components compete against each other. (After Papathomas et al., 1991.)

choices of stimuli. With their colleagues, they have applied their techniques to study motion (Gorea and Papathomas, 1987, 1989; Gorea et al., 1992, 1993a,b; Papathomas and Gorea, 1988, 1989; Papathomas, Gorea, and Julesz, 1991), depth perception (Papathomas and Gorea, 1989; Kovacs, Papathomas, and Julesz 1991), texture segregation (Gorea and Papathomas, 1993), and textural grouping (Gorea and Papathomas, 1991a,b). The results of their experiments can be used for improving existing neurophysiologically plausible computational models for motion extraction (Gorea, Papathomas, and Kovacs 1993a,b) and for texture segregation (Gorea and Papathomas, 1993).

I mention an example of applying their stimuli in examining the role of color in motion (Papathomas et al., 1991), an issue that has been debated over the last two decades. At equiluminance, directional performances fall to a minimum or even to chance level with random-dot cinematograms (e.g., Ramachandran and Gregory, 1978; Cavanagh et al., 1985; Troscianko, 1987). This was taken as evidence that the motion pathway is colorblind or, phrased differently, that color and motion are processed through entirely separate pathways (i.e., Hubel and Livingstone, 1987; Livingstone and Hubel, 1988). Experiments with the stimulus of figure 5, however, gave strong evidence that the chromatic contribution to motion is significant. In figure 5, the spatial variable *x* is horizontal, and time is quantized in frames and increases downward. Each frame (a horizontal row of targets in the figure) is replaced (i.e., erased and overwritten) by the next frame in temporal sequence, yielding one-dimensional motion along the *x*-axis. Targets are defined by a conjunction of values of color (R, G, and B standing for red, green, and blue, respectively) and luminance (low, medium, and high denoted by hatched, dotted, and open areas, respectively). In figure 5 luminance values are arranged to elicit motion to the right, whereas color values are arranged to elicit motion to the left. Papathomas et al. (1991) have shown that there is a significant range of luminance contrasts for which observers perceive motion to the left, indicating

that color-carried motion dominates and, therefore, that color does play a role in the perception of movement.

Having answered affirmatively the question "*Does* color contribute?," as described above, Gorea, Papathomas, and Kovacs (1993a,b) recently addressed the next important question: "*How* does color (and luminance) contribute?," i.e., how and at what processing level do the chromatic and luminance pathways interact with each other in eliciting motion perception? They obtained convincing evidence supporting the idea of two motion systems, offered earlier in quite different experimental contexts (Thompson, 1982; Murray, MacCana, and Kulikowski 1983): a "specific" system, dominant for high spatial and high temporal frequencies, and an "unspecific" one, dominant at the opposite end of the spectrum. Their results indicate that there are at least two separate motion pathways for the specific system, one for color and the other for luminance, which do not interact with each other until after the motion signal is extracted separately in each. The experimental data also show that there is a unique pathway for the unspecific system, which combines the chromatic and luminance signals at an earlier stage, before motion extraction. One other noteworthy development in their study is the design of a very efficient and accurate technique for assessing equiluminance, based on the luminance reverse-phi phenomenon. In essence, the scope of the research of Gorea, Papathomas, and their colleagues has expanded from merely examining the role of and the interactions among *attributes* in perceptual processing; their current scope is to study the properties of and interactions among the underlying *mechanisms*. Thus, their research not only addresses key questions in psychophysics, but also points to links in neurophysiology and in computational models in vision, which is the theme of this book.

Let me note, that in my first monograph *FCP*, I mentioned that RDS with one half pair having its polarity reversed cannot be fused; however, when they share the same color, then depth can be perceived. With Ilona Kovacs we called this condition "meta-isoluminance" and showed that color can yield both depth and can counteract reverse-phi in random-dot cinematograms (Kovacs and Julesz, 1992). So, color is certainly used by stereopsis and global motion perception, and the Gorea-Papathomas paradigm helps to clarify the role of color in early vision in great detail.

Finally, I want to include here an important insight about the preattentive-attentive dichotomy and the usual suggestion that texton gradients would grab focal attention, permitting identification afterward. However, with Braun we performed a concurrent paradigm (Braun and

Julesz, 1992). In concurrent tasks we loaded observers' attention with a difficult foveal task: to tell whether 5 Ts or 5 Ls were all the same and, simultaneously, to detect or identify certain other stimuli in the periphery. For instance, it was impossible to identify another character with a 120 msec SOA while attention was loaded. However, some simpler tasks could be done well, such as finding the location of needles having a different orientation from an aggregate of background needles. Interestingly, as the orientation gradient was reduced, performance was also reduced, yet it did not change performance of the concurrent (5 T/L) task. Therefore, we call these concurrent tasks that do not affect each other's performance "nonattentive." This nonattentive system can detect, even identify some simple tasks without the need of attentional resources. In a sense, some aspects of the stimulus can reach awareness without having to draw attention to themselves. This nonattentive system can do both "where" and "what" tasks, provided the stimulus feature is of a certain kind. Our nonattentive system, though similar to the "what" system, is simpler, since it cannot identify alphanumeric characters while attention is loaded down by the concurrent letter-identification task. Recently, Bart Farell (a former postdoc of mine) with Dennis Pelli showed, using the classic paradigm of George Sperling (1960), that for mixed scales identification is as good as for a single scale, while for localization mixed scales yield 75% poorer performance (Farell and Pelli, 1993). From this they conclude also that two different systems are processing the "where" and "what" information.

It would be tempting to speculate about the future of psychobiology, the more so because new noninvasive methods of brain scanning (e.g., magnetic resonance imaging) are becoming a reality. However, instead of speculating about the future, let me repeat the sage's words from the last paragraph of my *Dialogues: Life is only bearable for two reasons: Because everything changes; and because nobody knows the future!*

I hope that this brief chapter conveyed the flavor of *Dialogues* and expressed my gratitude to all the participants who found time and effort to celebrate with me and establish a memento with their contributions. Indeed, that I survived against all odds and reached this respectable age has been a miracle; that I stumbled into psychobiology—one of the last remaining intellectual frontiers of mankind—witnessing its amazing growth, and even contributing to it, was a special grace of fate, with the added bonus that I collected so many friends who share a passion for research with me. It seems that after all, it was worthwhile to stay optimistic.

I thought that I would end my thoughts with the previous paragraph, but I got a chance to add a few more (as I am correcting the galley proofs), as follows:

Indeed, a year passed and, as I am holding in my hands the conference proceedings, it is the first time I realize the huge scope of this undertaking. To begin with, this volume has now a title, *Early Vision and Beyond*, that nicely sums up the theme of my scientific interests. I also see the many edited manuscripts in their entirety, a most impressive corpus of work. In addition to this book, the editors of *Spatial Vision* surprised me with two *Festschrift* issues [1993(2) and 1994(2)] fully devoted to honor my sixty-fifth birthday. I thank the editors and the many authors who contributed to these three volumes for their time, effort, and thoughtfulness. My joy is tempered by the sad fact that two of my close friends Günther Baumgartner and Werner Reichardt died prior to the conference, and soon after, we lost Fergus Campbell, Gaentano Kanizsa, and Roger Sperry. It is, nevertheless reassuring that their scientific legacy is not forgotten and science is marching on.

As an example of how many things can happen even in my microcosm, I mention only some recent insights we gained with Ilona (Kovacs and Julesz, 1994b). The reader might recall how much I stressed the finding that closed curves made from Gabor patches would perceptually jump out from their surround composed of speckled Gabor patches in random orientations. Meanwhile we tested ellipses and found that perceptual contrast enhancements occurred now at two places on their longitudinal axes (but not in the focal points of the ellipses). Our psychophysical findings are in good agreement with the grass-fire model of Harry Blum (1973). It seems that closed curves exhibit strong perceptual sensitivity enhancement at points Blum called "skeletons," but of course the curves do not have to be closed in general. I quote this example merely to illustrate that the important thing is not that one is always correct; it is much more important that one should stumble on the right paradigm that can yield ever increasing insights. In my *Dialogues* I discuss how these ideas originated and developed into some unexpected directions.

I end this volume with some fireworks. Thirty-five years after I watched the first computer-generated RDS slowly emerge in vivid depth, a new fad started in Japan and now spread all over the world. Books and posters are now printed in the millions using "autostereograms" (precursors of which we experimented with Peter Burt in 1979, and called them "wallpaper stereograms" [Burt and Julesz, 1980]). Much credit must be given to Christopher Tyler (1983) and David Stork (Falk et al., 1986) whose work helped to popularize this format. What can be the nicest sixty-fifth birthday gift than to witness how the beauty of RDS is now shared by millions of people. Let us toast each other with a glass of wine, so our ocular muscles will relax, while looking at random-dot stereograms and then we will be able to fuse them without the need of a stereoscope!

References

Blum, H. J. (1973). Biological shape and visual science (Part I.) *J. Theor. Biol.* 38, 205–287.

Braun, J., and Julesz, B. (1992). Early vision: Dichotomous or continuous? Psychonomic Soc. Meeting, St. Louis, November 11, 1992.

Burt, P., and Julesz, B. (1980). A disparity gradient limit for binocular fusion. *Science* 208, 615–617.

Cavanagh, P., Boeglin, J., and Favreau, O. E. (1985). Perception of motion in equiluminous kinematograms. *Perception* 14, 115–162.

Falk, D. S., Brill, D. R., and Stork, D. G. (1986). *Seeing the Light: Optics in Nature, Photography, Color, Vision, and Holography.* New York: Harper and Row.

Farell, B., and Pelli, D. G. (1993). Can we attend to large and small scale at the same time? *Vision Res.* 33(18), 2757–2772.

Gorea, A., and Papathomas, T. V. (1987). Form and surface attributes in motion perception studied with a new class of stimuli: A Basic Asymmetry. *Bell Labs Technical Memorandum* 11223-870921-2TM.

Gorea, A., and Papathomas, T. V. (1989). Motion processing by chromatic and achromatic pathways. *J. Opt. Soc. Am. 6A,* 590–602.

Gorea, A., and Papathomas. T. V. (1991a). Extending a class of motion stimuli to study multi-attribute texture perception. *Behav. Res. Methods Instrum. Comput.* 23(1), 5–8.

Gorea, A., and Papathomas, T. V. (1991b). Texture segregation by chromatic and achromatic visual pathways: An analogy with motion processing *J. Opt. Soc. Am. A* 8(2), 386–393.

Gorea, A., and Papathomas, T. V. (1993). Double-opponency as a generalized concept in texture segregation illustrated with color, luminance and orientation defined stimuli. *J. Opt. Soc. Am.* 10A(7), 1450–1462.

Gorea, A., Lorenceau, J., Bagot, J. D., and Papathomas. T. V. (1992). Sensitivity to color- and to orientation-carried motion respectively improves and deteriorates under equiluminant background conditions. *Spatial Vision* 6, 285–302.

Gorea, A., Papathomas. T. V., and Kovacs. I. (1993a). Motion perception with spatiotemporally matched chromatic and achromatic information reveals a 'slow' and a 'fast' motion system. *Vision Res.* 33(17), 2515–2534.

Gorea, A., Papathomas, T. V., and Kovacs, I. (1993b). Two motion systems with common and separate pathways for color and luminance. *Proc. Natl. Acad. Sci. U.S.A.* 90, 11197–11201.

Hubel, D. H., and Livingstone, M. S. (1987). Segregation of form, color, and stereopsis in primate area 18. *J. Neurosci.* 7, 3378–3415.

Julesz, B. (1961). Binocular depth perception and pattern recognition. In C. Cherry (Ed.), *Proceedings of the 4th London Symposium on Information Theory* (pp. 212–224). London: Butterworth.

Julesz, B. (1971). *Foundations of Cyclopean Perception.* Chicago, IL: University of Chicago Press.

Julesz, B. (1978). Global stereopsis: Cooperative phenomena in stereopsis depth perception. In R. Held, H. W. Leibowitz, and H. Teuber (Eds.), *Handbook of Sensory Physiology, VIII: Perception* (pp. 215–256). Berlin: Springer-Verlag.

Julesz, B. (1981). Textons, the elements of texture perception and their interactions. *Nature (London)* 290, 91–97.

Julesz, B. (1984). Toward an axiomatic theory of preattentive vision. In G. Edelman, W. E. Gall, and W. M. Cowan (Eds.), *Dynamic Aspects of Neocortical Function* (pp. 585–612). New York: Wiley.

Julesz, B., and Miller, J. E. (1975). Independent spatial frequency tuned channels in binocular fusion and rivalry. *Perception* 4, 125–143.

Karni, A., and Sagi, D. (1990). Where practice makes perfect in texture discrimination. *The Weizmann Institute of Science Technical Report* CS90-02, January.

Kovacs, I., and Julesz, B. (1992). Depth, motion and static flow perception at metaisoluminant color contrast. *Proc. Natl. Acad. Sci. U.S.A.* 89, 10390–10394.

Kovacs, I., and Julesz, B. (1993). A closed curve is much more than an incomplete one: Effect of closure in figure-ground segmentation. *Proc. Natl. Acad. Sci. U.S.A.* 90, 7495–7497.

Kovacs, I., and Julesz, B. (1994a). Maps of global sensitivity change inside closed boundaries (abstract). *Invest. Ophthalmol. Vis. Sci.* 35, 1627. Proc. of ARVO meeting, May 1994.

Kovacs, I., and Julesz, B. (1994b). Perceptual sensitivity maps within globally defined visual shapes. *Nature (London)* 370, 644–646.

Kovacs, I., Papathomas, T. V., and Julesz, B. (1991). Interaction of color and luminance in stereo perception. *OSA Tech. Digest* 17, 202.

Livingstone, M. S., and Hubel, D. H. (1988). Segregation of form, color, movement and depth: Anatomy, physiology and perception. *Science* 240, 740–749.

Murray, I., MacCana, F., and Kulikowski, J. J. (1983). Contribution of two movement detecting mechanisms to central and peripheral vision. *Vision Res.* 23, 151–159.

Papathomas, T. V., and Gorea, A. (1988). Simultaneous motion perception along multiple attributes: A new class of stimuli. *Behav. Res. Methods Instrum. Comput.* 20, 528–536.

Papathomas, T. V., and Gorea, A. (1989). A new paradigm for testing human and machine motion perception. *Proc. SPIE-Int. Soc. Opt. Eng.* 1077, 285–291.

Papathomas, T. V., Gorea, A., and Julesz, B. (1991). Two carriers for motion perception: Color and luminance. *Vision Res.* 31(1), 1883–1891.

Poggio, G. F. (1984). Processing of stereoscopic information in monkey visual cortex. In G. M. Edelman, W. E. Gall, and W. M. Cowan (Eds.), *Dynamic Aspects of Neocortical Function* (pp. 613–635). New York: John Wiley.

Ramachandran, V. S., and Gregory, R. L. (1978). Does colour provide an input to human motion perception? *Nature (London) 275*, 55–56.

Sperling, G. (1960). The information available in brief visual presentations. *Psychol. Monog. 74*(11).

Thompson, P. (1982). Perceived rate of movement depends on contrast. *Vision Res. 22*, 377–380.

Troscianko, T. (1987). Perception of random-dot symmetry and apparent movement at and near equiluminance. *Vision Res. 27*, 547–554.

Tyler, C. W. (1983). Sensory processing of binocular disparity. In C. M. Schor and K. J. Ciuffreda (Eds.) *Vergence Eye Movements: Basic and Clinical Aspects* (pp. 199–295). Boston: Butterworth.

Werkhoven, P., Snippe, H. P., and Koenderink, J. J. (1990). Metrics for the strength of low-level motion perception. *J. Visual Commun. Image Represent. 1*, 176–188.

Contributors

Merav Ahissar
Center for Neural Computation
Institute of Life Sciences
Hebrew University
Jerusalem, Israel

Ulf B. Ahlström
Department of Psychology
Uppsala University
Uppsala, Sweden

Randolph Blake
Department of Psychology
Vanderbilt University
Nashville, Tennessee

Terry Caelli
Department of Computer Science
Curtin University of Technology
Perth, W. A., Australia

Patrick Cavanagh
Department of Psychology
Harvard University
Cambridge, Massachusetts

Leonardo Chelazzi
Laboratory of Neuropsychology
National Institute of Mental Health
Bethesda, Maryland

Charles Chubb
Department of Psychology
Rutgers University
Piscataway, New Jersey

Marvin M. Chun
Department of Brain and Cognitive Sciences
Massachusetts Institute of Technology
Cambridge, Massachusetts

Mary M. Conte
Department of Neurology and Neuroscience
Cornell University Medical College
New York, New York

Warren D. Craft
Department of Psychology
Vanderbilt University
Nashville, Tennessee

Robert Desimone
Laboratory of Neuropsychology
National Institute of Mental Health
Bethesda, Maryland

Barbara Anne Dosher
Department of Cognitive Science and
Institute of Mathematical Behavioral Sciences
University of California, Irvine
Irvine, California

John Duncan
MRC Applied Psychology Unit
Cambridge, England

Bart Farell
Institute for Sensory Research
Syracuse University
Syracuse, New York

Stacia R. Friedman-Hill
Center for Neuroscience
University of California, Davis
Davis, California

Jack L. Gallant
Department of Anatomy and Neurobiology
Washington University Medical School
St. Louis, Missouri

Andrei Gorea
Laboratory of Experimental Psychology
René Descartes University and CNRS
Paris, France

Zijiang J. He
Vision Sciences Laboratory
Department of Psychology
Harvard University
Cambridge, Massachusetts

Shaul Hochstein
Center for Neural Computation
Institute of Life Sciences
Hebrew University
Jerusalem, Israel

David H. Hubel
Department of Neurobiology
Harvard Medical School
Boston, Massachusetts

Bela Julesz
Laboratory of Vision Research
Rutgers University
Piscataway, New Jersey

Ephraim Katz
Department of Neurology and Neuroscience
Cornell University Medical College
New York, New York

Eileen Kowler
Department of Psychology
Rutgers University
Piscataway, New Jersey

Janus J. Kulikowski
Visual Sciences Laboratory
University of Manchester Institute of Science and
Technology
Manchester, England

Joseph S. Lappin
Department of Psychology
Vanderbilt University
Nashville, Tennessee

Jitendra Malik
Computer Science Division
University of California at Berkeley
Berkeley, California

Earl K. Miller
Laboratory of Neuropsychology
National Institute of Mental Health
Bethesda, Maryland

Ken Nakayama
Vision Sciences Laboratory
Department of Psychology
Harvard University
Cambridge, Massachusetts

H. Christoph Nothdurft
Department of Neurobiology
Max Planck Institute for Biophysical Chemistry
Göttingen, Germany

Thomas V. Papathomas
Laboratory of Vision Research and
Department of Biomedical Engineering
Rutgers University
Piscataway, New Jersey

Gian F. Poggio
Department of Neuroscience
Johns Hopkins University
Baltimore, Maryland

Keith Purpura
Department of Neurology and Neuroscience
Cornell University Medical College
New York, New York

V. S. Ramachandran
Department of Psychology
University of California, San Diego
La Jolla, California

Dov Sagi
Department of Neurobiology, Brain Research
Weizmann Institute of Science
Rehovot, Israel

Peter H. Schiller
Department of Brain and Cognitive Sciences
Massachusetts Institute of Technology
Cambridge, Massachusetts

George Sperling
Department of Cognitive Science and
Institute of Mathematical Behavioral Sciences
University of California, Irvine
Irvine, California

Steven T. Tschantz
Department of Mathematics
Vanderbilt University
Nashville, Tennessee

John K. Tsotsos
Department of Computer Science and
Canadian Institute for Advanced Research
University of Toronto
Toronto, Ontario, Canada

Christopher W. Tyler
Smith-Kettlewell Eye Research Institute
San Francisco, California

David C. Van Essen
Department of Anatomy and Neurobiology
Washington University School of Medicine
St. Louis, Missouri

Jonathan D. Victor
Department of Neurology and Neuroscience
Cornell University Medical College
New York, New York

Vincent Walsh
Department of Experimental Psychology
University of Oxford
Oxford, England

Roger J. Watt
Department of Psychology
University of Stirling
Stirling, Scotland

Daphna Weinshall
Department of Computer Science
Hebrew University
Jerusalem, Israel

Jeremy M. Wolfe
Center for Ophthalmic Research
Brigham and Women's Hospital
Boston, Massachusetts

Johannes M. Zanker
Max Planck Institute for Biological Chemistry
Tübingen, Germany

Index

Sutter, A., 10, 70, 89, 96
Symmetrical, 81, 150, 152, 162, 243
Symmetry, 50, 72, 81, 103, 147, 162
Synaptic weight, 210, 221

Tactile activation, 221, 241, 242, 245
Talbot, W. H., 44, 45
Tanaka, K., 216
Target, 21, 23, 38, 61, 71–76, 82, 111, 114, 115, 156, 168–170, 173, 174, 178, 181, 186, 187, 195, 199–203, 208, 209, 211, 216, 217, 220, 223, 224, 241, 254
Task-driven information flow 209. *See also* Data-driven information flow
Teller, D. Y., 18, 19, 122
Temporal frequency, 30, 128
Temporal lobe, 167
Temporal tagging, 209–211, 215–217
TENS, 242, 243
Teuber, H. L., 228, 241, 250
Texton, 56, 69, 80, 82, 181, 189–194, 196, 200, 203, 210, 250, 254
Texton gradient, 190, 192, 193
Texture
  adaptation processes, 56, 74, 79
  asymmetry, 73, 74, 81
  attention, 55, 56, 65, 66, 69, 71, 74, 75, 90, 99, 103
  border, 57, 69, 89, 90, 92, 96, 230
  boundary, 69, 106
  classification, identification, 56, 74, 75, 79, 80, 82–86, 96
  chromatic, color, 27, 30, 55–60, 90–93, 104–106
  definition problem, 55, 59–61, 63–64, 79, 99, 100
  discrimination, 69, 71, 76, 79, 81, 100–102, 146, 152, 252
  effortless/preattentive segregation, 59, 71, 74, 75, 90, 99, 100
  even, 100, 101
  first-, second-order properties, 70, 71, 80–83
  gradient, 70, 82, 92, 221
  learning, plasticity, practice effects, 55, 56, 74–76, 200–204
  local/global processing, 56, 62, 69, 70–72, 74, 80, 82, 100–105, 200–204
  models, 69–71, 79–86, 101–104, 106
  neural mechanisms/representation, 55, 56, 89, 90, 92, 100, 101, 104
  odd, 100, 101
  perspective, 86
  processing, 55–57, 59, 66, 79–83, 86, 89, 97, 102
  random, 100–103, 105, 106, 110, 250, 251
  segmentation, 57, 69–71, 73, 74, 76, 79, 82, 83, 85, 86, 89, 90, 178, 189, 190, 195
  segregation, 56, 109, 145, 152, 184, 186, 187, 252, 254
  viewer-centered representation, 92, 96
Thalamus, 239, 241, 243
Third-order statistics, 99
Threshold, 10, 13, 71, 74, 101, 103, 104, 118, 129, 141, 170, 199–204, 214
Tilt, and aftereffect, 13, 19, 37, 39, 92–94, 146
Todd, J. T., 89, 92, 139
Token matching, 156
Topography, 210, 215, 216, 227, 236, 237, 240, 241, 244–246
Top-down processes, 55, 69, 189, 190, 199, 205, 212, 214, 216, 217, 219, 220, 252
Touch, 221, 235–239, 242
Tracking, 23, 62, 110, 113–118, 139–141, 155, 156

Training, 75, 79, 82, 138, 160, 199–205, 231
Transcallosal, 244
Transcutaneous electrical neural stimulators. *See* TENS
Transfer function, 162
Transformation, 37, 38, 93, 103, 110, 136, 140, 145, 200, 205, 210
Transparency, 12, 34, 36, 37, 116, 117, 122
Treisman, A., 69, 71, 73, 90, 178, 181, 182, 189, 190, 195, 196, 199, 200, 219, 220, 224
Trichromacy, 60
Troscianko, T., 254
Troxler fading, 230
Ts'o, D. Y., 30, 103, 128
Tschantz, S. T., 111, 145
Tsotsos, J. K., 177, 178, 207–209, 211, 214–216, 220
Tuned-far neurons, 47
Tuned mechanisms, neurons, 1, 2, 9, 35, 45–51, 82, 92, 94, 96, 123, 125, 129, 158
Tuned-near neurons, 47
Tuning, 46, 49, 50, 57, 94, 96, 97, 103, 104, 128, 209–211, 213, 216, 217, 221
Turano, K., 110, 158
Turner, M. R., 70, 72
Tweedale, R., 236, 241, 244
Tyler, C. W., 1, 2, 5, 6, 8–13, 24, 31, 37, 47, 122, 231, 255

Ullman, S., 71, 92, 110, 133, 155–158, 163, 209, 211
Uncorrelated, 47, 49, 103
Ungerleider, L. G., 167, 205, 219, 220
Uniqueness constraint, 2, 11, 34–36
Unmasking, 236, 241, 245

V1 area, 2, 17, 30, 31, 35, 43–45, 47, 50, 57, 75, 76, 89, 90, 92, 93, 96, 104, 106, 175, 177, 187, 200–204, 210, 211, 216, 220, 251
V2 area, 43–45, 47, 96, 162, 167, 168, 200, 216, 220, 231
V3 area, 44, 45, 47, 48
V4 area, 57, 89, 90, 92–96, 111, 167, 168, 170, 173–175, 210, 211, 216, 217, 219, 220, 231
V5 area, 43, 44
van de Grind, W. A., 35, 157
van Doorn, A. J., 37, 39, 110, 133, 146, 157
Van Essen D. C., 6, 17, 24, 44, 45, 75, 80, 89, 90, 92, 96, 122, 128, 162, 167, 168, 182, 200, 202, 209, 210, 220, 251
van Santen, J. P. H., 110, 140, 157
Variance, 49, 56, 73, 82, 93, 136
  across textures, 56
  within texture, 56
Vector, 13, 35, 82, 83, 96, 147, 149
Velocity, 9, 47, 114, 146, 152, 158, 169, 173, 250
Ventral processing stream, 219, 222
Ventral prefrontal cortex, 222
VEP. *See* Visual evoked potentials
Vergence, 9, 13, 38, 39, 50, 51
Victor, J. D., 56, 57, 89, 90, 96, 99–106, 110, 145, 251
Visual attribute, 253
Visual cortex, 1, 2, 6, 30, 43–45, 47, 48, 50, 57, 82, 89, 100, 103, 104, 167, 177, 200, 203, 205, 209–211, 219, 228, 231, 251
Visual evoked potentials (VEP), 57, 100–105
Visual field, 6, 9, 64, 71, 75, 109, 110, 121, 168, 170, 173, 175, 178, 181–183, 189, 200, 210, 211, 219–221, 228–231, 234, 235
Visual noise, 69, 109, 231